ENERGY, SOUL-CONNECTING AND AWAKENING CONSCIOUSNESS

ENERGY, SOUL-CONNECTING AND AWAKENING CONSCIOUSNESS

Psychotherapy in a New Paradigm

Ruthie Smith

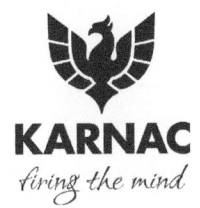

KARNAC
firing the mind

First published in 2024 by
Karnac Books Limited
62 Bucknell Road
Bicester
Oxfordshire OX26 2DS

Reprinted with minor corrections in 2026.

British Library Cataloguing in Publication Data

A C.I.P. for this book is available from the British Library

ISBN: 978-1-91349-467-4 (paperback)
ISBN: 978-1-91349-468-1 (e-book)

Typeset by vPrompt eServices Pvt Ltd, India

Printed in the United Kingdom

www.firingthemind.com

Karnac Books is committed to a sustainable future for our business, our readers, and our planet. This book is made from Forest Stewardship Council® certified paper.

To all on the path of awakening

*May we realise the open heart, and feel joy
relaxing in the stillness of our true nature
of spacious emptiness and compassion*

*TADYATHA OM GATE GATE PARA GATE
PARASAMGATE BODHI SVAHA*
The Heart Sutra

Contents

Part I
Introduction to energy psychotherapy

Part II
The practice of energy psychotherapy

List of illustrations and permissions

Acknowledgements

I am very thankful to all who encouraged me to write this book. First, clients and students who asked, 'what book can I read to tell me more?' which spurred me to write it, followed by promptings from the universe reminding me to get on with it. Then special thanks to Jane Ryan, founder of Confer who supported the development of my therapeutic ideas and interests by putting on events about energy psychotherapy at Confer when it was so new—not least, the one year postgraduate clinical training in 'Transforming Trauma: A Post-qualification online Clinical Training in Energy Psychotherapy' (https://energypsychotherapytraining.co.uk). I also thank Louise Smith who helped me get started, and those who kindly read manuscript drafts and offered their comments—Dinah Butler, Rebecca Cooper, Phil Mollon, Jean White, Dawn Wakefield, and John Reacroft, a dear friend from my Buddhist days whom I consulted about the Buddhist aspects.

I am also very grateful to those on the Energy Psychotherapy teaching team, especially Tessa Underwood, with whom I had lots of fun, laughter, and joy when we worked closely together writing the clinical training manual, and Paul Croal and Suzie Wood, who help in so many ways. I offer special thanks to family and friends—Karin, Carla, Lee, Robert, Mark and Emma, and my neighbour Vyv Matthews for her illustrations. And thanks for the joy and inspiration from wonderful musician soulmates too numerous to name—Stepney Sisters, The Guest Stars Jim Dvorak and others. And not least, the friends who have accompanied me on my path who I have not had space to mention here, but are an invaluable part of my life.

Much gratitude to Raquel Spencer for her personal help, and contribution to an updated understanding about the chakras which she wrote specially for this book; to Will Linville for his loving support and extraordinary insights; and to Sandi Radomski for 'Ask and Receive' and her wisdom and open-hearted generosity.

A very special thanks goes to Phil Mollon for all his support and advice in all sorts of ways over many years, and to all at Karnac, especially the Karnac/Phoenix publishing team for taking such care with producing and publishing this book.

Finally, tremendous gratitude to the Dzogchen Masters who introduced me to my true nature, especially Kabje Dilgo Khyentse Rinpoche, Kabje Dudjom Rinpoche, and Kabje Dudjom and Kabje Khandro Tséring Chödrön—and to all other helpers, seen and unseen.

About the author

Ruthie Smith is an attachment-based psychoanalytic psychotherapist (The Bowlby Centre) and energy psychotherapist with forty years' clinical experience in private practice, and ten years as a principal psychotherapist and supervisor in the NHS. She has taught extensively on psychotherapy trainings, speaks at various CPD conference events, has written several chapters and articles, and, after training in work with subtle energy and vibrational healing, founded The Flame Centre in London in 2009, specialising in trauma work. Alongside psychotherapy, Ruthie has a passionate interest in the 'shift' of humanity's awakening consciousness, and in integrating energy and spirituality within psychotherapy. Previously trustee and chant leader of an international Buddhist organisation where she compiled training manuals about Buddhism, Ruthie currently runs Flame residential retreats. She also has a parallel career, in which she has toured the world as a jazz musician (saxophone and voice) and sings in classical ensembles. Ruthie is currently Director of 'Transforming Trauma: A Post-qualification Clinical Training in Energy Psychotherapy' run by https://energypsychotherapytraining.co.uk. She is also a founding member of the Energy Psychotherapy Network (www.energypsychotherapynetwork.co.uk) and is invited to speak on various podcasts and at conferences such as the Masters International trauma conference in Oxford. She also writes various articles on attachment trauma, spiritual trauma, and is currently writing a new book which explores the nature of 3D and 5D reality. Ruthie's book, *Energy, Soul-Connecting and Awakening Consciousness: Psychotherapy in a New Paradigm*, introduces working with energy and the shift to the new paradigm to therapists, clients, and the general public.

Be careful what you water your dreams with.
Water them with worry and fear
And you will produce weeds that choke the life from your dream.
Water them with optimism and solutions and you will cultivate success.
Always be on the lookout for ways
to turn a problem into an opportunity for success.
Always be on the lookout for ways
To nurture your dream.

Lao Tzu, Ancient Text (1973)

Preface

*E*nergy, Soul-Connecting and Awakening Consciousness: Psychotherapy in a New Paradigm is contextualised within the multidisciplinary worlds of depth psychotherapy, working with trauma, and aspects of contemporary science and energy, against a backdrop of evolving consciousness. All this is taking place within a bigger shift into a new paradigm. The book provides an introduction to energy psychotherapy, a way of working which integrates energy psychology within relational psychotherapy, using the subtle energy system, the meridians and nervous system to relieve trauma, post-traumatic stress disorder (PTSD), and somatic stress. Easy-to-use self-applied energy methods are outlined which can regulate emotions, clear stress and trauma from the body, and help people find calm and balance. The reader may like to try these methods out for themselves.

There is so much that we don't know. While as a non-scientist I try to avoid making spurious links to other fields, we do nonetheless live in an age of synergy with increasing interconnections emerging between disciplines—for example, the ways that quantum physics interconnects with consciousness. This tentative exploration broaches humanity's evolving consciousness, the nature of the unified field and energy psychotherapy and how these come together. A lot of what is explored is subject to interpretation and not necessarily fact. Where it is possible to do so, I offer scientific backup, though such understanding may soon be superseded by new discoveries.

There are two main sections. The first part begins with a personal account of how I came to discover energy psychotherapy, and subsequent chapters look in more detail at overlaps with other disciplines, starting with an overall exploration of energy. We exist on a spectrum from matter (our bodies, or dense energy) to light (the higher frequencies of our consciousness).

The healing power and efficacy of frequency medicine is well-recognised in the medical field, where, for instance, laser surgery or infra-red treatments have been used for many years. Work with resonances and vibrations has also been developing within the field of psychology and psychotherapy since the 1970s and is becoming firmly established with an impressive evidence base and many benefits.

In the new paradigm, the book reflects on the changing therapeutic discourse which is expanding to include the idea of releasing the dense 'heavy' energies of trauma, to bring more light and well-being into what I term the *mindbodyenergy*. I use this word to acknowledge the multidimensional aspects of being human. Where previously psychotherapy tended to separate psyche from soma, science and ancient wisdom both show how the subtle energy system (our life force), our mind, body, and consciousness are completely interconnected.

Developmental 'maps' for our evolving consciousness include psychoanalytic, energetic, and spiritual frameworks for applying this work, and as a background thread throughout is my comparison between Dzogchen and energy psychotherapy—two experiential paths of energy and consciousness within the 'ease and grace' of quantum 'flow'.

The second section of the book describes a range of energy psychotherapy practices for working in depth, illustrated by clinical vignettes. This is accompanied by an overview of working with complex trauma and PTSD, and how to work safely with the *mindbodyenergy* so the therapy is appropriately grounded within relational work. The unique benefits of energy psychotherapy are explored, including its capacity to overcome therapeutic blockages, integrate and strengthen the fragmented ego, create healthy resilient 'energy boundaries', and work relatively easily to clear all forms of trauma including preverbal, attachment, transgenerational, and transpersonal trauma. Energy work offers many possibilities including depth archetypal and shadow work and working with a 'higher gauge' realm—or soul-connecting as I call it. Those working in this way report relief and an experience of real healing.

Underpinning the book is an acknowledgement of the radical change taking place on our planet where humanity is evolving towards a more heart- and soul-centred consciousness. As the idea of 'Awakening' becomes more mainstream, people seek spiritual practices such as mindfulness, yoga, and shamanism to open their hearts and experience the luminosity of their higher consciousness. In this paradigm of energy and vibration, the work of Eckhart Tolle and many others describes this change from the egoic world of the 'third dimension'—the world of Newtonian physics, duality, and cause and effect—to 'the fifth dimension', the multidimensional 'quantum' world of heart-based 'Unity Consciousness' and interconnectedness.

As we live through this 'Shift', we are witnessing the breakdown of outworn structures and hierarchies all over the world while, at the same time, prophets have foretold that humanity is giving birth to a humanitarian 'Golden Age', where new technologies and methods are manifesting in the service of the well-being of the planet. I see energy psychotherapy as one of these new methods and clients are very much benefiting from these ways of working.

In the evolving clinical terrain of the new paradigm, people increasingly come to therapy to explore confusing experiences as they 'awaken', and encounter such states as multidimensional timelines, transpersonal consciousness, or kundalini rising. We need to understand how psychotherapy might address this expanded remit in a grounded way, which avoids spiritual bypassing and provides a safe space for clients to work. Therapists may also need to consider their own experiences and what training might help, so that clients' 'altered states' can be held, accepted, and understood.

As our states of consciousness evolve, many are recognising how we are waking up from centuries of disconnection from our souls (our spiritual selves, 'higher selves', 'Source', or the 'Self'— or however we wish to name that numinous 'god within'). For me, expanded consciousness is not about going 'higher' but becoming more grounded as we connect deeply with the earth and bring our spiritual essence into our bodies. The simplest message of this book is that of finding our true selves—and helping our clients to find their true selves—through connecting with our hearts and souls and releasing any trauma which blocks us from our light.

Caveats

Glossary

To help you navigate any territory which is new to you, there is a brief glossary at the back of this book.

Energy psychotherapy and energy psychology tools

The book describes generic energy principles and methods you can try out which can easily be integrated within therapeutic practice. Many of these—such as energy balancing—can be used by both therapists and clients for regulating the nervous system and emotions. If you would like to explore further, you may like to experience this form of therapy with an energy psychotherapist. Since energy work is powerful, training in energy psychotherapy is recommended if you wish to deepen your understanding and practise safely with supervision (especially when working with complex trauma).

Evolving truths

Psychotherapy has changed enormously in the past thirty years as neuroscience and other disciplines have brought new understanding to light. Such discoveries are emerging rapidly, so our 'truths' are constantly being updated and my views may well have changed significantly in a few years' time. The book explores my perspective on a synthesis of different ideas including ones for which there may be no 'proof'. These are provisional speculations and wonderings in the service of locating psychotherapy in the New Paradigm.

Awakening consciousness

The perspective of this book is informed by issues concerning energy and consciousness, where quantum science and spirituality have converged at similar understandings about the nature of reality. Whether you are an atheist, agnostic, spiritual, or religious, the experience of 'awakening' the heart is applicable to all. I draw on examples from the Dzogchen teachings within Buddhism, a tradition with which I am familiar. Dzogchen feels relevant because it speaks of universal truths beyond concepts or doctrine in the field of energy and awakening consciousness, providing a bridge between ancient wisdom teachings, quantum science, and contemporary energy psychotherapy. However, any spiritual path which follows the heart share similarities, and so—for example—'Christ Consciousness' is another way of referring to the ultimate reality spoken about in quantum science and the Dzogchen teachings.

Language and terminology

People use different words to denote similar meanings, so my use of language is inevitably inexact. Where some speak of 'God within', 'Source', the 'Self', or their 'Buddha nature', others might prefer the terms 'Soul', 'Higher Self', or 'Presence'. Many treatises have been written about such things, so for the purposes of this book I use these words approximately and inter-changeably. For me, the term 'soul-connecting'—connecting with the spiritual self—has a personal resonance, but please use whichever words work for you.

Client examples

For the purposes of anonymity, all clients have been disguised and elements changed.

Repetition

It is difficult to take new things in all at once. Sometimes I introduce a concept and then return to it again to explain more—I hope this helps to absorb the information incrementally.

Generic principles for working with energy

This book focuses on the generic principles for working with the subtle energy system—meridians, chakras, thoughtfields, and intention. There are also numerous other excellent energy methods and 'brand' names which I have not had space to mention or explore which make a significant contribution to the field. I mean no disrespect by omitting them.

Choosing the path of joy

Throughout the global chaos of lockdowns, war, trauma, and much distress experienced by us all in the 2020s, we have been going through tumultuous change. Some named this the 'The Great Reset'—a New World Order run by a global elite; others, 'The Great Awakening'—which offers freedom to humanity. According to Lynne McTaggart, (2001), this radical 'Shift' which has been occurring on our planet, heralds 'a revolution … as daring and profound as Einstein's discovery of relativity'.

In birthing 'New Earth', we are seeing the crumbling of outworn structures and hierarchical top-down power, giving way to a new paradigm favouring egalitarian communities—a society based on co-operation rather than competition, an emphasis on personal sovereignty and self-responsibility, and exponential advances in science and technology.

Another aspect of this new world concerns a fundamental shift in consciousness. Eckhart Tolle's popular books *The Power of Now* (1999) and *A New Earth* (2005) attest to an increasing curiosity about heart and soul-based consciousness beyond ego, and the 'new energy'. These changes have been manifesting gradually, with previously fringe activities now considered part of the mainstream. For example, the practise of meditation for Western people only began to emerge in the nineteen-seventies, whereas now, fifty years later, mindfulness has become a component of treatment within the NHS and the large meditation apps 'Calm', 'Headspace', and 'Insight Timer' are standard on many phones. The public's appetite for various types of generic non-religious spirituality can also be seen in the burgeoning of all types of meditation retreats, such as mindfulness, yoga, and shamanism.

Amidst these changes we are seeing a flowering of new methods in psychotherapy and counselling. Developments in neuroscience, epigenetics, biology, quantum physics, and trauma have led to a greater understanding of the links between the body, mind, and consciousness—which I term *mindbodyenergy*—and a convergence of approaches in clinical work, resulting in radical change in the practise of psychotherapy. Energy psychotherapy is one such emerging method. For instance, acupoint tapping (EFT or emotional freedom techniques) calms the nervous system by tapping on points on the meridians to release traumatic stress. It is so effective that it is used in key statutory services such as the fire brigade, the police, and GP counselling practices and the self-help application of energy methods has become a normal part of daily life for many these days. Essentially, energy methods help remove trauma, conflicts, and blockages from our subtle energy system and their effects can often be quite astonishing.

Sceptical onlookers may wonder about this potential for bringing such wide-ranging healing to the body, mind, and soul. However, clients generally report significant feelings of relief and well-being, a finding corroborated by an increasing evidence base of research showing a lasting reduction in symptoms. All this may sound too good to be true—but I hope in introducing you to this work, that you might be interested to explore further.

After discovering and training in energy therapy and finding how helpful it was for myself and my clients, I decided to leave the security of my NHS job so I could further develop this way of working. This coincided with the end of a major relationship, when, during a period of depression and loss of heart, I experienced a 'death' of my old life. I knew I had to move on from the old energy and go it alone, so took a huge leap of faith into the unknown. Despite a fundamental sense of inner safety, I was shocked at suddenly being engulfed by visceral fear and part of me did not know if I would manage the 'rebirth'. I had made the change with a curious mixture of trust—certain of having to follow the truth in my heart—and terrifying anxiety in case the universe would not support me. While maintaining a semblance of normality, I suffered absolute terrors and am grateful that energy healing got me through and beyond this—and that I was indeed supported.

There are some principles in energy psychotherapy I would like to emphasise. First, these subtle energy methods are not an 'add on' because they are completely integrated within relational 'talking therapy'—hence the term *energy psychotherapy*. This is also not something therapists 'do to' clients. Healing is something which comes from inside us. We are our own healers—so the work is co-created, guided by the client's own healing process. Clients are facilitated in self-applied methods, an empowering process which brings greater stability, integration, and a sense of self. The energy 'tool kit' for working with thoughtfields, meridians, chakras, and the power of intention described in Part II provides self-help methods for both therapists and clients.

Second, working with energy is *experiential*, beyond words. The cognitive mind may doubt and want to understand 'why' but largely, we don't know, so these questions cannot easily be answered. Each person's experience is unique. As an example, my first experience of energy therapy came when clearing a preverbal trauma of which I had previously been unconscious. It concerned being shouted at when I was a baby. The energetic release of deep shock and fear—gently, painlessly, and naturally—was a complete revelation to me. I was amazed how my body remembered the trauma and how powerful and freeing it was to clear this. Afterwards, I went outside in the garden, stomping around on the grass, grounding the energy which 'fizzed' as it poured through my legs. This helped me know in no uncertain terms that energy therapy worked. It also helped me connect more deeply with my body and trust the process.

Third, energy work is very adaptable. We follow each client's unique preferences and *mindbodyenergy*. This even applies to the way we name the work itself. For instance, some people are attracted to the word energy, whereas others find it off-putting. A more scientific-sounding—and true—way of describing this work as 'clearing stress out of the nervous system' may feel more user-friendly for some. We can easily introduce energy methods by using some form of mindfulness, breathing, or 'felt sense' as a way in—so it is perfectly possible to practise energy psychotherapy without referring to 'energy' at all. This may be helpful for those therapists who might be interested to try this way of working but find the whole thing a bit 'woo woo' or worry what their clients or colleagues might think of them if they change their practice in what may feel rather radical ways. People understandably have a certain caution about things which don't necessarily make sense to the rational analytical mind.

My intention in writing this book is to build a bridge to support this new psychotherapeutic work, using some personal examples. So how did I discover the wonders of energy psycho-therapy? On a personal level, my search was for healing, safety, and authenticity. Despite many years of therapy, the deepest layers of trauma which had caused me to freeze and be unable to speak were only finally addressed when I came across energy psychotherapy. This method felt immediately 'right'. Its capacity to clear earliest preverbal traumas and its sensitivity and attunement to my body was transformative and has made a huge difference to my life.

More generally, I had been seeking to incorporate and integrate my personal interests and passions within psychotherapy—psychoanalytic and Jungian depth psychologies; resonance and vibration (I am a musician); trauma, and the ways it is held in the *mindbodyenergy*; energy healing; explorations in meditation, consciousness, and spirituality (I was a practising Tibetan Buddhist for many years); and my lifelong yearning to connect with my soul. Life's synchron-icities brought me via a somewhat circuitous route, providing interesting opportunities which ultimately led me to energy psychotherapy.

***

I thought carefully about how much to disclose in writing this book, and decided it was useful to share some personal experiences to illustrate specific points, starting first with a little about my family background. I will keep details to a minimum out of respect and love for my family, who, apart from one sister, are deceased. As with many psychotherapists, I was brought up in a family with its share of fear, anxiety, and trauma. My mother had an undiagnosed mental illness, and as her confidante, effectively, I became a therapist when I was very little. She was very busy going out at night to local committees, so, as children, we were often left alone in the evenings. I was close to my older sister who suffered agonisingly with paranoid schizo-phrenia, and after many years' struggle, she eventually took her own life in the late 1980s. My middle sister was somewhat overlooked by my mother in all this, although she had a particular place in the heart of my largely 'absent' father. He, with a double first from Cambridge, prized people if they were 'bright' or amusing and spent large amounts of time alone away from us all, developing his photos and binding books. Both my parents had terrifying tempers which, from time to time, would erupt out of nowhere. They also both had significant family legacies of trauma to contend with at a time when therapy barely existed. I am very thankful to them for giving me this life.

From 'common unhappiness' to joy

From an early age I carried family stresses on my face so road workers would call out saying things like 'lighten up love, it might never happen'. When I started exploring psychotherapy, Freud's well-known statement that

> much will be gained if we succeed in transforming … hysterical misery into 'common unhappiness'. With a mental life that has been restored to health, you will be better armed against that unhappiness. (Freud, 1895d)

seemed quite a realistic therapeutic aim.

Buddha also spoke about unhappiness ('dukka') as the fundamental human condition. However, his 'Four Noble Truths' offer hope for transcendence, describing how suffering occurs because we have not yet 'awakened' out of egoic reality. The first truth is that, as human beings, we all want to be happy but do things that bring suffering on ourselves. The second is that there is a way out of this suffering, because we all have 'Buddha nature'—our 'true' enlightened nature or whatever words you like to call your spiritual self. The third truth is that following the path to liberation offers a way out of suffering. When we 'awaken' out of ego, realise our true nature, and stabilise this state of unity—oneness-with-the-all—we arrive at the 'cessation' of suffering, which is the fourth truth. This is explored further in Chapter 6.

Energy psychotherapy offers another path for the healing of suffering, which uses remarkably straightforward methods. This will all be explained fully in Chapters 7–9, so for now, I trust the following brief outline of working with energy will suffice.

At the beginning we start with simple exercises/postures to balance and calm the body's subtle energy and nervous system. As with any relational psychotherapy, we talk together, and issues emerge. There are various indicators which help us know when energy work may be useful. The physiological disturbance when a person becomes overwhelmed or 'triggered' is one such signal. The free associations of the mind and body bringing out issues from the unconscious are another—these arise naturally in the work. Thirdly, kinesiology (otherwise called muscle testing or energy testing) is an invaluable skill, although it is possible to practise energy therapy without it. The body has its own wisdom and 'knows' things which we are not consciously aware of, so by testing such statements as 'This is correct issue to work with now' the Yes or No response helps guide the energy work (the therapist can use self-energy testing if it is not appropriate or possible to touch the client's arm).

Once we have ascertained that energy treatment would be helpful, client and therapist then co-create a simple 'clearing' phrase which sums up the issue. In the vignettes that I share, I focus on these phrases which indicate to 'intelligent energy' the precise nature of traumatic stress to be released via the neural pathways from the *mindbodyenergy*. These formulations may seem a bit stark, so I wish to emphasise that they don't at all convey the intimacy of the therapeutic relationship, nor the profound insight which emerges in the process of how we came to co-create the phrases together.

A useful feature of energy psychotherapy is that it can identify and clear 'reversed energy'—blockages or 'resistance' which get in the way of healing. Once we have attended to any reversals, we select the relevant energy method, and using the clearing phrase, might: tap on relevant meridian points; hold specific chakras or other parts of the subtle energy system whilst keeping the key issue in mind; or work with words and intention alone. These processes facilitate the discharge of the stressed energy from the body via the nervous and subtle energy systems, thereby transforming neural pathways and bringing about states of balance and calm.

I feel that my experiences—both of 'awakening' through Buddhism and of energy therapy—revolutionised my life. These pathways offer routes out of 'common unhappiness' and can bring us to states of peace and joy. Now, knowing as I do the potential for deep healing in energy psychotherapy, I feel Freud's therapeutic aims were rather limited.

I set my intention to choose the Path of Joy before either having had a glimpse of 'awakening' or of energy psychotherapy. I feel this intention played a key role in changing the trajectory of my life, gradually bringing circumstances to my path which helped transform my engrained outlook from one of gloom to that of joy.

From the old to the new—key themes

The so-called Aquarian Age has been coming into being for decades as several planetary cycles end simultaneously—the 2,000-year age of Pisces, the completion of a 5,000-year cycle of the *Kaliyuga* known as the 'Dark Age', and the ending of 12,000- and 26,000-year cycles (Perez, 2021) All this has profound implications for change and a new dawn.

It has been prophesised that the 'New Age' we are entering—variously called the 'Golden Age' or the 'Age of Light'—heralds a paradigm of energy, personal sovereignty, expanding consciousness, and freedom. 'Seeding' new earth involves the simultaneous building and creation of new structures inside the system, to replace dissolving outworn structures. In what follows, I explore the transition from the old to the new as I searched for balance and integration in the way I worked. This involved grappling with various themes and dichotomies (in no particular order) ultimately converging in energy psychotherapy:

- feminism—the personal is political
- the world of vibrations, energy, and music
- medical and holistic relational models
- traditional classical and free-flowing forms

- awakening consciousness—the rational and the mystical
- finding an authentic sense of self
- hierarchy and personal sovereignty
- connecting with soul—a search for something more
- the body

'The personal is political' was a slogan employed by feminism in the 70s to reclaim personal power and sovereignty. This trend was echoed in Scott Peck's *The Road Less Traveled* (1978) which blended science, spirituality, and personal growth. Peck invited people to free themselves from the pressures of conformity which stopped them from acting independently so they could find their own truth.

Another book of its time, Sheldon Kopp's *If You Meet the Buddha on the Road, Kill Him!* (1976) describes the necessary 'pilgrimage' of disillusionment we go through on our journey to individuation—a stage of growth where we recognise that others can't teach us what we need to learn for ourselves. When the therapist or guru turns out to be disappointing, just 'another struggling human being' like us, we stop idealising and depending on them and begin to find ourselves. The way to find truth is to go within and look within ourselves. Kopp's egalitarian stance made total sense at the time I read it, though it took many years of working with external and internal hierarchies of authority and self-judgement—overcoming 'shoulds', 'oughts', and acting out of 'duty'—before I actually found my sovereignty and stopped looking outside myself for answers. This path of discovery involved confronting ego, judgement, and shame, and learning to discern the difference between the soul's and the ego's voice.

Kopp's reminder that we are all 'struggling human beings' offers a humbling and cautionary note to therapists on our human fallibility. I have certainly made and continue to make many mistakes both in my life and as a therapist—though hopefully I am learning from it all.

In the following account I have written chronologically where possible, though some anecdotes do not always follow a strictly linear timeline because the strands of my life—of music, therapy, Buddhism, energy and so on—were operating simultaneously. Nonetheless, I trust that you can make sense of it.

A circuitous route

While there was pain and trauma in my family, I don't want to paint too gloomy a picture—we had many opportunities, including music, travel abroad, and adventures. On family holidays, quirky humour provided respite from family tensions. We sang in the car in harmony—a favourite was the hymn 'Guide me O thou Great Redeemer', where we substituted the words with the longest name of a village in Wales, (Llanfairpwllgwyngyllgogerychwyrndrobwllllantysiliogogogoch) to the tune Cwm Rhondda. This was obviously completely nuts. As children we constantly clamoured 'when are we going to get there?' as though 'there' was in the future, when actually, 'there' was each beautiful city, mountain, lake, historic site, or coastline that we visited on the journey. Similarly, I have come to understand that as we travel along our path in life, enjoying our experiences as we go along is as important as whatever destination we aspire to get to.

One of the legacies of having a hyper-rationalising father was a troublesome split between head and heart—he spoke the language of reason, and I, that of emotion. My father and sister used to discuss Kafka in German at the dinner table. As the youngest, I said nothing for fear of being stupid. I could never find words. I was sensitive and emotional and despite sometimes knowing things intuitively, I often fell into shocked traumatised states which blocked my brain, so I was unable to think. I was so terrified of being shamed for getting things wrong that I copied my sister's entire school project, word for word, picture for picture, because I didn't have a single original idea in my head. It wasn't until long after leaving my family that I felt safe enough to find the flow of my own creativity.

I became preoccupied by spiritual questions when, aged five, I sang at a church fete and developed a curiosity and passion for the heavens:

> What do the stars do up in the sky
> Higher than the wind can blow, and the clouds can fly?
> Each star in its glory, circle, circle—still
> As it was meant to shine, and set, and do its maker's will.

In Sunday school we were taught about compassion and Ruth in the bible who 'wept amidst the alien corn', though I wasn't quite sure what it meant. Like my namesake, I often wept, and one memorable experience as a toddler was of seeing little boys torturing crabs on the beach by pulling their legs off, one by one. I was inconsolable and screamed at them to stop, with tears pouring down my cheeks. I was distraught that they *enjoyed* being cruel.

As a child there were many different worlds– music, orchestra (I played the cello), swimming, living in the South (Surrey), moving up North (Liverpool), family, school, church, travel abroad. It wasn't safe to be the same person everywhere, so I adapted to my environment to avoid at all costs the shame and humiliation of being different. When in Rome. So, if I was with posh people, I had a posh accent and if I was with Liverpudlians I was a scouser. By the age of eleven I had learned to be a chameleon.

My soul always sought joy. There was much solace to be found in nature and I survived my family through finding space. Around ten I discovered meditation by swimming endless lengths on my own in the outdoor lido. This regulated my emotions and gave me peace and calm, and later, being in the swimming team necessitated attending regular training sessions which legitimised my escape from home.

Being a musician provided another escape—perhaps that was when I first really connected with 'energy'. My family often labelled me as too sensitive, but music, with its wide-ranging harmonies and vibrations, soothed my soul and allowed me to be me, to freely express myself. When I was thirteen, I played cello at an orchestral week at Attingham Park, the family seat of Sir George Trevelyan. The only child there, I was pleased to be invited to join seasoned musicians to play some chamber music one evening in his study. I still remember the energy of that room. Surrounded by beautiful old books, paintings, and period furniture, he and others smoked and drank fine wines while we played some of the most exquisite quartets, quintets, and octets late into the night. I was grateful that the other musicians put up with my inexperience and just let me get on with it. It was heaven—totally connected with the expansive resonances of the music and at one with my soul. Years later, I learned that George Trevelyan—in whom I had no particular interest at the time—was a proponent of the 'new energies', known as 'The Father of the New Age'.

In late adolescence I went through a depressive breakdown until Richard, my first proper boyfriend, thankfully came to my rescue saying, 'There's nothing wrong with you, it's your mother that is the problem'. I again found solace by singing in chamber choirs and playing in orchestras. I revelled in the glorious harmonies and vibrations of the great composers—from the transcendent vastness of works like Bach's B Minor Mass to Purcell and the delicate beauty of madrigal singing.

At the other end of the spectrum, in the early 70s at York University I did my fair share of 'turning on, tuning in and dropping out'[1] and went to psychedelic music festivals such as at Glastonbury, and the notorious 'mud bath' at the Bickershaw Festival. Seeing live bands inspired—when *The Grateful Dead* performed their well-known magic of playing the rain away into a spectacular sunset, it lifted all our spirits as we experienced that unity and oneness.

Rebelling against pressures to perform as a solo concert singer at York, I self-destructively gave up classical singing and turned down the role of Dido in *Dido and Aeneas*. I couldn't cope with having a 'big voice' and felt a fake in long evening gowns when I had no clue who I was. Instead, I joined a Motown-style band with two other girlfriends where the brilliant John Telfer (currently the vicar in *The Archers*) played piano and sang extraordinary boogie-woogie. I developed a totally different 'soul' voice. Our one claim to fame was to be the warm-up act to Bob Marley and the Wailers, who invited us to be their backing singers—we declined so we could finish our degrees.

At university, during another trough of despair about my sweet, gentle schizophrenic sister who was in excruciating pain I wondered, 'If there is a God, how can such suffering be allowed?' and made an aspiration to meet a spiritual being—perhaps like Jesus, but alive today?—who could help me believe that healing was possible.

All the twists and turns of this path outside the mainstream were contributing in their way towards my becoming an energy psychotherapist.

An uncertain identity

I left York after a brief sortie living in the countryside and running a community vegetarian café with friends. Our soul band came to London and aged twenty-five I took up the saxophone. The women in the band supported one another to compose our own songs and evolve from our

---

[1] Timothy Leary (1966), a key exponent of the 'LSD' experience, first coined this expression.

previous roles as 'chick singers' where only men played the instruments. Forming the Stepney Sisters, we became a feminist rock band at a time when there were few female rock musicians. I think the men in our lives must have had a difficult time.

Stepney Sisters was like a second family and a consciousness-raising group. We talked late into the night, angsting and sharing while we learned, laughed, and experimented together. In many ways this was a discovery about love. We were very co-dependent and not good at conflict. Apart from a couple in the band who were used to rows, most of us were too terrified to speak our minds, have good honest disagreements, or hold differences of opinion. It was a very different world then. *Hail Sisters of the Revolution* (Gilfillan & Scott, 2022) offers a vivid account of this time through poetry and photos. Despite our best endeavours to be feminists, we worried—'what will people think?'—to such an extent that on the way to playing at the National Women's Liberation Movement concert, we changed the lyrics of our songs to make them more PC, removing such words as 'baby' and other endearments characteristic of soul music. We hid behind the standard feminist uniform—short hair and dungarees, checked shirts and jeans—though I sometimes claimed some femininity by wearing flowery patchwork skirts. I was very pleased when I first met Susie Orbach to see her wearing bright-blue kitten heels.

We would be genuinely sisterly to one another overall, while suppressed undercurrents rumbled underneath. Ironically, although the women's movement empowered women to find themselves, there was a certain demand to think the same, because differences felt threatening. I spent a huge amount of time censoring myself and what I said out loud was often quite different from conflicting thoughts inside—I began to recognise just how 'split' I was. I didn't even know in those days that it didn't feel safe to be me.

Our world expanded when Stepney Sisters was invited to play at an international women's event in Rotterdam. We played our instruments (rather badly it has to be said, although we were keen to improve), and sang our repertoire, mainly of original songs penned by members of the band including a rousing number written by Caroline Gilfillan 'Sisters, hold up your heads, stand up and be counted'—while one of my songs was called 'Family'. Once again, I felt a bit of a fraud—writing songs about our lives, loves, and sexual politics, when I still didn't know who I was.

At the festival, we were somewhat shocked and affronted by a bizarre experiential 'happening' called The Charm School, organised by men. How, we wondered, could there be a Women's Festival with so many men involved? The Charm School invited visitors to have a consultation about their style and appearance. We were led through a curious, provocative installation full of challenging images, and then asked a series of questions. This gave the band much to think about and led to considerable confusion. To this day I still don't know whether The Charm School was a horrendous sexist joke subverting a Women's Festival, or an intelligent and thought-provoking art installation which really made everyone think and question themselves. Or perhaps both? The experience did however identify that there were a lot of judgements in my head, and that I lived life trying to work out what others felt was okay to think or feel, whereas I had absolutely no idea what I felt or thought myself. I also realised that a lot of my energy went into second-guessing, trying to fit in, and giving my power away to others, rather than being myself. Realising just how disconnected my internal world was from how I publicly presented myself was shocking for a so-called feminist.

This was the era of sex, drugs, and rock 'n' roll. One of the conference organisers called Franz took a shine to me, and guiltily 'forgetting' about Pete, my nice boyfriend back at home, I was thrown into a whirlwind love affair which completely blew me away. Franz was cool, sexy, and insightful, so he could see me much better than I could see myself, which was terrifying and exciting. With practically zero self-esteem and very little confidence about myself as a woman, I had absolutely no idea why he had chosen to be with me. His authenticity and emotional maturity taught me about realness, openness, love, and generosity. He spoke about the death of his father and his difficult experiences in adolescence which had led him into psychoanalysis. This helped me open up and speak of my own family's wounds. Franz normalised therapy (which, at the time was more or less unheard of in my circle). His self-awareness was a good advertisement, so I was able to let down my defences sufficiently to take the step of entering psychoanalytic therapy myself.

Therapy was initially spent either in withdrawn long painful silence or recounting florid dreams. My therapist helped me give voice to and grieve the trauma and distress. The validation of my perceptions and recognition of the reality of psychosis in my family was an important part of healing. As a traumatised client entering therapy, we have different parts operating simultaneously, with uneven levels of development. Our 'child' self longs to be looked after, fantasising about the ideal therapist who 'knows', to offer reassurance and support, all of which understandably gets played out in therapy. With intense trauma underpinning everything, it took time to work through such unmet need, especially with dissociated trauma that I wasn't aware of.

Stephen Mitchell (1998) in his book about relational psychoanalysis speaks of four different stages in the therapeutic relationship. I underwent several different therapies for various periods of time before I became resilient enough or felt worthy enough for a more real intersubjective exchange, as outlined in Mitchell's fourth stage. I kept my 'false self' going for a long time—we need to be quite strong to face the shadow elements of our psyches and heal our narcissistic wounds. It wasn't until years later that I was able to integrate the deepest fragments of trauma and resolve my internal splits through energy psychotherapy.

Medical and holistic relational models

Alongside playing in Stepney Sisters and being in therapy, I worked as a counsellor in a half-way house in London and went on to undertake a two-year full-time postgraduate Diploma at Middlesex, where I undertook psychotherapy placements at The Arbours Association Crisis Centre and one of their therapeutic communities.

When exploring what training to do, I remember a consultation with a psychoanalyst who greeted me with a powerful silence when I entered his room. It gave him such an air of authority, and not yet knowing the psychoanalytic 'rules', I sat squirming with anxiety and embarrassment. Subsequently I learned that this psychoanalytic method purposefully maximises anxiety. However, as someone new to psychoanalysis it felt shaming and uncomfortable, a repetition of my family trauma. I chose to go to The Arbours Association instead, who were welcoming and kind.

One of the things which attracted me to Arbours was their holistic view of mental illness. My sister had been an in-patient in psychiatric hospitals on several occasions, so I was keen to help her by finding other ways to understand her situation. At Arbours, Dr Joe Berke (Barnes & Berke, 1973) and Dr Morton Schatzman (1973), two psychiatrists and psychotherapists from the United States introduced a therapeutic sanctuary on similar lines to Laing's anti-psychiatry model (*The Divided Self* 1960), a trail-blazer at a time when the medical model and labelling was the norm. Arbours were pioneers in helping people in distress who might otherwise be in-patients in psychiatric wards. The treatment for guests was to live in therapeutic communities and understand themselves through individual therapy, family therapy, and community meetings. The centres were in ordinary houses which offered a normalising environment. Arbours prioritised relationship over psychopathology so although all residents were experiencing some form of extreme emotional distress, they were not labelled as mental patients. At the time I was a student at Arbours, the preference was for guests to be unmedicated.

The humanity of the crisis team (Sally Berry, Laura Forti, Andrea Sabbadini, and Tom Ryan, with Joe Berke as visiting team-leader from time to time) was key in creating a warm atmosphere. My first introduction to this way of working was to sit round the kitchen table making cakes with two very young children, while I tried to coax their mother into conversation. Recently convicted for murder, she stared blankly at the wall—the family was at Arbours for an in-depth assessment.

The balance between community—of preparing food, cooking, and eating together with the guests—combined with rigorous analytic thinking—created a heart-centred, depth approach. My feelings about that formative time of my learning might be summed up by a comment in one of Jung's letters: 'As you know, in olden times the ancestral souls live in pots in the kitchen'.[2]

During this period, I tried to come to terms with both my sister and mother being in psychotic states by immersing myself in therapy, studying psychosis, and undertaking a thesis on the Arbours Crisis Centre and its community model of treatment. I learned about the traumatic roots of Bateson's double-bind theory (Bateson et al., 1956), where people in families said one thing and meant another, making coherent response impossible. The 'damned if you do and damned if you don't' conundrum was pivotal in my understanding that *relational trauma* could be a causative factor in schizophrenia. Traumatic communications and misunderstandings mirrored my own family.

---

[2] Carl Jung (1973b, p. 168).

Arbours built a bridge with relatives in family therapy meetings, modelling non-judgement. This demonstrated how crucial it is to hold the therapeutic space compassionately without blaming mother or anyone else for the child's illness, which greatly helped me with my own mother. Writing my research dissertation about the Arbours Crisis Centre enabled me to think about, formulate, and make some sort of sense of my family. Reflecting on all this, I so value the soulful approach and therapeutic foundation which Arbours gave me in those early years. In terms of my views about medication however, after working in the NHS I came to see that when there is a chemical imbalance, contemporary medications can be very helpful in alleviating suffering, and on many occasions provide a lifeline for both clients and their families.

Fifty years ago, the medical model—both in psychiatric and psychoanalytic diagnoses— tended to define mental health conditions in terms of 'disturbance' and psychopathology, with little acknowledgment of underlying trauma. However, static labels, which fail to recognise the role of trauma, undermine the potential for recovery. A major diagnostic shift occurred when Harvard Psychiatrist Judith Lewis Herman (1992) and others redefined this, by bringing complex trauma, PTSD and developmental trauma within the International Classification of Diseases ICD-11.

The pivotal role that trauma plays in mental 'disturbance' has major implications. Quite apart from no longer pathologising the client, it brings hope. When trauma and PTSD became fully recognised in therapy, it helped me make sense of the traumatic PTSD-levels of triggering that I often used to experience. Today, energy psychotherapy and those therapies which specifi- cally work with the body, clearing PTSD and relational trauma, help regulate people's mood and emotion, and the increasing evidence base indicates that these methods bring significant and lasting healing and balance.

Connecting through a dark night of the soul

As a musician, soul music in all its forms—classical and popular—communicates a longing for and connection to spiritual essence. The word soul-ful pretty much sums this up. However, a significant trauma of our age is our disconnection from soul. While several therapeutic approaches include the soul, many don't, so one of the reasons for writing this book—apart from introducing people to energy psychotherapy—is to make a plea for the recognition of soul as a crucial aspect of our being.

Although the terms soul and higher self are often used interchangeably, I understand the soul to be our unique spiritual essence embodied in our individual physical being. Micheila Sheldan (2019) emphasises the eternal aspect of our soul, the divine spark of our spirit which is with us throughout all our lifetimes, whereas she sees the Higher Self as an energetic aspect of us which is interconnected with the wider *collective consciousness*—the keeper of our energy and 'seer' which holds an overview, supporting us while we live out our soul's path.

According to Ashbrook (1995) the 'meaning making' aspect of soul plays a significant role in integrating our human experience. At a time where for centuries our minds have been separated from our bodies, Moore (1992) highlighted how our loss of soul—the 'great malady'—manifests symptomatically in obsessions, addictions, violence, and loss of meaning, the root problem being that we have lost our wisdom about the soul, or even our interest in it. Moore recognised that we can't just think ourselves through this deep division because thinking itself is part of the problem. What we need is a way out of our dualistic attitudes—a third possibility, which he perceived as soul. Being soul-ful has to do with genuineness and depth. When we care for our souls, we appreciate 'the paradoxical mysteries that blend light and darkness into the grandeur of what human life and culture can be' (Moore, 1992).

Praying for light at the end of the tunnel

Despite the wonders of music, a fascination with psychoanalysis, and a positive first experience of psychoanalytic psychotherapy, my internal world still fell into bleak, disconnected states. During another bout of depression, I despaired that I couldn't help my sister out of her deep suffering, and everything felt completely hopeless. Although I had no specific faith, I prayed for light at the end of the tunnel and suddenly became aware of a neutral part observing me. Perhaps these depressions had some purpose after all? Rather than some form of punishment, for I know not what, might this depression—this dark night of the soul—be serving as some kind of 'training'? Who was this voice which challenged me? A new perspective opened, and I heard the words—'Choose the Path of Joy'. In that moment of guidance and clarity, even though I had no conception what 'The Path of Joy' might be, I chose joy and felt much better. This was when I first consciously connected with my soul.

As I reflect, I did not find this connection with my soul by looking outside myself. It was a deeply internal experience within my body, which happened simply through listening, trusting the information I received, and acting on what I heard. We all have this capacity. We connect with our souls through our hearts—the heartbreak about my sister had opened a gateway, bringing me to the flow of a higher dimensional reality, explored further in Chapter 6

Our soul carries us through our unique experiences in life, assisting us in expanding our consciousness and energy. Drawing on our infinite, limitless soul-self by accessing the highest dimension that our imagination can reach, lifts us up. This higher frequency then helps release our problems, conflicts, and disturbances.

Connecting with my soul, learning to tune in and follow its guidance, has been key in my path to healing. Our soul guides us via our intuition—something I used to ignore but have learned to trust—rather than by our thinking minds. When we connect up with the 'higher' aspects of our consciousness it helps us overcome, or at least accept our limitations, and deepens our experience. Thomas Moore (1992) brings this down to earth in a very human way—a life lived soulfully is not without its moments of darkness and periods of foolishness. He feels that when we drop the fantasy of salvation—of being rescued by another—it opens us to the possibility of deep self-knowledge and self-acceptance, which are the very foundation of soul.

A glimpse of awakening

Therapy was immensely helpful, but I ached for something more. In 1979, Jim Dvorak, my then trumpet-playing partner and soulmate, took me to hear a talk about 'Meditation and Peace' by his visiting teacher, a Dzogchen Master. As His Holiness Dudjom Rinpoche spoke, he transmitted an 'awakening' experience of love and compassion which changed my life. The *dharma* teachings offered a profound explanation of human suffering which revolutionised my understanding about my sister's pain. As I listened to the soft gentle lilt of his voice and felt the fine resonance of his energy, my heart opened, and in that moment, I experienced the light of my true nature—there was a sense of a dissolving of all boundaries as I merged into oneness with everything—a deep connection with 'the all'—or with 'God' if you like. This is known in Dzogchen as the 'Introduction to the Nature of Mind'.

Having felt plagued by a feeling of inner badness most of my life, I experienced for the first time my inherent goodness—a pervasive light and well-being throughout my *mindbodyenergy*. I had 'come home'. It was a tremendous relief. This was the best therapy I could imagine. I cried for—quite literally—hours. This life-altering transmission led me to regard Dudjom Rinpoche as my teacher or 'root guru'. However, as he travelled very little to the UK, I was advised to study with his translator, then a young Tibetan Buddhist 'Tulku'.[3]

I entered the Tibetan Buddhist Vajrayana (tantric) path of energy and transformation and later discovered this is sometimes called 'The Path of Joy'. Taking tantric vows creates a sacred thread or *samaya* which formally connects the practitioner with the spiritual path. Jamgön Kongtrül, a Tibetan mystic, described *samaya* as the way practitioners 'preserve the life-force of that empowerment within your being' (Padmasambhava & Kongtrul, 1998). Another teacher defined *samaya* as 'the truth within our heart', or one's inner wisdom teacher—what I refer to here as soul-connecting. Later, when I undertook a training in energy, sound, light, and colour, I discovered this spiritual link was called 'shoshona', a silver thread which connects our soul to our body, the vehicle through which we receive our intuitions and perceptions, and which animates our creative life force.

The women's therapy centre and feminist therapy

Around the same time in the late 70s, after being at Arbours, Sally Berry introduced me to The Women's Therapy Centre (WTC) in London. This was an innovative feminist collective founded by Susie Orbach, where I worked for twenty years, working variously as part-time

---

[3] Tulku is the name for a 'treasure holder' or reincarnate custodian of a specific lineage of teachings in Tibetan Buddhism.

administrator (a job I could do while touring as a musician), workshop leader, psychotherapist, supervisor, and teacher on the WTC training course. I greatly benefited from WTC's psycho-analytic attachment-based approach, which prioritised being client-friendly and accessible to women. I was fortunate to be there at a creative time amongst such an interesting group of women—too many to name. I learned so much from in-house training, continuous and enriching study groups, and excellent group supervision. There were also challenges when our unresolved aspects created certain dynamics. I feel rather embarrassed to look back and recognise my own contribution to these splits, as we first idealised and then projected all our maternal 'lacks' of the failing breast onto the Centre.

WTC was influential and empowering in many ways. A friend and colleague, Sue Krzowski, edited *In Our Experience* (1988), which explored themed workshops at WTC, egalitarian groups where women contributed and learned from one another. While the meaning we each ascribe comes from our own experience, it is very valuable to share and have support from others as we travel along our paths.

At WTC I began learning to trust my soul's guidance. Synchronicities seemed to confirm like a satnav when I was or wasn't on the right road, helping me distinguish between neurotic anxiety as compared with the very helpful steer of wisdom anxiety. For instance, during the early times of WTC as a feminist collective, one day I had a strong gut feeling that an Inland Revenue Inspector would come to the Centre and ask to inspect our books. I expressed my concern at our feminist collective meeting. We had started to receive grants from public funding and our bookkeeper was having problems balancing the accounts, so in many ways this was quite a rational concern, though the other therapists clearly thought I was rather batty. As my anxiety wouldn't go away, I knew I had to listen to and act on my instincts. Taking the matter into my own hands, I asked an accountant friend to help and took the books home that night. We pored over them the whole weekend, staying up late into the night, going back over months, until she eventually found the anomalies and got the figures to balance. It was quite extraordinary when on Monday morning, there was a knock on the door at the WTC—it was an officer from the Inland Revenue asking to look at our books! This taught me never to ignore my gut feelings, which I now totally trust as my soul's guidance—something that we all have, if we tune into it.

Spirituality in the closet

While playing music felt expansive, I tended to contract within the psychoanalytic world. In those days, *mindfulness* as we know it today, did not exist and hardly anyone I knew practised meditation. It felt a bit weird using my annual leave for meditation retreats while others went off on 'normal' holidays. It was also somewhat embarrassing to be following a guru, which did not fit in at all with left-wing feminist culture. I ignored this conflict and kept my worlds apart because I so valued the extraordinary learning at the WTC and the Dzogchen teachings. To avoid the disapproval of some fellow therapists (who dovetailed into my judging inner mother), I tried to conform to the group norm.

One day in a study group about diversity, a therapist was discussing an Asian client who had been struggling with her faith when someone said, 'Surely people don't still believe in God these days?' Sadly, I lacked the confidence to protest, either at the racism or the religious prejudice. In those years I generally froze in such situations, not feeling safe enough to publicly own my differences or speak my truth. Since many of the therapists frowned on spirituality, I kept quiet and put myself firmly in the spiritual closet—I had a long way to go towards individuation. With so little integration between the separated worlds I inhabited, this incident did however crystalise my desire to write something about 'psychotherapy and spirituality' and see how they might fit together more inclusively.

Later, a small reading group from the WTC and associates comprising Sue Krzowski, Mary-Jayne Rust, Jean White, myself, and one or two others decided to investigate contemporary spiritual writings and their relevance to therapy, from an exploration of the 'sacred feminine', to ecology and quantum physics.

'They'll do much better if you offer them love'

In the eighties and nineties, the relational approach of the Women's Therapy Centre was my clinical foundation. Theoretically Bowlby's concept of a secure base was fundamental; personally, I found it easier to open up when a relationship feels safe, so I liked Winnicott and Kohut who honoured the client's experience and were gentle with people's defences. Experiencing anxiety was—and still is—encouraged by many analytical schools. However, having lived in states of persecutory anxiety myself for tranches of time, and feeling dogged by the harsh inner judgement of what Kalsched terms the 'persecutor/protector' (1996), I knew such an approach was not helpful for me because it caused me to disintegrate and fragment.

I was somewhat relieved when I came across Margaret Little's account of her analysis with Winnicott (1977) where she explored her psychotic anxieties and deep wounds while simultaneously working as a psychoanalyst. I had always hidden such shameful states and it wasn't until much later when I discovered energy psychotherapy that I was able to clear and be free of my own preverbal psychotic anxieties stemming from a traumatic infancy. Subsequently, several therapists have come for energy psychotherapy to address their traumas of extreme anxiety, exacerbated by 'old school' psychotherapy trainings. While the fantasy that someone else has authority and 'knows' is comforting, it is easy to feel infantilised and for our sense of self to be overridden by interpretations from powerful analysts.

Against WTCs theoretical backdrop, I was taken aback in my early days at WTC when a client commented that therapy was like 'beating a bruise'. 'Hilary' had come for therapy to find healing from the core belief instilled in her by her father that 'You're rotten to the core'. This powerful message had dogged her life but focusing on it in therapy made her feel worse.

This led me to question the nature and intentions of therapeutic work—what is the most effective way to help clients?

Around that time, by chance—if there is any such thing—a friend wanted to consult 'Gladys' about her boyfriend troubles and egged me on to go along with her. Gladys, an archetypal clairvoyant with mysterious objects around her, quite literally peered through her crystal ball and looked at me rather seriously. My heart sank—was she going to tell me something terrible about my love life too? Gladys said (I remember this vividly,) 'Well dear, you seem to be seeing some very unhappy miserable, fearful people—they all look rather anxious and depressed. But it looks as if you are rather hemmed in, having to toe the line and say things to them you don't really believe in. They all want love dear—just trust yourself, they'll do much better if you offer them love.'

Gladys' advice about the importance of love hit home. Having grown up feeling fundamentally 'bad', it wasn't until I awakened that I experienced my own inner goodness and wholeness. Buddhism teaches that our inherent nature is the Buddha and that without exception, we all have the potential to become enlightened. Since, at our core, we are already whole, our spiritual essence cannot be distorted or contaminated by any event in our lives. A classic Buddhist metaphor describes our true nature as being like the sun—always there, shining, even if at times it is hidden by the clouds of our emotions.

Starting out from an assumption of fundamental wholeness in therapy—for instance, that we all have Buddha nature—brings confidence that it is possible to work with brokenness and that trauma can be healed. The task in therapy becomes that of clearing away the dense clouds/energy of trauma which obscure this light, rather than trying very hard to be good enough or better. A perspective of innate wholeness and dignity makes a big difference to our sense of self-esteem. Anyone can feel silted up by the heavy energy of trauma, but when we clear away the layers, it brings in light and well-being. If our true nature is whole, it is much easier to love ourselves and integrate our shadow elements.

Balancing traditional classical with free-flowing forms

Finding a balance between tradition and innovation—between classical and more free-flowing forms—has been another theme which occupied me. Playing classical music from an early age involved a certain amount of discipline to achieve a 'high enough' standard, along with all the judgement, pain, and disappointment that entails. When I later became a jazz musician, it was a relief to let go of the safety net of 'form' and learn free improvisation with its expansiveness and inclusivity. Similarly, in psychotherapy in general, and more specifically, energy psychotherapy; there is sometimes quite a dance between the flow of free associations which open up 'the field', as compared with more structured and containing ways of working.

In some ways, my preliminary training in working with energy was through playing music. When in my late 20s, Jim helped me learn about jazz, I found the expansive realm of improvisation freeing and unblocking for an introvert like myself. Learning to trust the free flow of energy helped me break out of the inhibitions of a classical training where one can get stuck in 'form', too scared of being judged for playing a 'wrong' note. Jim's version was that there is no such thing as a 'wrong' note—instead you just repeat it and improvise around it and make it part of the music. At the same time, I was, and am, appreciative of the discipline of a classical music training which helped me apply myself to learning the saxophone. It also offers exquisite attention to form, detail, and tonality when singing or making music in classical ensembles.

I am grateful to Jim, who not only introduced me to *dharma* and taught me about jazz, but also took me to see his astrologer friend. Astrology—which I speak of more later—made sense of my inner contradictions. I discovered that my placement of the planet Saturn (often associated with structure), showed a cautious, inhibited nature and a strong sense of form, whereas my Jupiter, (representing freedom, spirituality, and expansiveness) indicated my potential for excess. Touring with various jazz groups—particularly with The Guest Stars—and chanting mantra within Buddhism gave me space and time to expand and explore sound and improvisation. The power and reach of music's energy, frequencies, and 'flow' provided a wonderful vehicle for pure emotional expression which helped create a balance between a more creative, playful self and a somewhat traditional, inhibited aspect of me.

Similarly, I was exploring where I stood on a spectrum from orthodox psychoanalytic models to more integrative relational approaches. Arbours had managed to combine a mixture of the two. When starting out as a novice therapist, I am afraid that to borrow a sense of authority I put forward my best analytic blank screen. This was met with short shrift by the WTC client who said, 'Is that your brick wall impersonation Miss?' This reduced the two of us to laughter—something which was not supposed to happen—and in that moment, I realised how being human, natural, and real was important in facilitating a relaxed connection. Offering a blank screen to a potential sufferer of trauma creates an unknown threat, so my preference has been to hold the therapeutic space with a softer energy field.

Subsequently I undertook a project alongside two Black psychotherapists at the WTC, Carol Mohamed and Rosamond Grant, to help make psychotherapy more accessible to minority groups. Being accessible involved inducting clients so they were not shamed or alienated by unfamiliar 'rules' or starkly triggered by the intensity of their trauma—being responsive facilitates regulation and holding.

I really enjoy psychoanalytic theory, finding its depth, structure, and clarity of clinical thinking incredibly grounding. Personally, in terms of therapeutic practice however, I found the more traditional classical models of psychoanalysis similar to the more stringent approaches within classical music. While I learned so much from many compassionate analysts, I also struggled with what I experienced as a certain snobbery within the psychoanalytic world. Some seminars seemed rather dry, with intensely head-oriented analysis. As my personal tendencies veer towards feelings, the heart, bodily countertransferences, and the felt sense, I sometimes felt like a fish out of water.

The mid-1980s saw a trend away from the hierarchical classical models of analyst as authority and the 'one-person psychology' model, in favour of more relational intersubjective approaches (Stern, 1985). In recognition of the neurological importance of attachment and connection as a means of establishing safety and attenuating trauma, over the last few decades, therapists have been developing more embodied and attuned ways of working. An attachment-based approach supports clients gently—especially those who have experienced trauma—in finding autonomy and a sense of self. These days, the greater emphasis on inclusion and diversity, which recognises cultural, social, and power differentials, invites more of the whole person of both client and therapist to be seen and acknowledged in the room.

As energy psychotherapy emerges as another therapeutic form, it too is working out its relationship between structure and flow. The NICE guidelines recommend a structured approach when working with complex trauma, something I explore in Chapter 9. Some energy therapy methods are structured—for instance, going down the energy centres/chakra repeating a phrase such as 'All my anxiety when x happened', or the 'Tearless Trauma Techniques'. Such protocols are containing and help ground and embody the work. Alternatively, we can follow the flow of the energy which arises through the free association of the body's sensations, words, and images. This approach tends to open up and unblock things, with the caution that we may access deep material very fast. The beauty of energy therapy is that one can work easily with both structure and 'going with the flow', and they complement one another.

From 3-D to 5-D—the rational, the mystical, and awakening consciousness

As a young woman I was fascinated by states of consciousness, exploring the differences between rational and mystical states of mind—states which are sometimes unhelpfully polarised. The rational world of ego operates in the third dimensional world of Newtonian physics, our consensus everyday reality, whereas the intuitive/sensate states pertain to the soul and 'quantum'—the awakened fifth dimension. As we evolve into awakened consciousness, we move between these states, which are both important dimensions of reality.

At the turn of the twentieth century, when Victorian society lauded rationality over the mystical, William James (1902, 2010) explored the dichotomy between the rational and the experiential and the importance of 'making proper connection with the higher powers'. His drift was towards a common-sense, non-conformist approach of personal experience of 'God within yourself'. James' influence was far-reaching: he validated the embodied, sentient nature of individual spiritual experience, and helped launch the explosion of awakening consciousness which manifested in the 1960s. His human approach created a foundation for developing new therapies which prioritised the client's personal experience, such as Carl Rogers' person-centred therapy. These trends provide a foundation for placing energy therapy within a wider historical context.

Aldous Huxley's ground-breaking *The Doors of Perception* (1954) provided another avenue for bringing mystical states of consciousness into public awareness. The 'veil' of ego was lifting, which continued throughout the psychedelic era of the 60s and 70s with The Beatles' *Sergeant Pepper* occupying 'number 1' on the mainstream music charts for twenty-seven weeks. I took LSD myself on several occasions—thankfully without any damage to my psyche—which opened my awareness to 'altered states', though I am not sure I would be so gungho now. During the 70s, I was also fortunate to have LSD-assisted therapy which was very beneficial—a form of treatment which has gained considerable credence these days.

New therapeutic approaches have continued to emerge which support the different work required of us these days, extending towards deeper concerns and questions traditionally considered more the preserve of religion. This includes 'soul-based' therapies (Dent, 2019); angel healing; spirit release; shamanism, and psychedelics; and of course quantum and energy therapies (Hover-Kramer, 2002; Mollon, 2008; and many others).

Dzogchen—the path of liberation

My personal quest led me to Dzogchen. After the life-changing awakening with Dudjom Rinpoche, I joined the local Buddhist group who were studying The Longchen Nyingtik tradition of Tibetan Buddhism. This graduated path to enlightenment culminates in Dzogchen—the 'direct path' of liberation. Dzogchen's special feature is that it operates beyond mind and concept in the fifth dimensional state of pure awareness and light-consciousness—the realm of energy.

Practising Tibetan Buddhism was in some ways a continuation of therapy but at a different level. Tantric visualisation practices work directly with emotions including the shaming, frightening, and split-off shadow-aspects of the psyche's energy. 'Purifying' energy (as it was termed) increasingly made space for glimpses of expanded consciousness. Dzogchen practice helped me find a deep underlying peace—'the ground of being'—even if emotions fluctuated on the surface.

I felt at home in the world of mysticism and followed this devotional path for thirteen years. Being a musician, I ended up as the umze (chant leader) which allowed me to express my soul-self. A number of enlightened masters visited, so chanting in the presence of their refined energy was like bathing in blessing—people sometimes used to fall asleep because their transmissions resonated at such high frequencies.

After my sister died, I went on a pilgrimage, visiting the sacred Buddhist sites to honour her, including visiting His Holiness Dilgo Khyentse Rinpoche in Nepal, asking for blessings and practices to be done for her. Then, shortly before his passing, Dilgo Khyentse gave a special Dzogchen transmission high up in the Pyrenees. He had written a new form of 'Guru Yoga' so I sang him the chant I composed for it. We were in an open-sided marquee, looking out directly over the mountains—it was a vast, glorious location where it was easy to dissolve into oneness with the space, exploring the furthest reaches of the sound and its vibrations. Later, when recording the chant, the studio engineer said the wide range of frequencies were difficult to capture—perhaps this was because of all those years connecting with the wider whole while chanting.

Body

Energy work—which includes all aspects of the *mindbodyenergy*—requires that we are properly embodied. It has certainly helped me link more meaningfully with my body. At the simplest level, we can at least be aware when we are operating from our heads as compared with from our hearts.

As a young woman, I was rather disconnected from my body, going through my first experience of psychotherapy without even realising I was more-or-less dissociated from terrifying early trauma. It was when I had my first glimpse of awakening that I realised just how much spirituality was an embodied experience.

As a therapist, my bodily countertransference always provided me with information. Years ago, when working with—or even supervising—the work of clients with early unmet needs, I would start yawning. I later came to understand this indicated that I was connecting energetically with the client. It wasn't until a consultation with Hans King, who named my clairsentience, that I fully recognised that my sensitive body was a conduit for communicating and picking up information about others. I then began to own and care for my body differently. I became increasingly aware of my habit of overriding my body's needs, or unknowingly 'taking on' others' energies. This would deplete and exhaust me energetically, until I learned through energy therapy how to have better energy boundaries, a process described in Chapter 8.

My body sometimes communicates to me through illness. Once I was flat on my back for three months unable to do anything at all. In one of the universe's synchronicities, I came across Raquel Spencer through a webinar. An energy and 'body technician', Raquel was enormously helpful. She recognised my need for specific antibiotics and defined this 'healing crisis' as my body needing to take 'time out'. Raquel told me I was going through an 'energy upgrade' of my subtle energy systems which required a period of complete stillness as I went through 'ascension symptoms'. She worked with my body energetically via remote healing using sound to activate the dormant mind/body pathways and 'multidimensional cellular codes of light' to help me better access what she terms the 'quantum self'. I am so grateful that my soul found her—and other such people—at critical turning points when I needed help.

During this new dawn of 'New Earth', our planet and all beings are being bathed in fine vibrations of photonic light from the photon belt. This light it is like an etheric plasma, a golden space dust or 'aurora network' (Pixie, 2022[4]). As it touches our field, we take in directly a golden

---

[4] Dee Taylor-Mason and Friends presented Magenta Pixie 'New Earth Enlightenment', https://www.youtube.com/watch?v=W4Xnij-G9zU (webinar, accessed December 2022).

knowledge from the collective library of all experience from the beginning of time, which is held in the morphogenetic field.

Since humanity is considered to be 'genetic royalty' (Perez, 2021), our DNA is important. It was thought that we have just two strands, with the remaining vestigial ten strands being considered 'junk DNA' by scientists. However, when we absorb the photonic particles pouring onto earth, our being recognises these 'codes of light' which activate and light up our vestigial DNA strands as part of the awakening process. This upgrades us spiritually and brings increased creativity. These days many children are born with several strands already activated—it is said we have the potential for up to 144 strands of DNA, and even more.

The awakening process requires that we take good care of our bodies—our spiritual 'temple'. I have learned to listen to my body and am responsive to natural remedies. At different times I have had specific needs for vitamins, minerals, good-quality water, and electrolytes, which help the electromagnetic aspects of our energy. Adding Himalayan sea salt, with its wide range of trace minerals, and lemon is a good start.

I am completely indebted to allopathic medicine in times of clinical emergency. However, I have also learned to take charge of my own body and well-being. For example, standard blood tests—such as checking thyroid—do not always identify my conditions. One time, exhausted with my hair falling out, my doctor said, 'I don't care what the blood tests say, I am putting you on thyroxine'. On account of the overlay between *mindbodyenergy*, viewing ourselves holistically is important and I have learned to keep myself informed about health and medical issues.

Vibrational healing

Fascinated by archetypes I debated training as a Jungian analyst, but at the same time, an opportunity arose to undertake a three-year training in the vibrational medicines of sound, light, colour, and energy. Buddhists habitually seek divinations and blessings from Lamas when undertaking new projects. Surprisingly, the divination favoured the course in energy, which was quite 'out there' in those days, and entirely different from the world of psychoanalytic therapy or analytical psychology. I undertook this training from 1989 to 1992. It taught on subtle energies; *Ta Yin Fa* (a qigong-like practice which connected us with the energy of the stars); working with the energy field or aura doing 'etheric massages' using colour; working with the chakras using 'aura soma' essences connecting with 'Ascended Masters'; using sound and Tibetan bowls; and discovering the subtle energy of meridians using tuning forks. I loved this training and felt totally at home in the world of energy.

Astrology, soul maps, and archetypes

Lots of people are sceptical about astrology, but various Jungian analysts have offered tremendous insight into depth astrology which has nothing whatsoever to do with superficial horoscopes. Birth charts provide energetic blue-prints for the soul. Studying my chart significantly expanded my understanding, helping me identify multifaceted aspects of myself, so I was better able to accept and integrate them. I had previously struggled to manage my energies but astrology helped me recognise the contradictions of my character—beneficial, shadow, and stressful aspects—laid out clearly and objectively. I spent years devouring astrology books, grateful to understand more about fulfilling my soul's purpose and the archetypal energies (represented by the planets) inherent on the journey. At times of personal crisis, astrological transits clarified specific archetypes I needed to work with. For instance, Pluto transits often involve a painful dive into the underworld to plumb the depths—which also brings its own healing gifts. These archetypes also bore similarities with Tibetan Buddhist 'deities'.

Integration

My lives and worlds remained separated. At the Women's Therapy Centre, I was a young psychoanalytic therapist, developing my practice. As a Tibetan Buddhist, I was the chant leader on retreats, taught foundational courses, and wrote practice manuals on Buddhism. A third part of me was a musician—my jazz self went abroad on tours, playing at jazz festivals. (Later, in terms of classical music, I was accepted on a postgraduate training in opera singing. My mother developed dementia so I could not follow this through, but I did nonetheless find an excellent teacher who helped my singing feel the freest I had ever known.) A fourth part of me taught psychoanalytic theory and spent a lot of time writing training manuals. A fifth part was exploring 'energy'—the cosmos, astrology, energy healing, colour, light, and the chakras.

My worlds started coming together. Aspects from one fed into another, so that, for instance, in 1989 I presented a paper entitled 'Dzogchen and Psychotherapy' about the 'awakened state' and the dangers of splitting and projection for those who did not have healthily functioning egos at a conference in Amsterdam on 'Psychotherapy and Buddhism'. Meanwhile in The Guest Stars, I was writing songs about awakening consciousness, such as 'Wake It Up' whose lyrics concerned working with energy and emotions—'Love, Joy, Pain and Anger—all emotion—it's energy in motion … wake it up … keep it light'.

Disillusionment

The hierarchy of Buddhism started to feel problematic. In the early 90s, the Tulku with whom I had been studying (who had become an international best-seller) increasingly emphasised 'subjugating ego' and frowned on autonomy. He used judgement, public shaming, and angry outbursts as vehicles for teaching his students. The devotional path of Vajrayana requires that one perceives the Vajra Master with 'pure perception' as a Buddha. However, the teacher's erratic temper became increasingly abusive. While initially ignoring my doubts, my psychoanalytic understanding compelled me to acknowledge that the teacher had a narcissistic personality disorder—we were unhealthily co-dependent students, idealising the Vajra Master in debasing servitude.

Despite the benefit from connecting with other realised Dzogchen Masters, studying with this Lama was no longer viable. During those thirteen years, I became a bit of a door mat, re-enacting early subservient relational patterns. Unfortunately, playing the role of Echo in relationships with Narcissists has happened more than once in my life.

When you enter the *dharma*, which essentially means truth, you take Refuge vows 'until enlightenment'. However, I was perceiving untruth all around. The Master was abusing his power and exploiting students—sexually, emotionally, physically, and financially—and I had to take action. The temporal responsibilities of being a Trustee helped me confront the situation and speak out against the oppressive culture in the organisation. My attempts to speak directly with him were to no avail, so I wrote to the Dalai Lama, left the group (viewed by all as a pariah), and reported the teacher to The Charities Commission. It was my connection with my soul which gave me the courage to overcome my fear and withstand the backlash both during and after this debacle.

That the Lama had feet of clay was profoundly disillusioning. Spiritual betrayal is agonising and losing a devotional spiritual path which had been the foundation of my life felt deeply traumatic—which of the Buddhist teachings could I still trust? Which ones were distorted by the Lama and needed to be discarded? Although I knew in my heart of hearts that I had not lost my sacred link because the truth of the teaching is inside us, it was time to grow up and rely on myself. In fact, as the Buddha himself taught, 'You are your own master. No one else is your master.'[5]

I had drawn a line in the sand concerning the Buddhist hierarchy and there was no going back. I was now on a fast track to individuation to recover my autonomy. On telling my family what had happened, my father was remarkably sanguine. I was surprised when he told me he admired me for going my own way in search of myself—something he hadn't been allowed to do himself. I was grateful for these perceptions and a positive perspective.

Still grief-stricken at the losses—both of my sister who died in 1987 and leaving the Buddhist community in 1992—I maintained a front to the external world and decided to continue exploring energy by studying the chakras in depth. I also returned to the idea of training as a Jungian analyst, which would help me process what had gone on. The training analyst—fortuitously a musician, and sensitive—attuned well. His experience in pre-natal and early infant trauma meant that when I lay on the couch, he recognised my attachment needs to see his face, so he turned his chair to face me. It was very upsetting when, through ill health, he was unable to see me through my training and needed to end with me prematurely. 'The universe' seemed to be pushing me out on my own again. Nonetheless, I set out to find another analyst.

---

[5] Article posted on 14 August 2017 in Buddhist Facebook group called 'What's Now?' written by Dzongsar Khyentse Rinpoche.

At my assessment, the analyst—who wore a tight pencil skirt and extremely high white stilettos—interpreted my spiritual path as an avoidance of dealing with trauma about my mother. This was definitely not a good fit. I eventually found an analyst who, I knew instantly, was a safe pair of hands. I am not sure whether it was helpful—or not—that she had a Thangka (spiritual image) of Guru Rinpoche on her wall. This was an image of the same Buddha whose mantra I had chanted for years. It was a strange piece of synchronicity. I cried non-stop four times a week as I went through the shellshock of all that happened. Preferring to have face-to-face contact, I hadn't yet lain down on the couch with this analyst. However, the rules of the Jungian organisation required that to enter the next phase of training, after eighteen months all analysands should be lying on the couch with the analyst sitting behind the patient. I had already lost time when accumulating this prerequisite with my previous analyst.

Although the analyst genuinely didn't want to push me, these were the rules. Perhaps the energetic presence of Guru Rinpoche—a powerful symbol in her consulting room—made it impossible for me, like a re-enactment having to submit to The Master. Having already accumulated one hundred thousand prostrations as a Tibetan Buddhist, my body would not allow me to submit again. It just wasn't doable. (Incidentally, the true meaning of doing prostrations is in essence to bow down to one's own Buddha nature and is actually quite an amazing practice.) My analyst was kind and generous. While encouraging me to stay on and train, she recognised that I knew my own mind and respected my decision. I was grateful she did not pathologise me.

This encounter with institutional power was another opportunity to reflect. Submitting to rules can prevent people from being themselves—a man in training as a psychoanalyst went through his entire five-times-a-week analysis without coming out as gay since it wasn't safe to do so. On the other hand, the discipline of training can temper character and be useful. The structure and framework of rigorous trainings both as a musician and in Buddhism had helped me, and I had benefitted. However, I did not need to put myself through a similar process again.

Jung in *The Red Book* speaks about re-finding the soul, and one of his key points is that we must each find our own path:

> Who knows the way to the eternally fruitful climes of the soul? You seek the way through mere appearances, you study books and give ear to all kinds of opinion. What good is all that? There is only one way, and that is your way. You seek the path. I warn you away from my own. It can also be the wrong way for you. May each go his own way. (Jung & Shamdasani, 2009, p. 241)

After years of following others, spiritual sovereignty—growing up, and being fully responsible for my choices—was challenging. It was a question of trusting my soul and following its guidance. Step by step this involved listening to gut responses, or the feelings in my heart—does this feel right?—and then choosing the next step. Obvious as this may sound, having overridden and doubted the quiet promptings of my inner voice for a lifetime, learning to trust myself took time. The paradigm of hierarchical authority really was at an end for me—it was no longer an option to give my power away with false-self compliance.

As I look back, it wasn't until my debacle with the Buddhist organisation where I had to stand up to those 'above me', that I shifted the internal hierarchy of my inner judgemental parents and started to fully trust myself. The truth of Sheldon Kopp's idea that 'the Guru is Dead' was finally sinking in. It is empowering when we stop idealising the 'other' or expecting them to know, or to be perfect. There is no one to tell us what to do—we are our own arbiters—it is up to us.

As I went forward in life it was hard to bear other Buddhists feeling sorry for me, perceiving that I had lost my way, especially when I so loved and longed for the Dzogchen teachings. I still had a nagging doubt. To be spiritually realised, Dzogchen requires that one follows a Master, so when the possibility of entering a classic three-year retreat, overseen by a different, rather radical Lama, came up, I was tempted. The retreat was doable because it had been arranged to fit in with people's daily lives.

Part of me already knew the answer but perhaps I just needed support in confirming this, so I consulted a spiritual director called Hans King to talk this through. I was about to engage in discussion, when Hans made short shrift of my question by saying that I was already 'on my own path'. He then abruptly changed the conversation with 'When are you going to get on with that book?' I was astonished because I had made no mention of this. After various attempts to write 'Psychotherapy and Spirituality' I had given up because it seemed too daunting. Having known deep down it was not right to undertake the retreat, I was glad for the clarity, and returned to thinking about the book.

All this—eventually—was leading me to energy psychotherapy.

Energy therapy training

From 1989 to 1992 I undertook a three-year training in energy, sound, light, and colour and afterwards continued studying about energy and the chakras with various people. Alongside being a psychoanalytic therapist, I practised colour healing, using etheric massage as a separate discipline. My consultation room was literally split in two—on one side was a colour healing area—on the other, my chairs and couch. One day, a private analytic client was very traumatised, so I offered her colour healing to ground her—she felt the calming results immediately, and thereafter generally asked for colour work rather than talking therapy. It struck me just how powerful energy work could be, and I yearned to find a holistic approach where I could integrate energy work within psychotherapy.

I eventually left the Women's Therapy Centre in 2000 and worked in the NHS for ten years as a principal psychotherapist, supervising the work of a tertiary psychoanalytic psychotherapy service with complex trauma and so-called 'personality disorder'. I also taught at The Bowlby Centre and other psychotherapy training organisations.

In 2005, my different worlds converged. I was invited to give a presentation in the United States at the Hershey Research Medical Centre, Pennsylvania State University, a neo-natal unit for premature, sick, and traumatised new-borns.[6] Michal Levin was training a group of doctors and medical professionals in energy work and had invited me to contextualise energy in relation to psychoanalytic/attachment theory, Dzogchen, and consciousness—a synthesis was beginning to happen.

Around the same time, I helped plan a training day in the NHS where we invited Phil Mollon to teach about trauma. He agreed, as long as he could speak about energy psychology. After his training session which used tapping, I was hooked—this was what I had been looking for. I spent many years travelling backwards from the USA to study various energy modalities including Asha Clinton's Advanced Integrative Therapy (AIT), Jo Dunning's 'Quick Pulse' Technique, and Kenji Kumara's 'Quantum Lightweaving'.

I am very grateful for the weekly energy psychotherapy I had on the phone with a lovely woman from the States (we didn't have zoom in those days). Margaret had a 'light touch' and was very sensitive. She was a good role model. I learned that it is more helpful to spend most of the session time clearing traumatic stress rather than overly talking about things, something I had already done for years. When we focused on my mother's terrifying angry volatility, using clearing phrases such as 'Her angry eyes' my body gradually came to a place of peace and calm as all the shocked energy and stress was released while I breathed out through each chakra. I was astonished at the speed and thoroughness with which Margaret helped me clear anxieties, stresses, triggers, and frozen traumas which had been buried in my body all my life. I became stronger and more resilient and noticed huge changes in my well-being. Where previously I erred on being easily triggered by things, clearing traumatic stress transformed and integrated my ego so that life felt calmer and smoother. I also noticed that when the trauma is thoroughly treated, it really is gone.

I also met Sarfaraz, a Sufi, in upstate New York, who kindly invited me to stay with her during trainings. She became a dear friend and training buddy. The work we did together addressed archetypal, transpersonal past life, and transgenerational trauma, and accessed deep splits and unpleasant, ugly shadow elements in my psyche. One day, when she was challenging my passivity, Sarfaraz declared: 'You're not a mouse, you're a lion' and was intent on getting me to 'roar'. The transpersonal work unblocked (as I discovered) lifetimes of traumas at my throat, of being persecuted for speaking my truth which had contributed to difficulties in finding my voice. Interestingly, there is a teaching in the *dharma* about 'The Lion's roar'—which means the 'fearless proclamation of truth'.

I began integrating energy work into my private therapy practice, attended an online supervision group in the USA, and went on to train in how to teach energy therapy and supervise others.

---

[6] Dr Charles Palmer, MD, Head of the Neonatal Unit had invited Michal Levin to teach about energy as a contribution to the development of the work of his department.

Then after a second dark-night-of-the-soul experience, I left my NHS post to set up the Flame Centre in London so I could focus on developing energy psychotherapy and working with trauma.

I continued to drag my feet about the book. 'Life' had intervened for many good reasons. Together with psychoanalytic and integrative therapy colleagues who had also trained in energy work, we began offering peer support to one another as we honed our skills in working with trauma and expanded our study of energy methods. There was much new in the 'field' about the neurobiology of trauma, *The Biology of Belief* (Lipton, 2010) epigenetics and so on, and we began integrating these ideas. We developed an informal network, (now known as the Energy Psychotherapy Network), taught 'Converging Streams' trainings in energy psychotherapy, spoke at conferences, and introduced ways of using energy methods in psychotherapy. Most of my writing about energy went into training manuals.

Then one day, listening to a webinar from the USA on contemporary spirituality, the webinar leader saw my name in the 'chat', and out of the blue called out to me saying 'It's time you stopped procrastinating and wrote that book now'. I was utterly startled because I had never seen this teacher before, nor he me. This confirmation from the universe provided further impetus for writing. At the time, I was working with Jane Ryan, the founder of Confer, devising a weekly programme entitled 'Psychotherapy and Soul'. Writing my introductory lecture helped me get going again with this book.

The rollercoaster of awakening

This path of learning to live from my soul rather than my ego has been a rollercoaster. I had to stop going against my inner truth to fit in with others. Instead of following a guru—or placing intermediaries above me—there were many ups and downs before I started properly believing in myself and embedded 'going direct' to source.

Valuing our own experience—what Buddhism terms our 'inner teacher'—involves honouring and loving ourselves and seeing ourselves as worthy to be our own guide. In the shift from ego to the 'Great Awakening', the head-based effort and drive of ego—of not feeling good enough—sets 'self-improvement goals', whereas the soul sets intentions and trusts in the flow of life which is a gentler path of 'ease and grace'.

That said, if we wish to fully avail ourselves of the precious life we have been gifted with, the path of awakening does require a certain commitment to 'work' on ourselves. As well as enjoying life as much as we can, there are certain challenges and upsets to face on the path. The 'rollercoaster of awakening' for me has been concerned with finding balance—letting go of the trauma-based pressures from childhood where I was constantly striving to be better, learning to relax and accept myself, and aspiring to make positive choices in each moment. One measure I use to check if I am still being driven by duty and/or a stressed nervous system, is to enquire if my energy is moving forward with enthusiasm, inspiration, and joy.

Reflections

Looking back over the last few decades, there have been considerable shifts in psychotherapy. While the therapeutic relationship remains central, there is increasing recognition that the states of fear, terror, and shame associated with trauma require work with the body. Books such as *The Body Keeps the Score* (Van der Kolk, 2015) and *The Body Remembers* (Rothschild, 2000) have led us to understand the vital role played by the body in therapy, so these days there is considerably more emphasis on integrating the body and 'the felt sense'.

As a therapist and client, I feel energy psychotherapy offers a relatively comfortable approach for those who have been fragmented by trauma. It facilitates autonomy and integration, prevents and lessens re-traumatisation, and offers balm to ease and soothe. It is relational, respecting the client's needs, and pacing the work in a way that can help people rebuild themselves and find their self-possession. When trauma is cleared thoroughly and completely, it brings an end to dysregulation and triggering, and helps us find calm and balance. In so many ways we can say that energy psychotherapy is about healing rather than therapy. The natural simplicity of this work helps people feel present, embodied, and connected with themselves. And as we connect with our bodies, feelings, mind, and spirit—in turn we connect more easily with others.

Choosing the Path of Joy set a healing trajectory in my life that I could not have imagined. We all receive the same light—the same 'Source'. However, it depends for each of us, where we are on our soul's journey. When we can get our egos out of the way and transform our pain into peace, we can experience our light, allowing it to blossom and radiate—naturally, joyful, and spontaneously. In the new world, in our search for happiness, freedom, balance and so much more, may the development of heart and soul-based wisdom be one of our key therapeutic aims.

I hope you will find this introduction to energy psychotherapy whets your appetite to go on and try it out for yourself, and if you are a therapist, undertake further training and experience the wonderful 'grace and ease' offered by these quantum methods.

Part I

Introduction to energy psychotherapy

Introduction to Part I

P eople will be approaching this book from various perspectives and backgrounds, and with different interests. With this in mind, please treat this book as a resource, exploring the various sections as suits you.

Part I introduces the reader to the wider context of energy psychotherapy. It considers the multidisciplinary fields of depth psychotherapy, working with trauma, and aspects of contemporary science and energy, against a backdrop of awakening consciousness. After sharing how I came to discover energy psychotherapy, Chapter 1 offers an exploration of energy. Chapter 2 then looks at the new paradigm of working with the energetic spectrum of vibration and frequencies from matter to light, and how raising our vibration becomes another way of viewing the therapeutic and awakening process. Chapter 3 considers aspects of science which are relevant to energy psychotherapy—neurobiology, cellular biology, and epigenetics—while Chapter 4 offers speculations about quantum science, energy psychotherapy, and awakening consciousness. In Chapter 5 I explore the relational practice of energy psychotherapy with its experiential therapeutic focus 'beyond analysis', emphasising that this is an integrative way of working following the free associations and the quantum 'flow' of *mindbodyenergy*. Chapter 6, 'Psychotherapy in the quantum era', explores ways of understanding our development and evolving consciousness, starting with psychological and soul perspectives, and then outlining two energetic 'maps', one of the chakra systems, and another, an overview of the Tibetan Buddhist path in relation to awakening consciousness and Dzogchen.

Many therapists will be considering how they might like to try out and put this work into practice for themselves and their clients. Chapters 7 to 10, which are outlined in the introduction to Part II, provide an overview of the practical applications of energy psychotherapy and the energy methods we use.

Naturally, if you would like to deepen your understanding, you may wish to undertake an energy psychotherapy training, try out energy therapy for yourself, and enter specialist supervision to help you to practise safely.

CHAPTER 1

Everything is energy

Introducing energy psychotherapy

'My mother wants me dead'

Perhaps it is easier to introduce energy psychotherapy by describing some work rather than jumping straight into 'energy' and its rather nebulous concepts.

I once had a client, Alys, who demonstrates just how powerful is the interconnectedness and synergy between our body, emotions, mind, and spirit/energy—or *mindbodyenergy*. Although I am no specialist in somatisation, Alys' situation shows clearly how the psyche, comprising the mind and emotions, profoundly interacts with the body's nervous systems and both form an essential link with our defences. While energy psychotherapy makes no claims to treat physiological illness, and it is important, ethically, that therapists don't work outside their spheres of competence, nonetheless we do occasionally work with psychological causes of somatisation and, sometimes, physical symptoms are successfully removed.

Psycho-neuroimmunology is the science of the interactions of mind, body, and the indissoluble unity of emotions and physiology throughout life, in both health and illness. I found Gabor Maté's ideas (2003) particularly helpful in singling out self-repression as a major cause of stress and a significant contributor to illness. Maté highlights how illness can be the body's way of saying 'no' to what the mind cannot or will not acknowledge. This was very relevant with Alys, who became ill on account of deeply repressed material. I have abbreviated the following account to pull out key issues.

EXAMPLE

Alys, a Welsh woman, had been signed off sick from work for three months with a case of life-threatening tachyarrhythmia. This condition combines a fast, racing heart rate (tachycardia) with an irregular heartbeat (arrhythmia), a potentially serious medical problem, which had necessitated her being put into a clinically induced coma. So volatile was her condition, there was concern she might not be able to work again. Once out of the coma, having heard about energy work from a friend, she contacted me and asked to do some short-term work to see if it was possible to get to the roots of this condition on a psychological level. Her husband brought her down to London for four intensive sessions which took place over two days.

Alys' crisis had been triggered by the breakup of a close friendship. This had been a very traumatic ending where she felt totally betrayed by her friend who had suddenly and destructively invaded areas of her private life. Alys was experiencing feelings of shock and terror as it dawned on her that the person, who had seemed a solid, safe, 'friend for life', might be as crazy as her manipulative and sadistic mother. This shook Alys' sense of reality—had she trusted someone who was totally unbalanced? There was nowhere to run to. Nowhere was safe, so her heart was racing and beating in a chaotic, life-threatening way.

Further exploration in therapy reminded her of a similar instance in her early life, where her mother had completely invaded her boundaries, denying her any privacy so Alys had no protective boundary or 'emotional skin'. In the panic of all the recent events, and on account of the strong malicious energy she felt from both her mother and her friend, everything felt evil, dangerous, and unsafe. We hypothesised that she was suffering from toxic emotional shock.

At this realisation, Alys was feeling a great deal of emotional and energetic 'charge', an indicator that it was time for some energy work, so we started using meridians on which to tap, using the phrase:

This toxic emotional shock.

This produced a profound sense of her connecting with all that had happened, coming back into her body, and strong memories of her earlier life experiences, and, also, a greater calmness.

Alys recounted that following the trauma with her friend, she started experiencing extremely high blood pressure. Her mother then phoned her out of the blue from hospital with the bombshell that she had had a heart attack and wanted Alys to visit straight away. Alys felt very angry and upset. 'As usual' her mother was competing with her to have 'the same drama'—it felt like a total psychic invasion that her mother should be experiencing heart problems at the same time as Alys. Aware of the contradictions that her mother needed Alys' care while simultaneously feeling malice and envy towards her, Alys' immediate physiological responses to her mother's phone call were of revulsion, disgust, and weakness in the legs. In energy psychotherapy we understand this to be a 'flop' reaction of the vagus nerve, where her system was collapsing. She was in the relational trauma of a double bind, because she knew it wasn't safe to have contact with her mother, yet she did not know how she could avoid going to see her.

When her mother came out of intensive care, perhaps not coincidentally, Alys' sister was also too 'deadly ill' to help. Alys thereby felt obliged to go and visit her mother, though her husband urged her not to because Alys' own blood pressure was dangerously high.

The final trigger which induced Alys' tachyarrhythmia was when she felt compelled to lie to her employers, pretending she was going to visit her mother and then not doing so. She felt terrible shame that her mother was so ill and that 'no one should know what a bad daughter I am'.

A key aspect of this way of working is to follow the flow of energy which arises in the moment. Alys' triggered state was a clear indicator for more energy clearing so I guided her on how to tap on her feeling of shame, which reduced the intensity of her distress. We then spent more time talking until we formulated her problem as:

> I feel toxic shock at realising both my mother and friend are mad and unpredictable, and as there is nowhere to run to, and nowhere is safe, I have tachyarrhythmia.

Alys went on to work with her chakras (clients self-apply this work) to clear the traumatic stress from her body depicted by this phrase, which was repeated at each chakra as she moved down her body. She felt release as we did this, and we also followed the free associations which emerge from mind and body during clearings, or from triggered states. While undertaking the clearing, Alys was reminded of her coma, where she saw terrifying pictures of hanging upside down and having to give birth to a big baby bull with horns. Her whole body was torn by emotional pain and physical torture, which, she felt, represented the sadism and evil of her mother, who was constantly attacking her femininity and creativity. We then went on to clear the next trauma with a new phrase:

> Because of the life-threatening toxic shock, my defences were pierced by disbelief at the evil of my mother when I was in a coma, and I have no resilience or protective layers to deal with it, so I have developed high blood pressure and tachyarrhythmia.

The insight which emerged was that 'I know my mother is fighting death and she is trying to draw me in to die with her'. Alys recognised that her life-threatening heart condition was actually her defence, trying to protect her from having to be subjected to visiting her mother and her murderous wishes. After this we then continued with the final piece of our work together, the realisation that:

> My mother wants me dead.

Alys felt considerable relief after using energy work to clear this trauma. Working with this last phrase gave her permission to acknowledge this repressed truth. Following these sessions, she reported a big shift, her blood pressure and tachyarrhythmia returned to normal within a week, and she was able to return to work with a clean bill of health after her time off.

This vignette illustrates how closely linked *mindbodyenergy* is. What we undertook was, on one hand, quite straightforward psychoanalytic work, following Alys' unconscious process. Stress and trauma create a complicated cocktail of physical and biochemical responses to powerful emotional stimuli. Physiologically, emotions are themselves electrical, chemical, and hormonal discharges of the human nervous system. Emotions influence—and are influenced by—the functioning of our major organs, the integrity of our immune defences, and the workings of the many circulating biological substances that help govern the body's physical states. When emotions are repressed, this inhibition disarms the body's defences against illness. Repression—dissociating emotions from awareness and relegating them to the unconscious realm—disorganises and confuses our physiological defences. These defences go awry for some people, becoming the destroyers of health rather than its protectors.

When we work with energy psychotherapy, psyche, soma, and stress are relatively easily linked in energy clearings, and many find significant relief from physical symptoms. Although therapists assist their clients in this work, the release occurs as a direct result of the client working with their own body and healing process, clearing their own energetic blockages. I am constantly amazed by the elegance of the *bodymindspirit* and the ways that, given the right support, apparently miraculous recovery can occur.

Everything is energy

My earliest memories are of lying in my cot as a baby, enjoying the pleasure of vibration as I brushed my fingers across my bottom lip making a 'broom broom' sound while light danced across the curtain. Then when I was four, the fragrance of roses was so captivating I decided to make rose-petal water. Using my mother's exquisitely fine, thin-cut crystal glasses as fitting vessels for the delicacy of the scent, I poured in some water and crushed and mashed with a metal spoon—totally delicious! I didn't bargain on the furious repercussions when I broke one of these precious glasses, but nonetheless the waft of roses is still one of my greatest delights—and roses, by the way, resonate at a very high frequency. These memories of the early sensory delights of energy and vibrations to this day remain totally vivid and present.

Everything that exists is energy: all the senses—smell, touch, sound, taste, and sight—solid objects such as rocks, as well as the invisible world of feelings and emotions. We exist on a spectrum of frequencies, from the slow dense vibration of matter to the faster vibration of light—and this is science.

Although we may not have clear beliefs about how the universe or multiverses work, most people broadly accept some notion of 'source' or 'universal' energy:

> The idea that the essence of reality is a non-material spiritual quality is one of the oldest and most common cross-cultural concepts in the history of the world. It's an idea that almost every one of the world's indigenous cultures has developed independently, and one that each of the world's mystical or spiritual traditions has also independently incorporated. (Taylor, 2018, p. 31)

However, contemporary views on the nature of reality still differ. Notably, a strand in science, known as 'scientific materialism', believes that what cannot be seen or tested with existing scientific tools simply does not exist. Richard Dawkins (*The God Delusion*, 2006) is the most well-known sceptic of the idea of an energy-basis of reality, where the universe itself is considered to have a consciousness, a meaning, that can be discerned and worked with. Perhaps Dawkins' hostility to the parallels between God and quantum physics may be driven by a frustration with the oppressive excesses of organised religions. History, if you like, has not taught him to have any faith in the application of the materially unknowable. In contrast to this is the philosophical tradition of pragmatism, exemplified by William James (1902, 2010) which argues that matter (energy), which is ultimately 'sensed', reveals more about ultimate reality than mind (words and thought) can. The debate continues, but any scepticism you may have about an unseen, but still felt, reality will certainly not prevent you from experiencing the real benefits of energy psychotherapy and learning to help others heal their own embodied trauma with this method.

Let us now explore the notion of energy and the role it plays in many everyday aspects of our lives.

Energy transmits

We are all affected by the energetic transmission of frequencies, whether it be from the earthly environment around us, such as nature, people, places, technology, and the media, to the celestial bodies like the moon and the planets in our solar system. Animals are highly sensitive, and readily pick up if they like or dislike the energy of a person or a place. Energy is transmitted in both positive and negative ways—so just as trauma can be thought of as being the result of the absorption of negative energy to which we are especially vulnerable in childhood, so too, joyful experiences—such as my baby memory which began this chapter—can have a lasting benefit.

Transmission is a dynamic aspect of energy. We are interconnected in 'the field', so energy moves between people and things, and we are all affected by different resonances. The impact goes both ways. Psychoanalysis holds that the energy within and around us is felt, stored, and as such, is largely unconscious. These depths may remain unknown unless we have the curiosity to investigate. In dynamic psychotherapy, the concepts of intersubjectivity, transference, countertransference, and attunement are part and parcel of the work. This acknowledges unconscious energetic processes such as Melanie Klein's projective identification. These therapeutic concepts are essentially referring to the same idea—the transmission of energy.

Through the intersubjective exchange of field energy, the unconscious mind is brought more into conscious awareness. The psychoanalytic method (and its psychodynamic derivatives), whilst enhancing cognitive awareness, may also bring out stored traumatic energy. If old memories are triggered without bringing relief this can feel very painful—'brutal' was the word one traumatised client used.

The sum is also greater than individual parts, so energy transmission is amplified in groups, and their 'fields' are especially powerful. Lynne McTaggart's *The Power of Eight* (2017) denotes eight as the optimum number for a group's healing intention. Perhaps it is no coincidence that this is also considered the best size for therapy groups. Whether talking, sharing ideas, learning, or meditating together, interconnecting energetically in groups amplifies the experience so everyone's learning becomes exponential and 'fractal'. The group process also helps to raise—or lower—the vibration, depending on the group's intention.

Chopra (1989) explains this phenomenon in terms of 'biofields' and compares going into a stressful room where you can 'cut the atmosphere with a knife' with the peaceful atmosphere in a holy temple. Every part of our body—every cell—has a magnetic field that transmits, and we can biologically measure this. These magnetic fields are somewhat like Jung's concept of the 'collective unconscious' and what Rupert Sheldrake terms 'morphogenetic fields'.

The energy of the collective is very powerful and shapes our reality. For instance, an experiment in Washington DC studied the effect of a large group of meditators. Led by quantum physicist John Hagelin (1993), this major social study set out to show how easy and simple it is to reduce crime and social stress by using meditation to intervene from the field of consciousness. The project rapidly reversed the violent crime trend by 23.3 per cent, and the police, who were initially sceptical, also joined in with the meditation.

Rupert Sheldrake's research on morphogenetic fields has a delightful study of the telepathic communication which takes place between pets and their owners (the ORF experiment). Although physically located miles apart, the dog Jaytee moves to the front door to wait expectantly for his owner at exactly the moment when she decides to return home from having coffee with a friend. https://www.youtube.com/watch?v=aA5wAm2c01w

Energy and consciousness are intertwined—all aspects of our experience are recorded and held as encoded information in our subtle energy. In energy psychotherapy we connect with this information in our 'biofields' (often termed 'thoughtfields') to release trauma. Our entire history—all the data and information about what has happened to our soul throughout all existence—is registered in what are termed the 'akashic records'. This soul dimension provides a vast library of information which everyone has the potential to 'tap' into. This highly sensitive energy field provides a repository of all our past lives/previous experiences, including the transpersonal. Through the akashic records we can access the wisdom of our soul and draw on previous experience to help us change and transform in the present.

Energy is universal and communicates beyond language

The nonverbal communications of energy provide an important sensory means for negotiating life, relationships, and the world. Energy operates at an experiential level beyond thoughts, concepts, or constructs of mind where all beings can sense energies communicating something. For instance, what is it that a dog senses when it whines and backs away from a particular corner in a house? When we are looking for a place to live, how do we just 'know' that we have 'come home'? Is this our 'gut feeling' talking to us?

We are surrounded by symbols, nonverbal conveyors of meaning which communicate potent energy. A symbol—a sign, mark, or visual image—is a conduit for energy whose resonances energetically affect us, serving as motivating forces for groups of people. National flags evoke passionate feelings at sporting events and religious symbols evoke equally powerful responses. Some symbols are universal in their nature, creating links with archetypal human experience, though we may not be fully conscious of their meanings. The images in a deck of Tarot cards constellate strong energies and archetypes, just as metaphors and mementos are strong carriers of energy which communicate directly with the psyche.

Different cultures have innumerable ways of connecting with 'energies'—Indigenous Americans invite in their ancestors as conduits of energy, shamans work with spirits and power animals, Buddhists visualise and integrate the energies of different 'deities', and Christians take the Eucharist to symbolise Christ's flesh and blood.

Our thoughts and emotions resonate at specific frequencies, and each of us transmits our own unique vibration or energetic 'signature'. People receive these signals and unconsciously 'read' the energy field, naturally sensing the difference between 'low' energies such as negativity, fear, anxiety, and depression as compared with the 'high' frequencies of elation, love, or joy. In everyday language, colloquial expressions such as 'she really lit up the room' or 'he seemed a bit low' assume that people intuitively understand the vibrational world. Such phrases are saying something quite literal and real in energetic terms. Psychics have finely honed senses which they use to 'read' energy in various ways, with clairvoyants seeing images and clairsentients feeling and sensing the energy around people and things—we all have this potential if we choose to develop it.

Energy is intelligently responsive to language

Energy therapy is flexible and can communicate energetically without words or images but it is also wonderfully responsive to language. Even when someone is in a coma, their bodies can signal receptivity to words/sound. Words are signifiers, indicating our intentions to 'intelligent' energy. So, when we use specific phrases as part of the process of trauma clearing—whether via thought or speech—the energy held and transmitted in words is communicated. For instance, a simple phrase such as 'My terror when mum left' informs our brain's neural pathways that the specific traumatised energy associated with this abandonment trauma needs to be released from the body. Conversely, intelligent energy also recognises when we wish to bring positive frequencies into our *mindbodyenergy* with which to resource ourselves. Masaru Emoto's research clearly demonstrates the transformative power of words and energy's responsiveness to language in Emoto's photographs of frozen water crystals (see also Chapter 2).

Energy flows and transforms

Energy also flows and transforms. Just as water changes between ice, water, and steam, so too, by clearing trauma, we can transform ourselves in energy therapy. This is achieved through a process of activating subtle energies—namely, the meridians, energy centres (chakras), and thoughtfields. When subtle energy flows through our channels, free associations of the mind and body arise and take shape in images, feelings, memories, and physical sensations. These bring insight and deeper understanding, transforming our *mindbodyenergy* on all levels. Our thoughts, emotions, and beliefs gradually change, and stress is reduced, all of which can result in transformation. For instance, someone who has suffered months or years of sleeplessness may suddenly find themselves able to sleep, or a person may develop new insights and gradually shift their perceptions about themselves and others. Research on war veterans shows extensive recovery from post-traumatic stress disorder (PTSD), where after years in constant states of 'hypervigilance', sufferers feel calmer and more relaxed. The Association for Comprehensive Energy Psychology (ACEP) has a substantial data base of research showing positive outcomes. https://www.energypsych.org/

Energy and consciousness operate together

Dawson Church's *Mind to Matter* (2018) synthesises hundreds of studies in the fields of biology, physics, and psychology, confirming how we are literally creating our reality—an idea which brings strong reactions. We are all 'creator consciousness'—we create all the time with our thoughts and emotions. Regardless as to what we believe about reality, our consciousness has tremendous creative power. When we understand this, free will and our power to choose becomes very significant.

Our capacity to choose how we view and interpret complex experiences positively is an important tool, transforming our energy and consciousness to a 'higher' frequency. However, for those who are cut off from a positive sense of themselves, the idea of choice may seem like a luxury. When we feel stuck in our traumatic histories, reality may feel negative and oppressive—from this perspective 'bad things always happen to me'. The adage 'be careful what you wish for' is to be taken seriously however—despite our best, sincere, and conscious efforts to change, such 'script's will manifest painful re-enactments, where history unconsciously repeats itself.

Energy, the heart, and breath

Essentially, we are talking about vibrations. Until recently, the brain was viewed energetically as our primary driver. However, the heart is a more powerful electro-magnetic field generator in the human body. The electrical field measured in an electrocardiogram (ECG) is about sixty times greater than the brain waves recorded in an electroencephalogram (EEG) and the magnetic component of the heart's field is also around one hundred times stronger than that produced by the brain (McCraty, 2004). This is important, because the physical world—as we know it—is made of those two fields: electrical and magnetic fields of energy. Physics now tells us that if we can change either the magnetic field or the electrical field of the atom, we literally change that atom and its elements within our body and this world. The human heart is designed to do both.

'Heart rhythm meditation' (Redington, 2019) speaks of the interconnection between energy, breath, the heart, and intention. Our breath is our life force, connecting us directly with 'source' energy, and plays a helpful role in energy work. Redington refers to Sufi Master Puran Bair (1998) saying that 'Energy rides on the breath'. Physicist William Tiller (2004) says that 'Energy follows intention' and Joe Dispenza (2019) says that 'Where attention goes, energy flows'.[1]

---

[1] Redington, H. (2019). 'Energy psychology and heart rhythm meditation: An illuminating convergence?' This is taken from an article by Heather Redington on 'Heart rhythm meditation using breath', written for the clinical training in Energy Psychotherapy Course, which provides an exploration of the quotations. Heather also runs online workshops training people in this method. For further information about the HeartMath Institute see https://www.heartmath.com

'Heart rhythm meditation' serves as a gateway to elevated states of consciousness, with the HeartMath Institute noting that when the heart resonates harmoniously, it creates a beneficial energy flow between people. We can use the magnetising and transformative power of the heart's intelligence to shift our perceptions and direct the flow of our emotions to help magnetise towards us that which we wish to create in life (Childre, Martin, Rozman, & McCraty, 2016).

Since breath is a catalyst for changing our energy 'field', breath, presence, and intention are key elements in energy psychotherapy. Breathing techniques help us access energetic potential and are useful self-help tools for both clients and therapists. Heart-centred meditations facilitate the entrainment to our own breath and heartbeat, helping to calm and balance our systems. Change in our electromagnetic field produces transformation at an atomic level, and changing our energy changes our bodies (matter) at a cellular level. In this way, breathing with awareness can help us maintain balanced energy in a state of heart-centred presence. Moreover, because we transmit energy, as we transform ourselves, this beneficially affects everyone we encounter.

Energy—sound and colour

Sound and colour exist on the spectrum of energy frequencies measured in Hertz (Hz) and hold a significant place in the category of 'energy therapy' and 'vibrational medicine'. Cymatics—the study in physics of wave phenomena, sound, and its visual representations—shows how sound creates different patterns and shapes on sand, according to the frequency emitted, illustrating vibrations at work. The human body is profoundly impacted by frequency for good and ill. For instance, sonic forces—such as lasers—can be used for healing pain in the body. On the other hand, sonic weapons were used as control mechanisms during the Covid pandemic when the Australian police blasted out painful frequencies on crowds who were protesting about the lockdowns, which quickly dispersed people.

More subtly, people have been adversely impacted by a change in the universal tuning of the musical scale. Scientists report that the 'older' tuning of the note 'A' had a more beneficial resonance than the new harsher tone.[2]

---

[2] For some reason, which is not clear, the tuning pitch for the note 'A' in the scale was changed from A432 Hz to A440. People argue that the lower pitch has more healing properties, whereas the higher-pitched Hz has a less harmonious impact on the body, mind, and spirit. As shown by musician Brian T. Collins, the Schiller Institute, and various physicists and scientists, the 440 Hz frequency not only lacks mathematical or scientific significance, but it is also actually out of tune with the natural world and wider universe. For this reason, many believe that the 440 Hz pitch doesn't just make music less pleasant and enjoyable, but has a negative effect on our mind, our consciousness, our natural energies and vibrations, and our spirituality. https://www.mindvibrations.com–432 Hz

Many famous musicians, from Jimi Hendrix and Bob Marley to Mozart, used to tune their music to the older frequency of 432.

Horowitz discovered an astonishing frequency, which he named the 'Universal LOVE/528 Constant' (2011), with revolutionary new healing applications. He describes this solfeggio frequency as the love energy radiating at the heart of everything—'Life Force' 528 nm/Hz is fundamental to everything including the sun, pyramids, circles, squares, rainbows, pi, Phi, the Fibonacci series, buzzing bees, and snowflakes and the reason that grass is green. We can beneficially reprogramme our subconscious mind while we sleep by listening to recordings of such high-frequency harmonic resonances.

Have you ever listened to music and felt it throughout your whole body, or opening your heart? Music strikes a chord within us that resonates with our heart, mind, and soul, expressing at times what we cannot vocalise ourselves. Ludwig van Beethoven spoke about music as the mediator between the spiritual and the sensual life. Evelyn Glennie (2015), a musician who, like Beethoven, has hearing impairment, can nonetheless feel music's vibrations.

The sonic energy of music helps us connect with our feelings, transporting us into the sensual/spiritual in a variety of ways. Music therapy is widely used with those who struggle with words. Relaxing vibrational 'sound baths' are also becoming popular these days using instruments such as gongs, Tibetan bowls, and crystal bells. Chanting a mantra emanates specific frequencies which resonate throughout the body, bringing healing and balance. Once, when I went to an acupuncturist for my regular 'tune up', she was surprised she had no work to do because my energies were completely balanced. She asked what I had been doing—I had been chanting literally thousands of mantras on retreat.

Colour, too, affects us in everyday life and has major therapeutic uses. Having trained in colour healing I find this area fascinating. All colours—not only medical infrared or ultraviolet treatment—can be used for healing. For instance, research by The Forest Bathing Institute (https://tfb.institute/scientific-research/shows) that the green of forest bathing is highly beneficial, bringing improvements in the ability to access more supportive emotions, and helps people connect with nature, reducing mood disturbance, slowing excessive rumination, and aiding the development of compassion. It also stabilises heart rate, which is, perhaps, what makes these other benefits possible.

People generally belong predominantly to a particular ray or colour family (Wood, 1989) and tend to be attracted to specific colours. While it is true that certain colours tend to suit a person, it is not wise for those who have had colour analysis consultations to get fixated on the idea that (for example) 'I always go for blue'. If you do, you might be denying yourself colours which you really need. When we suffer from a deficit of energy, colours feed and nourish us. We can replenish our energy by simply having colour around us in various forms—flowers, clothes, jewellery, paintings, our environment, and the colour schemes we choose—or eating foods of the colour we crave. Our attraction for and need of colours changes over time depending on the state of our energy, so it is good to pay attention to our cravings.

Colour 'readings' identify colours and frequencies that we need at specific moments in time. Before training in colour therapy, when on tour with The Guest Stars in Egypt, we visited the souks and saw fabulous arrays of gems on display. There was quite an overwhelming choice, but I was surprised to find myself particularly drawn to and 'hungry' for deep lapis lazuli beads, pale amethyst, and coral, whereas the turquoise—a feature of Egyptian gems—didn't attract me at all. I was surprised later when indigo, lavender, and orange came up for my first colour reading—colours which I was not normally attracted to at all. And then I made the connection. My body had known it needed the energy of those gemstones before I did.

When we have a strong desire for a specific frequency, that colour will undoubtedly enhance our energy. This too is energy medicine. Red was not usually a colour I'm drawn to, but after a scary operation which traumatised me and my body, I couldn't get enough red and had the impulse to buy a very bright red sweater. This significantly boosted my energy levels and several people remarked, 'that colour really suits you, you should wear it more often'. On reflection I realised that red governs the root chakra, which is the energy centre concerned with survival and fundamental safety (colours and chakras will be explored further in Chapter 6). Similarly, on another occasion I couldn't stop wearing pale pink—and I later discovered that it is the frequency of unconditional love, something I really needed at the time.

People perceive colours differently. The segment of the electromagnetic spectrum that can be seen by the human eye is called 'visible light'. However, perception varies among cultures, with the Himba culture being able to see green but not blue (Wood, 1989). At school we learned the classical 'rainbow' with the phrase 'Richard of York Gave Battle in Vain' to designate red, orange, yellow, green, blue, indigo, and violet. But where were turquoise and magenta? Today these are known as the 'New Age' colours, which did not appear to exist in England a few hundred years ago—although they were well favoured amongst the ancient Egyptians. What might be the cause of this phenomena? According to Braden (2009), this has something to do with the rhythmic flow of time, mirrored in fractals which loop back in spirals and cycles. There is therefore some correlation between the cycle of the Ancient Egyptian age with its use of colour and vibrational medicine and the current spiritual awakening of the 'New Age' (Farrer, 2002) which features similar vibrational technologies and colours.

Energy fields: (biofield, energy body, aura, light bodies, thought fields, the field) NB Energy bodies will be explored further in Chapters 2 and 8.

We referred previously to Chopra's term 'biofields' (1989), an energetic 'field' surrounding all living things, including plants and animals. This term was popularised by Redfield's novel and movie *The Celestine Prophecy* (1994) which brought the notion of energy fields into popular awareness. I introduce here various words—energy body, aura, light body, thought fields, the field—so that if you come across them, you will know they mean more-or-less the same thing.

Since Roger Callahan was the originator of Thought Field Therapy or TFT (1995), which is a significant modality in energy psychotherapy, so energy therapists frequently used the term 'thought field'—though I also have a personal liking for the terms energy body and light body.

'Energy bodies' (plural) create an energetic field comprising layers of energy around the body. Different traditions variously consider that there are between four and seven layers, and some perceive even more. Empaths often become overwhelmed by all the energy they pick up in the field from the 'mass collective'. Other sensitive people may have 'porous' personalities (Mollon, 2015), an indicator that their energy field is compromised in some way. Energy psychotherapy has the facility to strengthen the weak energy boundaries of the energy bodies, so that people can become more resilient and less vulnerable to energetic intrusions from others. (Energy boundaries will be explored in Chapter 8.)

The energy field reflects the state of a person's consciousness, with colour and frequency giving a unique vibrational picture of each soul. Some people can 'see' the nature of people's energy and when the aura radiates with a high vibration, the person will tend to emanate a sense of 'Presence' and people will be drawn to them. 'Halos' in spiritual pictures attest to the radiance of those whose spiritual consciousness is highly developed.

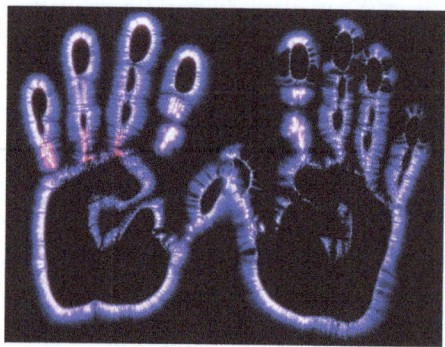

Figure 1 A Kirlian photograph of healing hands

Kirlian photography has made it possible for us to photograph our energetic state showing how colours and energies change depending on our feelings, emotions, and mood. I knew a healer who had her hands photographed at a Mind Body Spirit Festival, which showed wonderfully clear bright light extending evenly all around her fingers. She was amused that her partner was somewhat miffed because despite having been on his spiritual path for much longer than her, his Kirlian photograph showed his energy to be in less good shape, with gaps and 'holes' in his 'field'.

Why work with 'energy'?

An opening to 'rich, new dimensions from within'

My reasons for writing this book introducing energy psychotherapy are many. I wanted to share its benefits, both in terms of its practical usefulness, and more broadly, its capacity to bring deep healing into the realm of psychotherapy.

I feel energy therapy is important on different levels.

First, it is very effective in addressing a wide range of conditions and therapeutic issues in straightforward practical ways. Energy psychology was first noted for its effectiveness in treating phobias such as a fear of flying, which can generally be routinely cleared in one or two sessions. I remember once when Sue, one of the NHS secretaries, asked me about energy therapy over lunch, wanting an example of how it worked. I asked her if she had any specific issues in mind and she replied that she hated spiders, needing her husband to take them out of the bath for her. I demonstrated a chakra waterfall clearing, inviting her to join me as we both went quickly down the sequence of our respective chakras saying 'My fear of spiders'. This was not at all a 'proper session', just a casual sharing of what happens. She was astonished to report the following week that not only had she managed to remove a spider from the bath on her own, but had also, without flinching, run the gauntlet of the mass of spiders sitting in their webs along the path to her front door. The methods of energy psychotherapy can also easily be integrated within most therapeutic disciplines, so they are applicable in all types of counselling and psychotherapy, from psychoanalytic therapy to cognitive behavioural therapy (CBT), and in clinical psychology, psychiatry, family therapy, couple therapy, and with children.

Within the field of psychology and psychotherapy, the value of working with resonance and vibration is gaining recognition. A significant evidence base, compiled by the Association for Comprehensive Energy Psychology (ACEP), an international body for energy psychotherapy,[3] demonstrates that this work is remarkably effective. Tapping is increasingly used by mainstream and student counselling services, and in the USA, it is used for treating PTSD in war veterans. The National Institute for Health and Care Excellence (NICE) guidelines in the UK, also noting the beneficial results, advocate further research. There are many energy methods, and sadly there isn't space in this book to include them all. Apart from the practices I share, I at least wanted to mention Donna Eden's wonderful Energy Medicine, Tapas Fleming's TAT, and Asha Clinton's AIT as examples of transformational approaches.

Second, energy is an invaluable bridge between psyche and soma. In medical fields, the healing power and efficacy of frequency medicine is well recognised in laser surgery, infrared treatments and other sonic approaches. The convergence of multidisciplinary approaches within psychotherapy in recent years includes the recognition that when treating trauma, the body needs to be included. As therapists, we choose methods that work for and best suit our clients—experientially and evidentially, energy work with the subtle energy and nervous systems facilitates interconnection between *mindbodyenergy*, releasing stress and pain from the body, mind, and emotions in surprisingly easy ways. This brings heartening relief and healing to people who may have struggled with their issues for years.

---

[3] Research in energy psychology methods has increased considerably in recent years. The Association of Comprehensive Energy Psychology (ACEP) is compiling extensive resources. See www.energypsych.org/research to view and access a comprehensive list of studies.

Energy therapy also fosters a natural, intimate therapeutic alliance. Energy work is integrated seamlessly within relational psychotherapy, taking us into a different 'domain', an experiential realm which facilitates an embodied connection with ourselves. The collaborative sense of therapist and client working intimately together also fits well with attachment theory. There is often something light and playful (key ingredients in healthy attachment) about the process of energy work which helps clients feel safe enough to be real and authentic. In this open state, egoic defences gradually fall away and the work flows effortlessly—we are 'in the zone'.

Third, is to convey something about the 'flow' of quantum energy methods. 'Ease and grace' is a phrase summing up the gentle way that energy work cuts through mind chatter—the incessant thinking and wanting to be in control—that blocks peaceful states. Quieting the mind helps take people out of the fight/flight survival modes into states of relaxation and tranquillity in their bodies and also brings them clarity. When therapist and client are working soul-to-soul it brings transformative holistic healing into psychotherapy. This might sound 'too good to be true', and undoubtedly there will be those who don't have such experiences. However, the numbers of clients who, once they have tried these methods return to them and want to work with them, makes energy psychotherapy a very rewarding way of working.

Experiencing energy therapy for myself showed me that it works. When clearing early infant trauma, I felt the powerful visceral release of energy coursing through and out of my body into the ground, which provided tangible proof of the reality of the depth and effectiveness of this way of working. I needed no further convincing. When we experience how freeing this is—both for clients and therapists—and how transformative it can be in bringing a greater sense of peace and balance, it is very rewarding to integrate this approach within psychotherapy.

However, it is also understandable that some may be hesitant to change their ways of working, being uncertain about what this might mean in practice. Actually, energy therapy employs quite down-to-earth and easily appliable skills which can facilitate transformation in seemingly effortless ways. It is sometimes a little astonishing when psychotherapists and counsellors first experience the natural release of long-standing blockages and difficulties that were not previously helped by 'talking therapies' alone.

In 'Choosing the path of joy', the drive of my story was essentially concerned with the desire to find liberation from suffering and to find my true self. By introducing you to energy psycho-therapy, I hope to convey how these methods are very much aligned with both these aims and can facilitate an expanded state of consciousness, leading people to an experience of their 'true' self, bringing considerable relief from suffering. As Dorothea Hover-Kramer (2002) writes:

> When we see our therapeutic interactions with clients as communication between biofields and watch our clients heal, we increase our sense of the numinous and the transformative. In addition, the energy therapies seem to facilitate the alignment of both therapist and client to the resources of the higher self, the transpersonal perspective, and the pervasive qi of the universe. Alignment with intuition allows accessing of potentials for the highest good of the client, an opening to rich, new dimensions from within both healer and healed. We come to see therapy as the creative blending of both science and art.

CHAPTER 2

From matter to light: working with frequency and vibrations

From matter to light

The first chapters in this book are largely concerned with theoretical speculations rather than clinical practice. Some of this may feel new or a bit 'heady' and absorbing material about energy, matter, and light without yet knowing how it fits into therapy can feel a little intense. You may wonder, how on earth could this apply to my practice? If you are not particularly interested in these more abstract aspects, it is fine to go straight to Part II to look at the practicalities—whatever is the easiest way for you to take in the information. Please see this book as a resource which you dip into and use as suits you.

In the meantime, I would like to provide a brief clinical context. Dawson Church, in *Mind to Matter* (2018) cautions against extremes. In everyday life, some things are manifestly true, and others manifestly untrue and in between there is a 'wide middle ground' which is the subject of our applications in energy psychotherapy.

There are contradictions in this work—it is simple and complex; one size by no means fits all. It is easy to learn and in fact energy psychology techniques are accessible to everyone on the internet regardless as to whether they have had any therapeutic training. Certainly, these can be very helpful as self-help tools for clients and therapists. At the same time, it takes time to deepen clinical experience and understand the complexities. Crudely applied ideas may be counterproductive and even therapeutically harmful. In recognition of the vulnerability of clients who have experienced trauma, and the power of energy methods, it is recommended that you train in energy psychotherapy after qualifying in your therapeutic discipline, so you are experienced in holding and grounding clients and practising safely. This is especially the case where complex trauma is concerned.

Understanding conceptually about working with frequencies is one thing—bringing such ideas into clinical practice is another, requiring subtlety and skill so we are sensitive to people's needs and meet them where they are. There has been much justified criticism about facile interpretations of 'positive thinking' and how we 'create our reality'. Years ago, a book called *The Secret* (Byrne, 2006), which claims that thought alone can influence objective circumstances within ones life, disappointed many who found it 'didn't work'. A client who has suffered severe abuse would feel re-abused by crudely delivered suggestions of 'mind over matter' or 'matter to light'; others might feel they are 'failing' to manifest their positive desires, where others still might feel superstitious about their obsessive negative feelings and thoughts, fearing they might be dangerous and 'make bad things happen'. I remember one survivor of trauma being deeply affronted when she was told by a counsellor to 'just think of the glass as being half full'.

While the paradigm of working with energy and frequency may seem foreign, please be assured that emotions and relationships are equally attended to, as in conventional therapy. Energy psychotherapists continue to use their core therapeutic skills and the heart-to-heart connection between therapist and client creates a holding therapeutic relationship where all the ups and downs of life, emotions, and relationships are explored. A significant part of the work concerns creating safety so that people's grief, fears, anxieties, struggles, anger, resentment, traumas and so on can be attended to—and sometimes, the client may wish simply to talk about and be with their feelings.

Integrated within this frame, at certain points we undertake energy work, where the client self-applies energy methods to release stress, trauma, and stuck feelings. This brings considerable relief and clarity, while the collaborative process of the *mindbodyenergy* of both client and therapist increases the attunement and intimacy of the therapeutic relationship.

Working with energy takes us beyond the cognitive, to experiential, embodied aspects of psychotherapy. My aspiration is to find balance between 'taking it lightly' and being grounded. If there are people reading this book who have experienced considerable degrees of trauma, please take care of yourselves—although I do wish to emphasise that energy psychotherapy is an inherently gentle way of working.

Awakening out of 'the matrix'

The world of psychotherapy has explored the mind a great deal but spent relatively little time on the body and energy, which also include spirit and consciousness. This chapter explores the relationship between matter, mind, consciousness, and energy. In the new paradigm, energy psychotherapy is essentially concerned with releasing the dense energy of trauma from the body to bring in more light. Once free of fear and trauma, we have more possibility of raising our states of consciousness—hence the title 'Energy, Soul-connecting and Awakening Consciousness'.

Many will be familiar with the film *The Matrix*. It is not until we awaken out of the 'matrix'—a metaphor for our egoic third-dimensional consciousness—that we realise that we have been in it and that there are other dimensions/realities. Working with energy can help take us outside the matrix and give us a taste of ultimate reality beyond ego. This glimpse of unity consciousness, (fifth-dimensional consciousness) is a universal experience which anyone can have—a non-conceptual state beyond mind, religion, or dogma. I learned to access this through Dzogchen, a path of the heart which brings us to the awakened state by purifying energy and consciousness—so energy psychotherapy, in focusing on 'clearing energy', shares some similarities.

The experience of the awakened heart is known as 'emptiness' in Buddhism, or 'zero point'—the 'still point' in the quantum world. It is a transformative experience which changes our entire world view.

Dzogchen describes this natural state as 'pure awareness':

> Pure from the beginning, free and empty,
> Not falling into the concept of an 'empty' emptiness,
> Instead, in the luminosity of its self-existing energy it is fully accomplished.
> This is the very ground for the manifestation of compassion's Rigpa,
> Rigpa is beyond designation and verbalisation,
> Out of it arises, as its display, the variety of appearances of Samsara and Nirvana.
> Manifestation and manifestor are not two –
> In this state of oneness, naturally remain.
>
> Jamyang Khyentse Chökyi, Lodrö 'Heart advice in a nutshell'[1]

For most of us, our 'true' nature of pure awareness lies hidden under layers of trauma, 'dense' energy, and unresolved painful experiences. The quantum world, Dzogchen, and energy therapy all operate in a state of 'flow' characterised by peace, simplicity, grace, and ease. I hope I manage to communicate in this book that energy psychotherapy, in common with Dzogchen, can help us to access this depth, profundity, and naturalness.

'Form is emptiness, emptiness is form'—the *Heart Sutra*[2]

At the ordinary level of our lived experience, we feel things are solid and real. However, within the absolute (quantum) nature of reality, when we 'awaken' through the heart of compassion, we see the 'empty', dreamlike, illusory nature of reality. This is the profound realisation of the Heart Sutra.

Albert Einstein's equation $e = mc^2$ 'proved' what these wisdom traditions have known all along—the empty nature of reality—that matter doesn't solidly exist but only appears to do so. Even the apparently solid form of a rock is just pulsating energy and holds as much energy

---

[1] Jamyang Khyentse Chökyi Lodrö, a twentieth-century Dzogchen Master, uses this phrase to describe the ultimate state of mind in his 'Heart advice in a nutshell', one of the first Dzogchen teachings I came across. These teachings were originally secret.

[2] One of the 'turnings of the wheel of *dharma*', 'Form is emptiness, emptiness is form', known as the Heart Sutra. The Heart Sutra was taught by Avalokiteśvara in the presence of the Buddha.

within it as the ocean waves. The waves arising in the solid rock cannot be seen because they are very subtle—but the rock *is* waving, pulsating.

The universe is one indivisible dynamic whole in which energy, matter, and consciousness are so deeply 'entangled' it is impossible to view them as independent elements. We have learnt from quantum physics that physical atoms are made up of vortices of energy that are constantly spinning and vibrating. Everything is interconnected in a sea of continually emerging and disappearing particles and waves, in which normal assumptions of time, space, and location do not apply—and this realm appears to be, in certain ways, entangled with our human consciousness. Mind itself seems startlingly similar to the vision of the quantum world revealed by conventional science. Meditation perhaps allows a disentanglement so that we are no longer tied to the same fixed repeating patterns—a flow is enabled that allows new connections and synchronicities to form.

In quantum science, the question that then arises is, how do objects (things we see as held in a form) become so? Eddington helped confirm Albert Einstein's general relativity theory in 1919 with his astronomical measurements of light bending as it passed the sun in eclipse. He also discovered that whereas scientists used to think of matter as a form, 'matter is more like a thought than a thing' (Mayers, 2018).

Nobel Prize–winning physicist Max Planck, discussing this phenomenon from the perspective of quantum physics, says:

> There is no matter as such. All matter originates and exists only by virtue of a force which brings the particle of an atom to vibration and holds this most minute solar system of the atom together. We must assume behind this force the existence of a conscious and intelligent Mind. This Mind is the matrix of all matter. (Planck, 1944)

Lanza (Lanza & Berman, 2008), in a book about biocentrism, posits that consciousness is at the core of the universe:

> Without consciousness, 'matter' dwells in an undetermined state of probability. Any universe that could have preceded consciousness only existed in a probabilistic state. … Life creates the universe, not the other way around. (p. 160)

Jude Currivan, in *The Cosmic Hologram* (2017) explains how:

> The fractal in-formational patterns that guide behaviour at the atomic level also guide the structure of galactic structures in space … consciousness connects us to the many interconnected layers of universal in-formation, making us both manifestations and co-creators of the cosmic hologram of reality. (Back cover of the book)

Church elucidates that: 'Our consciousness affects the material reality around us. As our consciousness changes, so changes the world' (Church, 2018). Hence, in this conversation about energy, information, and matter, matter is seen to be a physical expression of thought. Your brain interprets the light waves and energy you are seeing as a physical object.

A world of frequencies

In our vibrational universe, energy exists on a spectrum measured in resonance and vibrations along with consciousness, matter, sound, colour, and light. The Universe is energy just as our *bodymindsoul* is energy. The difference between the two is only that of rhythm and wavelengths—of frequencies. On a physical level, the body's energy functions in an obvious way and is only immediately understood as matter. However, mind is more subtle. Thoughts are only privately experienced (unless one is clairvoyant and can sense and interpret the subtle energy of thoughts). Consciousness, which is the purest, fastest, and most subtle vibrating energy, is invisible and therefore can never take objective form. It can only be experienced subjectively.

In terms of our lived human experience, how does this continuum of energy, from matter to light, and conversely from light to matter (energy flows in both directions along this polarity), express itself? How do the slowly vibrating dense frequencies at one end of the spectrum and the fast vibrating 'light' frequencies at the other end affect us?

In a very ordinary sense, 'feeling low' or being in 'high spirits' tells us something about the state of our energy. When dense energy blocks us, it can manifest at the physical level as physical and mental symptoms. Feeling 'high' might be a sign of the medical diagnosis of mania but it more usually signifies something of spiritual significance, manifesting as a surge of happiness and joy.

Refining our energy and 'raising our vibration' involves the process of shifting from unconscious to conscious awareness, from dense to fine, and from gross to subtle energies. In practice, this requires that we attend to issues as they arise in our lives—our emotional and relational difficulties, problems about our beliefs, anxiety and stress, or trauma and events which trouble us and throw us out of kilter. When we clear 'heavy' energies using energy psychotherapy, the fortunate biproduct is greater insight. As our frequency rises, we become more intuitive, evolving towards greater alignment with 'Source'.

The energy/light bodies—from matter to light

The energy/light bodies introduced in Chapter 1 are part of the subtle energy system, described fully in Chapter 8.

All our happy and unhappy experiences reside as information within our energy bodies. The densest vibrations are in the etheric body, closest to the physical body. As the field extends outwards, vibrations become higher, faster, and more refined.

From the dense to the fine

A simple structure of the energy bodies comprises:

i.   *Etheric body*

Our etheric body, the layer closest to our physical body with the densest energy, permeates the meridian system and chakra system serving as the interface between the physical body and our light body.

The three 'main' energy bodies which are part of personal human experience are the following.

ii.   *Emotional body*

Our emotional body carries cellular memories of our negative and positive experiences. Work with the emotional body involves releasing the stressful dense emotional energy stuck inside the body—such as fear, guilt, blame, hate, shame, depression, anxiety, destructive forms of anger and so—which helps raise our vibration. Energy psycho-therapy can clear the emotional trauma and blockages residing in our cellular memories, and once free of these, we become stable and are able to operate in a non-judgemental space of equanimity and peace. Part of this work involves becoming more aware of how we are feeling in a given moment—such as 'I'm feeling really resentful'—so we have more choice to change, and are fully conscious.

iii. *Mental/cognitive body*

Our mental body holds our thoughts, core beliefs, and conflicting patterns at a cellular level. Again, awareness is an important tool—when we catch ourselves unconsciously using a negative turn of phrase like 'I always make that mistake', we can step back and make a different choice by reframing with a new intention such as 'I learn effortlessly'. High vibrational thoughts cut through limiting beliefs and help to create positive outcomes. Learning to master our thoughts is good preparation for entering higher states of consciousness where our capacity to create manifests more quickly. The adage 'be careful what you wish for' is therefore very relevant. When working with our thoughts, the power of breath can bring a pause which activates the soul and gives us space to recalibrate.

iv.   *Spiritual body*

People have all sorts of spiritual trauma—often unrecognised and largely unconscious.

Being disconnected and separated from our spiritual selves/souls is an obvious and very significant one.

v.   *'Causal' body—'source' energy*

At the transpersonal level, the 'causal' level of light resonates with fastest finest vibrations. Some might name this as 'God', others, the 'Unified Quantum Field' or the 'Fifth Dimension'.

My neighbour Vyv drew a picture to represent these ideas, with the pink, yellow, and blue strands representing the emotional, mental, and spiritual bodies.

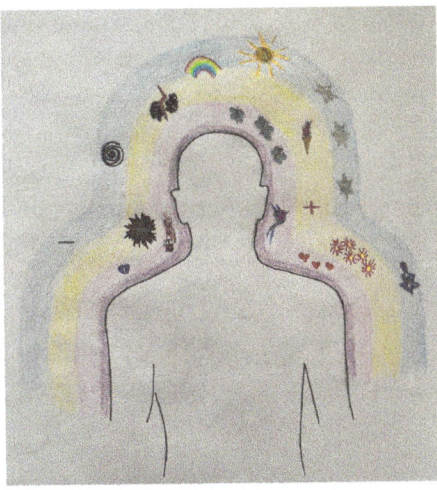

Figure 2 The energy bodies—emotional, mental, and spiritual experiences

Eckhart Tolle in *The Power of Now* speaks about what he calls the 'pain body' which is similar to the energy body. For those whose sense of self is habitually invested in pain, it perpetuates an unhappy self (Tolle, 1999).

Manifestation from light to matter

The process of manifestation involves energy flowing down from 'Source'. As it flows through the different energy bodies, the vibrations become slower and denser. Eventually, the energy vibrates slowly enough to manifest in physical form—matter—as the physical body.

The continuum of vibrations moves[3]

- from LIGHT/COLOUR imperceptible and perceptible—(photons)
- to SOUND (imperceptible and perceptible)
- to PHYSICAL MANIFESTATION, FORM, and MOVEMENT

Our energy 'field' is the zone of subtle energetic exchanges between people and their environments. People's energy fields radiate out to different distances from their physical bodies, some extending just one or two feet, where those with expanded states of consciousness will radiate out much further. When someone is 'radiant' it means something energetically. We can expand our radiance by visualising rays of light, extending to the furthest reaches of the universes and multiverses to infinity. There is no limit when we visualise 'limitless light'.

Our energy—how true and authentic we are—can be seen by the energetic state of our field. If the different layers of energy bodies surrounding us are clear or blocked, this will also be reflected in the state of our meridians and chakras. These in turn are determined by the state

---

[3] The scientific debate about which comes first—light or sound—continues. They are not on the same spectrum. Light belongs to the electromagnetic spectrum but sound does not, but they can both be measured in Hertz.

of our thoughts and emotions. When we are in a state of coherence and integrity, our energy is quite radiant and the 'line of the light' of our chakras is straight.[4] When we are out of alignment, and our energy feels unclear or murky, we are usually carrying unresolved mental/emotional/issues. In short, our energy reflects our truth and most of us usually have a mixture of light and shadow in our fields.

Energetically, our emotional, mental, and spiritual bodies offer useful tools in the service of our evolution as we raise our vibration. Each emotion or thought connects with the entire subtle energy system, with the power to either create density or raise our vibration. If we have made a decision to be on an evolving path, a core question when dealing with challenging situations might be to ask: 'How can I bring in a new frequency to raise this experience to a higher level?' When the emotional and mental bodies become clear, it allows for the unimpeded flow of the energies of our 'higher levels'.

From *Homo sapiens* to *Homo luminous*—the rainbow body

Various esoteric traditions emphasise the capacity for the miraculous transformation of the human body. The energetic principle of 'matter to light' is inter-cultural and universal. White (2018) speaks of enlightenment ('God-realization') as not purely a psychological event, describing how bodily changes occur, most dramatically, in the higher, final phases of enlightenment. According to various sacred traditions and hermetic schools, White says, the body becomes alchemically changed from flesh into light, to become immortal. Shri Aurobindo prophesised that 'supramental light' would pour onto earth in our current times to assist us in evolving from *Homo Sapiens* to *Homo Luminous* (Sri Aurobindo, 1950).

The transsubstantiated body is referred to by different names—the resurrection body, light body, solar body, diamond body, and rainbow body. Christianity's sacred purpose, for example, is to enable people, through the resurrection of the body, to become Christed. The Diamond Path within the Sufi tradition offers a similar path of light. In the Dzogchen tantras, the practices of Anuyoga and Atiyoga offer a comprehensive path to enlightenment through the 'path of luminosity'. The great Dzogchen masters realised enlightenment by going into rainbow body. Their bodies became so purified and refined they were no longer visible, their beings dissolving into rainbow light, leaving nothing behind except hair and fingernails.[5] When studying Tibetan Buddhism, I was fortunate to meet several realised traditional Dzogchen Masters and witnessed something of this phenomenon.

---

[4] 'The line of the light' (Levin, 2001) refers to the vertical column of the light going up the spine where the chakras are located. It was also the name given to a series of monthly spiritual seminars and meditations which Michal Levin gave to a small group over a period of approximately ten years.

[5] The ultimate fruition of the Dzogchen *tögal* practices is a body of pure light. The dissolution of the physical body at death is called a rainbow body (*'ja' lus*, pronounced ja lü.) If the 'four visions' of *tögal* are not completed before death, then during death, from the point of view of an external observer, the dying person starts to shrink until he or she disappears. Usually fingernails, toenails, and hair are left behind. The attainment of the rainbow body is typically accompanied by the appearance of lights and rainbows.

When I was in Nepal, I heard about the passing of His Holiness Dilgo Khyentse Rinpoche (for whom I used to chant) and I was keen to pay my respects. Synchronicities—or perhaps we could say the blessing of the Lama—came to my aid on a challenging journey. Against all odds, somehow tickets materialised for flights across Nepal and India which were supposedly sold out or cancelled, and the universe helped me make difficult connections where flight delays worked in my favour. When I eventually arrived at my destination, lost, and wandering through the narrow higgeldy-piggeldy streets, 'by chance' I walked straight into His Holiness's funeral procession en route to his *dung shuk* (sacred cremation). Dilgo Khyentse had been a mountain of a man in life (both in terms of his achievements, and literally—he was 6ft 7 inches) yet his *kudung* was remarkably small, demonstrating that most of him had already transformed into light. Holding onto the rail of the open carriage which carried his *kudung* (square box coffin),[6] I chanted the mantra, streaming with tears.

Similarly, the *Parinirvana*[7] of the female Master Khandro Tsering Chödron was also completely humbling. Khandro taught me the chant, and the dedication of this quiet modest woman, who had practised all her life and achieved such great realisation was awe-inspiring. I am incredibly grateful to have met these extraordinary beings who showed the reality of enlightenment, and moreover, within one lifetime.

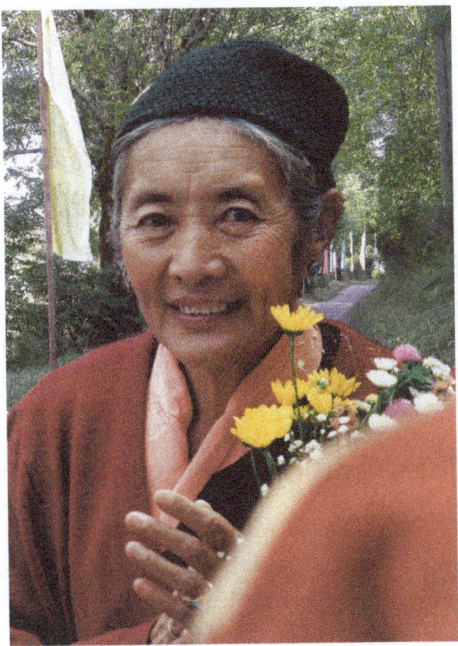

Figure 3 Dzogchen master Khandro Tséring Chödrön—'flowers'

---

[6] A *Kudung* is a square box-type of coffin, where the Master sits in mediation after death as their dissolution process continues.
[7] *Parinirvana* means 'final nirvana'. This is the final passing beyond suffering, manifested by buddhas and highly realised masters at the end of their life.

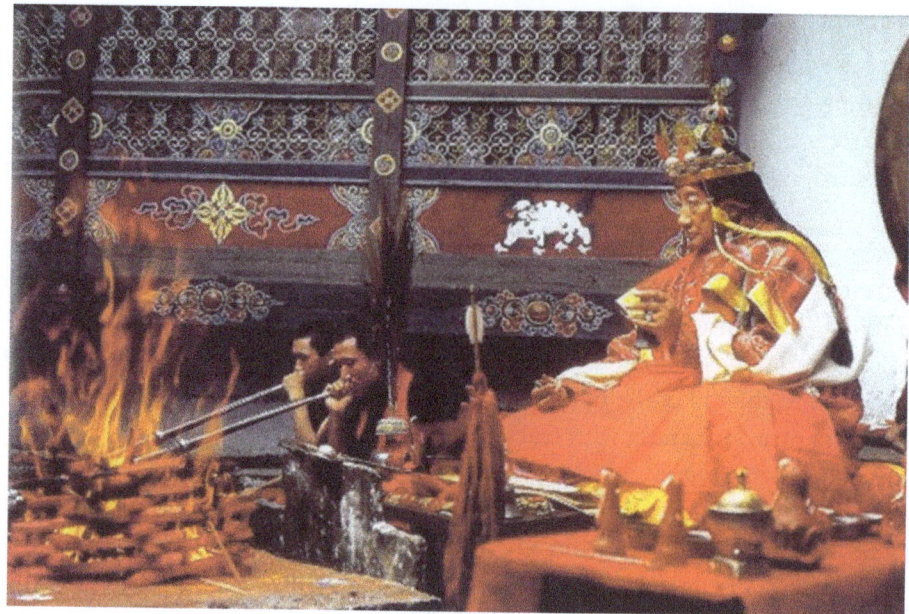

Figure 4 Dzogchen master Dilgo Khyentse Rinpoche conducting a fire ceremony

I find it very inspiring that it is possible to purify one's energy and dissolve into light. So why am I juxtaposing this with energy psychotherapy? In our busy lives, very few of us have the time, resources, or dedication to meditate in caves for thirty years or so, like the great masters who undertook the complex tantric practices of *Tsa Lung Tiklei* (subtle channels, inner air, and energy) to purify their energy. I hold that at this time in the evolution of our consciousness, humanity has been gifted with easier, faster methods which are accessible to everyone. Whether or not we can arrive at enlightenment—who knows?—but we can most certainly transform ourselves and become happier more fulfilled people by working with the subtle energies of our energy bodies, meridians, and chakras, refining our energy, changing our neural pathways, and raising our vibration.

Energy, vibrations, and consciousness in the unified field

In *Mind to Matter* (Church, 2018), Church speaks of our connection to the expanding universe and its energetic 'fields', where vibrations and information are transmitted. Though these fields are invisible, they are efficient conductors of information:

> Genius inventor Nikola Tesla said: 'If you wish to understand the universe, think of energy, frequency and vibration'. We use invisible energy fields such as cell networks to transmit information every day. When we originate an idea in consciousness, we send signals into the field. Transmission requires hardware, in the form of the brain, as well as software, in the

form of the mind. Signals traveling through neural pathways create energy fields, and those fields change, depending on the content of consciousness.

Another interesting view on Tesla and vibrations can be found in Michael Tellinger's fascinating video.[8] Healing involves 'field effects', whether local or distant. These have been explored by scientists in a myriad of ways, and Church cites seemingly miraculous contemporary research, demonstrating the impact on the 'field' of biofeedback; biophoton emissions; quantum coherence; communication through quantum frequency emissions; clairvoyance; remote intention; collective intention and consciousness and more.

The secrets of the power of vibration have been known about and practised by many indigenous and Eastern traditions for thousands of years. For instance, many African cultures use rituals involving dance and powerful drumming as an invitation to spirits or gods to help with a good harvest, and the Ancient Egyptians used energy healing with the frequencies of colour, crystals, and advanced technologies (Kaehr, 2019).

Quantum healing

Today, we are seeing an increase in vibrational healing, (naturally, all sound and colour healing comes under this category). Many, including some energy therapies, refer to this as 'quantum' healing. Meg Benedicte (2019) who created 'Quantum Access' says on her website: 'All healing begins with vibration—subtle vibration rules all matter.' Her method accesses the quantum field, using high frequencies of subtle energy to release dense energy. Mashhur Anam's *Life Harmonized* (https://lifeharmonized.com) has made it his life's work to bridge the gap between science and spirituality, creating 'revolutionary holographic tools for humanity' which use intention to create specific resonances and harmonies. I mention Benedicte and Anam to illustrate how the quantum world is gradually becoming part of the mainstream. Anam advocates that rather than the old-style approach of doing things 'the hard way' via space and time, we align with our 'divine self' (what I call soul-connecting) using quantum tools in the 'holographic playground' of the unified field. He compares the world of quantum play and its holographic properties (sets of 'codes', and projections of light and sound) with computing analogies. Just as we download an app for the iPhone, we can connect with 'plug-ins' from the field and reprogramme our consciousness with 'divine' algorithms and because we control these 'codes', all of us have the power to change. Transforming ourselves by tapping into the 'source code' is in fact very similar to the energy therapy of Callahan's Thought Field Therapy (TFT).

'Quantum tools' provide access to higher planes. In the vibrational world, like attracts like, with the universe responding to our energy frequency output. The higher the vibration we resonate with, the easier it is to realise our intentions, almost as quickly as we can imagine it.

---

[8] https://www.youtube.com/watch?v=Br5Qik1-spA Michael Tellinger's video about sound and 'God Lives Here'.

In Chapter 7 I talk about Sandi Radomski and Tom Altaffer's wonderful work 'Ask and Receive', another quantum method using intention which is incredibly transformative.

A general feature of energy psychotherapy is the idea of 'quantum leaps'—the speed of change which is possible, and the 'grace and ease' with which this is accomplished 'in the flow'. Results happen very quickly when working with high resonances. Dzogchen acknowledges this phenomenon using such phrases as: 'Perfectly and spontaneously accomplished, as soon as you think of it'. We might also use the term synchronicity.

One client who had previously been in psychoanalysis five times a week for many years was somewhat put out to discover how quickly trauma can be released using these methods. However, while it is true that quantum methods—if we can call them that—work rapidly, most of us vibrate at lower frequencies, and struggle to maintain states of higher consciousness. While we can clear trauma relatively quickly, we easily fall back into habitual limiting beliefs such as 'I'm not good enough' which stem from trauma. Maintaining consistently high frequencies takes practice, discipline, and steadfast application. It involves mindfulness to recognise when we fall back into negative core beliefs. For those who have experienced long, enduring, or complex trauma, just as with any psychotherapy, this work takes time, requiring long-term depth energy psychotherapy over many years. Nonetheless, we can transform ourselves more easily than in previous times.

Language and vibration

The vibrations from positive or negative thoughts, beliefs, and emotions send strong energetic, chemical signals to our bodies (explored further in Chapters 3 and 4). How we use language is therefore significant. Compare the contracted sense of energy when we say things like 'I am stupid', 'I am bad', 'I hate myself', with the expansive energy of 'I am grateful', 'I am joyful', 'I love and accept myself'. Emotional frequencies are significantly more powerful electromagnetically than cognitive thoughts, so 'stupid' not only resonates with the low frequency of the word itself but also with a 'cocktail' of underlying emotional responses to it such as shame, self-hatred, and revulsion. Becoming conscious of the strong, repetitive, and often largely unconscious messages we give to ourselves and our bodies provides the possibility of choice that we can change such messages.

Emoto's inspiring book *The Healing Power of Water* (2008) offers scientific evidence of the vibrational nature of words and their power to create chaos or harmony in the energy field. In it, Emoto shows photographs of water crystals which had been charged with the respective vibrations of positive and negative words and intentions. The beauty and harmony of the crystals infused with 'love' and 'gratitude' in the image are radically different from the chaotic images of water crystals infused with words such as 'hate'.

Different sources cite that our bodies are comprised of anywhere between 50 to 70 per cent water, averaging at approximately 60 per cent, so Emoto's images remind us just how powerful is the vibrational nature of our internal programming and self-talk. We are impacting our bodies and energy field with every word we think and speak, so to have healthy bodies, it makes sense to speak lovingly towards ourselves. This is why mantra is so powerful—for instance, if we constantly repeat the mantra 'infinite love, infinite gratitude', or 'all is well', we help the cells of our bodies to open and resonate with harmonious patterns. Gratitude and compassion practices now have substantial research support for their effectiveness and have become NICE-accredited/mainstream therapies.

The creative energy of words, language, and 'mind'

> In the beginning was the Word, and the Word was with God, and the Word was God. (John 1, *King James Version of the Bible*)

Emoto's powerful images showing the dramatically transformative impact of words for good or ill affirm this quotation from the Bible about the creative power of the word and of language. Similarly, Buddha taught that:

> We are what we think. All that we are arises with our thoughts. With our thoughts we create our world. (Buddha, *The Dhammapada*)

In the Sufi, Hindu, and spiritual traditions generally, great honour is given to the sublime power of words and creativity. Poets such as Rumi and Tagore enable us to experience the beauty of art, where 'beauty is truth', transcending the human condition and facilitating a direct, lived experience of the sacred.

Words and their energy play a significant role in energy psychotherapy. We manifest our lives through the power of our imagination, through images, thoughts, emotions, words, speech, and intention. Thoughts arise at the imaginal creative level of our mind and are then expressed in words. The emotion behind words has a stronger energetic 'charge' than the words or thoughts themselves, so it is the power of emotions which drive thoughts. Spoken words provide the bridge between the inner world of our feeling and thought, and the outer world of visible reality.

Since creativity is happening all the time, awareness is an essential tool, so we are conscious of whether we are creating a loving vision of health and happiness, or a negative vision of fear, doom, and gloom. The Hicks' *Law of Attraction* (2006) explains the science of how this all works, and how what we repeatedly affirm—positively or negatively—creates neural pathways from which our reality manifests. The process of creation involves holding a steady vision in our mind of who we are or wish to become. Prayer, positive intentions, and affirmations are simple ways of doing this, providing a valuable aspect of our energy healing 'tool kit'.

To summarise, resonance and vibration is a key aspect of creativity. To shape and create what we desire, we need to emit sympathetic resonances to match the desired-for outcome. Rather than grasping after the result, this involves setting intentions, trusting in the outcome, relaxing, and letting go. We set intentions from a space of peaceful neutrality and non-judgement, and then let it happen. If our trust falters, there is a balance to be found between having an open, neutral attitude of unknowing, and an acceptance of whatever is the outcome. 'In this suspended state of mystery, miracles transpire with divine timing' (Ward, 2021).

Understanding the science of manifestation is fine when we are in a positive frame to be able to work in this way. However, for those who are really struggling with a negative sense of self and lack of self-love, we can still use words creatively to heal trauma, and gradually introduce the solution focused energy of working with intention.

Working with intention and the difference between conscious and unconscious drivers is explored further in Chapter 7.

Working definitions of 'mind'

When we talk about humanity's innately creative power, the words 'mind', 'consciousness', and 'awareness' are sometimes used interchangeably. However, when different terms are used to describe similar things, it can be quite confusing. The nature of mind and consciousness has occupied philosophers and religions for thousands of years, with a myriad of contemporary books exploring this subject. For now, I include some working definitions of various aspects of mind, although these overlap and are not discreet separate entities.

One Mind (non-local mind)

Larry Dossey sums up the multiplicity of various subdivisions of mind:

> In the 20th century we were introduced to several subdivisions of mind, such as the conscious, the pre-conscious, the subconscious, the unconscious, the collective unconscious. The One Mind is an additional perspective in our mental landscape. The difference is that the One Mind is not a subdivision. It is the overarching, inclusive dimension in which all the mental components of all individual minds belong. I capitalize the One Mind to distinguish it from the one mind that is possessed by each individual. (Dossey, 2013, p. xxii)

Dossey also refers to One Mind as 'non-local' mind, since mind is free, beyond space and time and cannot be pinned down to one location.

Creator consciousness

William Linville (2021) describes the mind as our 'Creator Consciousness' whose nature is to think, perceive, vision, and dream. Each of us has the power to create, and what we manifest in our life arises out of the visions we choose to focus on, where thoughts and emotions are creative and shape our visible reality. So, the thoughts and emotions we think and experience, both consciously and unconsciously, matter.

The mind is an embodied process that regulates energy and information flow

If thoughts come from mind, what is mind? With the added complexity of including the brain in defining mind, Dr Daniel Siegel (2016) gathered forty scientists from a variety of disciplines (neuroscience, anthropology, sociology, etc.) to ask, 'What is the connection between the brain and the mind?' Differing perspectives emerged about what the mind is:

- neuroscientist: the mind is what the brain does
- psychologist: the mind is our subjective experience
- anthropologist: the mind is what's shared in culture
- sociologist: mind is what shapes how people behave in groups

The common denominator was energy flow, and all could agree on the definition that: 'The mind is an embodied and relational process that regulates energy and information flow.'

Cognitive/ordinary mind

The cognitive mind is the ordinary thinking conceptual mind which operates within the realm of ego. It is generally associated with the logical, rational thinking of the left brain and a 'head' state of consciousness. Ego operates in a space of separation and is generally disconnected from our spiritual self.

Pure awareness/'unity consciousness'/presence

I find Buddhist definitions helpful, though other traditions, will, I am sure, have equally useful explanations. In Dzogchen, the heart-centred state of non-dual consciousness is termed 'pure awareness' ('Rigpa'). This expansive state is in the realm of energy, beyond conceptual, cognitive mind, residing in an embodied state 'in the present moment'. In the 'now' there is no subject/object duality, and no past, present, or future. This pure awareness is a peaceful state of light consciousness which observes everything directly 'as it is'—unaltered, unbiased, with compassion, wisdom, and clarity—without getting caught up in what is being observed. There is a purity and simplicity in this state of consciousness, which in Vajrayana Buddhism is known as 'pure perception' or 'sacred outlook'. In contemporary language, this is the same as 5-D 'unity consciousness'. Eckhart Tolle refers to this as 'presence'.

When we say, 'everything is energy', mind, consciousness, and energy are all one—unity consciousness (non-dual consciousness) is one with the unified field.

'Mind', 'thought fields', and 'mindbodyenergy'

The Dzogchen definition of 'mind' is like Einstein's idea of the 'Field' and Callahan's concept of 'thought fields', where 'mind' denotes the energy, information, and intelligence of our entire *mindbodyenergy*. This pervades our physical body, the subtle energy systems (chakras and meridians), and all the subtle bodies, (or biofields/thought fields), including the mental, emotional, and spiritual bodies, extending far beyond our physical body, and expanding out to the universe.

'Love and above'

The psychiatrist Dr David Hawkins' famous 'Map of Consciousness' provides an interesting adjunct to working with feelings and emotions in energy psychotherapy. Copies of this energetic map, based on a logarithmic scale which spans from zero to a thousand, can be found in Hawkins' books, providing a serviceable measure of specific emotions and aspects of consciousness. In one book (Hawkins, 2015) he refers to this map as a 'Stairway to Enlightenment'. Shame is at the bottom of the scale, and it moves up to enlightenment at the top. Several of the emotions are missed out of the scale, which is incomplete, and there are many anomalies, but nonetheless, it is still a useful therapeutic tool, not least because the scale alerts our attention to the higher or lower frequencies of different states of mind.

The scale is divided into various bandwidths of consciousness. The 'higher' aspects of 'love and above' include enlightenment, peace, joy, and love, and the band below this includes acceptance, willingness, and neutrality. Then the scale descends in order of vibrational resonance from courage, pride, anger, and desire, down to fear grief and apathy, with guilt and shame right at the bottom of the scale.

Shame features strongly in trauma. Resonating at only twenty, it is one of the most debilitating of all emotions—we feel on the floor, wanting the earth to swallow us up. Phil Mollon (2002) talked about shame's 'toxic' quality—a sense of being inadequate as a human being, unworthy of love and rejected by others. While shame is a universal experience which needs to be accepted, energy psychotherapy can considerably alleviate this. I used to experience intolerable shame relating to early trauma and went to Phil Mollon for some energy sessions. I am so grateful that I no longer feel persecuted by this excruciating state. Guilt is another persecuting emotion which resonates at thirty, a similarly low frequency.

Some emphasise the value of raising our vibration to 'love and above'—the so-called 'enlightened' emotions. Dawkins places love right in the middle of the scale, resonating at 500 MHz, with joy, gratitude, and peace above love, leading up to enlightenment. If one studies the scale in depth, it is easy to see that it takes a considerable amount of emotional work to rise to a level which aggregates at the frequency of love.

We know from neurobiology and biochemistry that our bodies are directly impacted by emotions. Fear, for instance, is a significantly low frequency, a 'separating' emotion which disconnects us from our true sense of self, and from our soul nature. When driven by fear, people can become very stuck, living from their stressed and traumatised nervous systems, and find it hard to envision more hopeful possibilities. Love helps to overcome this fear and illusion of separation.

Connecting with the harmony of higher frequencies makes it easier to connect with the unified field—the multiverse. Naturally, it is desirable to be able inhabit the upper part of the scale on the higher dimensional planes, so that we can master our human bodies, our life force, and thrive, rather than merely survive. This is why this book emphasises the idea of connecting with our souls—because this helps us access the higher frequencies and therefore the joyful emotions.

The universe responds to our frequency

Understanding frequency—the power of our mind, thoughts, and emotions—will become increasingly significant in the new paradigm as human consciousness continues to evolve.

Energy in its natural state has no form—how it takes shape is determined by our thoughts and consciousness.

> The universe responds to your frequency. It doesn't recognise your personal wants, desires or needs. It only understands the frequency you are vibrating at. For example, if you are vibrating at the frequency of fear, guilt, or shame you are going to attract things of a similar vibration. If you are vibrating at the frequency of love, joy, and abundance, you are going to attract things that support that frequency. It's like tuning into a radio station. YOU have to be tuning into the music you want to listen to, just like you have to be tuned into the energy you want to manifest into your life. Change your mindset—it will change your life. (Eisenhower, 2022)

The frequency we broadcast correlates directly with the world we create. During the tumultuous times of the early 2020s, our minds were bombarded by a fear-driven media. It was contagious, and challenging, to step outside the power of a fearful collective consciousness to resonate with a more peaceful, loving vibration. However, we have the power to raise our frequency by clearing our denser emotions, which makes space in our bodies for 'light' and positive feelings. This in turn radiates out, attracting more loving encounters with others.

With the gift of free will, we can choose, take responsibility for, and be conscious of our thoughts and emotions. This helps us determine our path—the more we develop positive thoughts, emotions, and actions on a daily basis, our bodies start to transform. Actions based in love lead to beneficial outcomes, which create new vibrations and positive neural pathways.

On the other hand, if we become stuck in bitterness and resentment it can feel difficult to change. Naturally our lives and emotions do not unfold in a neat linear scale—life is more often like a game of snakes and ladders, full of ups and downs. Healing is possible, however, when we resonate with compassion or love—even if we can't stay there for long—so, setting the intention to live in the energies of 'love and above' gives us something to aim for.

The four immeasurables

In the Buddhist teachings, the 'lighter' feelings in Hawkins' scale are termed 'noble qualities'. When we have an 'awakening' experience—such as at the birth of a child, or we are amazed by the beauty of nature—our hearts expand and love naturally flows. This state is called *bodhicitta*; *bodhi* means the seed of our natural enlightened nature (Buddha nature) and *citta* means our awakened heart.

A beautiful Buddhist prayer/intention which arises from awakening is as follows:

> Mesmerised by the sheer variety of perceptions, beings wander endlessly astray in samara's vicious cycle. In order that they may find comfort and ease in the Luminosity and all-pervading space of the true nature of their minds, I generate the immeasurable Love, immeasurable Compassion, immeasurable Joy and immeasurable Equanimity of the Awakened Mind of Bodhicitta. (From the Longchen Nyingtik *Ngondro: Preliminaries to Vajrayana practice*)

These 'Four Immeasurables' resonate at frequencies beyond the coarser emotions, leading us up the scale towards freedom, self-liberation, and enlightenment. When we consciously cultivate them, it helps us rise to a state of 'love and above'.

Clearing dense energy from our *mindbodyenergy*

Energy psychotherapy provides a significant vehicle for raising our frequency. As we clear our distorted perceptions and remove blocked energy, the 'veil' of ego, which prevents us from seeing clearly, is gradually dissolved.

Detailed energy clearing methods are found in Chapter 7. The subtle energy system is discussed in Chapter 8.

The principles of the energy clearing process are as follows:

Removing dense energy resulting from unresolved traumatic experiences
Unresolved traumatic experiences, emotional distress, and negative core beliefs are recorded as dense energy and 'information' in our subtle energy system. This creates blockages in the

meridians, chakras (energy vortexes), and thought fields, impeding the flow of energy. Energy psychotherapy 'clears' this blocked energy by facilitating the flow of energy and information throughout the cells of the body. This releases trauma through the neural pathways and out of the body, naturally giving rise to free associations of the *mindbodyenergy*. Memories, feelings, and images come to the surface. As we release these traumatic experiences, our perceptions gradually clear, like cleaning a dirty mirror, or clearing the distorted lens or 'filter' through which we have been perceiving the world. This process of unblocking makes space to bring more light into our subtle channels.

Energetic blockages: traumatic patterns held at physical, emotional, mental, and spiritual levels

Since our body holds our history, it registers the repetitive patterns of experiences—or 'repetition compulsion' (Freud 1920g)—in our *mindbodyenergy*. Physically, we struggle with the fight/flight/freeze/flop aspects of our nervous system; emotionally, we can be repeatedly triggered by reminders of distressing events; mentally, ruminating thoughts go round and round in our heads; and spiritually, at the level of our souls, we are often disconnected and not fully 'present' in our lives. All this distress—'perturbations', or 'dense' energy—is held at a cellular level in our bodies (Pert, 1999) and presents challenges for living our lives. When there has been significant transgenerational transmission of trauma, energy psychotherapy is very effective in bringing change and a more hopeful, resilient outlook.

Blockages distort our perceptions and skew development

Unresolved stressful experiences result in negative self-perceptions and core beliefs about ourselves—we become unbalanced. Clearing this energy helps us develop insight so we understand how our beliefs become biased when looking at life through the lens of trauma. For instance, a person who was abandoned in childhood may have a profoundly distorted sense of themselves—a limiting belief that 'I am unlovable'. When trauma remains unprocessed, it can also manifest in our physical body as physical illness.

By recognising and releasing this traumatised energy and limiting core beliefs, we gradually return to the 'natural organic template' (Mollon, 2022) of who we truly are. Over time, clearing these perturbations in the field enables us to overcome the 'false self' (Winnicott, 1960) and become real and authentic so we can develop and become who we truly are. Then our perception and understanding will be at its most expansive.

Co-creating phrases designates the energy to be cleared

Issues emerge while talking in therapy. To guide the work safely, we energy test to see if it will benefit to use energy therapy. If it tests positively to do so, client and therapist co-create phrases which carry the potency of the energy to be cleared. This traumatised energy is cleared through the subtle energy system by tapping on meridians, holding chakras, or using intention in the thought field, while repeating these phrases out loud, or simply thinking them.

Clearing using electrical/electromagnetic energy and the subtle energy system

Broadly speaking, two distinct forms of energy are involved in energy psychotherapy:

Electrical and electromagnetic energy is relatively well understood and can be detected by suitable instruments. Our cells contain hundreds of billions of neurons that each connect electrochemically creating a complex electrical system of pathways. Wherever there is an electrical current, it creates and is surrounded by an electromagnetic field.

Subtle Energy—our life force has long been recognised in other cultures. In China, 'Qi' is the basis for acupuncture, and 'prana' is referred to in Eastern religions. Freud (1922g) used the terms *libido* to describe the 'love' energy—*Eros*[9] a forward-flowing life force with intelligent intention which releases trauma when we work with energy methods. Reich developed the idea of libido further with his concept of 'orgone energy', and Neville Symington in a less physiological way, uses the term 'the life giver' to describe life-affirming intent (Symington, 1994, p. 137).

Abreaction—releasing blocked energy

When blocked energy is released, abreaction occurs so the energy can flow forward positively again. Understanding the flow of energy is key in the releasing techniques of contemporary energy therapies. People experience this uniquely—some have strong abreactions, whereas others barely feel anything. There may be yawning, sighing, laughing or crying, gurgling and so on, showing that the energy is moving. Some experience the energy moving through their bodies and down their legs. Energy releases are generally gentle subtle experiences, and the process works, regardless as to how much people actually feel anything is happening—a common reflection is that people feel calmer after clearings.

Reversed energy

Sometimes however, there may be a 'reversal' of this energy flow which is akin to Freud's idea of the 'death instinct' or *Thanatos*. When people struggle with thoughts such as 'I don't deserve to get over this problem', this literally blocks or 'reverses' the energy system and inhibits its flow. Psycho-energetic 'reversals' are explored further in Chapters 7 and 9. They are extremely common and can be cleared relatively easily.

---

[9] Freud's concept of libido has been hotly debated. It went through various definitions, and up until 1914, Freud considered that 'libido' related to manifestations of bodily sexual tensions. Subsequently he redefined this to the manifestations of sexual energy in the psychic field though this was disputed by those who felt it missed out on the 'affective' aspect of the discussion (Zepf, 2008).

Subtle energy: ancient wisdom, quantum healing, neuroscience and energy psychotherapy

Energy psychotherapy inhabits similar territory to the holistic ancient healing arts of the wisdom traditions which draw on the subtle energy system of the chakras and meridians. Quantum physics is bringing this ancient spiritual wisdom to the contemporary world. These days many books are bringing spiritually and quantum science together. Bohm's *Wholeness and the Implicate Order* (2002), McTaggart's *The Field* (2002), Taylor's *Spiritual Science* (2018), Sheldrake's *A New Science of Life* (1981), Lorimer's *Whole in One: The Near-Death Experience and the Ethics of Interconnectedness* (1990)—and many more.

There are many similarities between the ancient wisdom traditions and energy psycho-therapy. Tantric yogic practices purified energy through the psychophysical system—a dynamic network of subtle channels, winds (or inner air) and 'essences', somewhat like the Chinese meridian system in acupuncture, and the chakra system in Eastern traditions. These long-established healing arts unblocked, purified, and balanced energy, allowing its free and unobstructed flow. However, the methods that we have been gifted with in energy therapy are simpler and easier to use than esoteric tantric practices.

The liberating current

Anodea Judith (1987) in her study of chakras speaks of 'the liberating current' (p. 32) which brings personal liberation. It is the pathway through which slow-moving constricted energy gradually gains new freedom, liberating us from outdated or constricting habits, and from our egoic perception, otherwise known as 'the veil of Maya'. Through the process of clearing trauma and unresolved issues at the chakras along the central column, or 'Line of the Light' (Levin, 1998), this frees the flow of energy up and down the spine and the central nervous system, creating the conditions for 'awakening' our kundalini energy. Once the blockages in the chakras and energy channels (*nadis*) are cleared, the life force (*prana*) starts flowing unobstructed in copious quantities through the energetic spine (*Sushumna*). This provides direct access to 'Source' energy—or 'universal consciousness', if you like—opening the 'third eye' which helps us gain access to the intuitive wisdom of our soul. Some, who have been deeply traumatised, may also experience 'kundalini rising' despite—or even because of—their trauma.

Neuroscience, the chakras and meridians

There are significant links between the synergy of neurobiological discoveries and our ways of working energetically with chakras and meridians. The nervous system links with both the physical nervous system of the spinal cord, brain, and nerves, i.e. the ('gross') physical body (*anamaya kosha*) and the subtle body (*pranamaya kosha*) of chakras and subtle channels (meridians or 'nadis'). The former is visible to the surgeon's naked eye when the body is cut open, whereas the latter are visible only when the third eye opens. In Western countries we tend to use the term 'nervous system' as a common term for both the subtle and gross systems.

Neuropeptide-enriched nodal points within the neurons along the spine

The chakra system corresponds to the location of neuropeptide-enriched nodal points within the neurons along the spine. These nodal points are key nerve centres, like energy junction boxes of the nervous system which can release blocked energy and help us enter relaxed states of mind, where natural recuperation and recovery can occur.

According to many spiritual practices there is a strong linkage between the two bodies, the physical and the subtle, with none of our feelings, sensations, or emotions getting communicated to the brain unless they first go through the subtle body or psychic nervous system. Spiritual practices tend to work directly with the subtle or psychic system, since, according to the ancient traditions, that is where all 'blockages' caused by our past and continuing karmas (experiences) and samskaras (patterns) are lodged.

Clearing our energy brings our energy system back into balance and alignment. This process of understanding the energy around and within us and learning about our biases is crucial to awakening our spirituality, intuition, and creativity. It helps us to be fully human, deeply conscious, whole, and connecting to a multi-layered universe.

A further note on 'raising our vibration'

As a means of reflecting on the state of our consciousness, Hawkins' scale provides an approximate measure of where we are. However, people react strongly—in positive and negative ways—to the idea of this scale and there can be misunderstandings about its use. Aspiring to 'Love and Above' does not imply that energy psychotherapy aims to cover up painful feelings by 'being positive'. Nor do we adopt a judgemental attitude about 'higher' or 'lower', 'better or worse'. People are at different places in their lives, so a holistic approach to working with emotions and experiences respects each individual. Things occur in timely ways. It is not a question of being competitive (ego's way) and seeing how high up one is on the scale. As new circumstances arise to help us evolve, we might rapidly fall to a low vibration as we face a new challenge as part of our journey of healing.

People bring wounds and trauma to therapy which involve suffering and grief. Sitting with and bearing pain is a significant aspect of therapeutic work—as Eisenhower puts it (2022), 'feeling it to heal it'. Energy therapy, far from avoiding the task of working with painful emotions, enables us to go into pain while at the same time offering the energetic release which heals it. A significant use of energy methods lies in integrating dense 'shadow' energies including the lower frequencies. When we get stuck in repetition compulsion patterns and complexes such as that of the 'Martyr', 'Scapegoat', or 'Abuser', archetypal work facilitates ways of taking back and owning our projections (explored further in Chapter 9).

Naturally, change occurs in all therapies. However, one of the reasons I find energy psycho-therapy so rewarding is because it can transform complicated complexes. When I compare the slow painstaking work of my previous practice as a psychoanalytic therapist, I am amazed at how energy psychotherapy can facilitate deep work in much shorter spaces of time.

Choosing our perceptions

It is commonly said that 'it is not what happens to us, but how we perceive our circumstances' which affects our state of mind. Being aware of the energetic reality of resonances can inspire us to make more nurturing choices so we move beyond ego's habit of judgement and polari-sation. 'Victim consciousness', for example, by its very nature, will keep people resonating at a low vibration, whereas those who take responsibility to transform their experience will inevitably access higher frequencies. The free will we have as human beings offers a significant power to choose. When we chose heart-based intentions, connect with our souls, and aspire to awaken our consciousness, it becomes easier to accept our life's circumstance as a path of transformation. At this level we have the 'sacred outlook' of the 'Five Perfections' (explored in Chapter 6), where we view all as sacred beings who are playing their part in helping us to evolve. This lightens our view of reality and we increasingly experience well-being, happiness, and 'flow' in life.

There are some helpful quantum methods for consciously creating positive outlooks on life using energy. The practice of *Ask and Receive* created by Sandi Radomski and Tom Altaffer offers a wonderful way of setting positive intentions and transforming our beliefs about ourselves (mentioned further in Chapter 7) and Phil Mollon's 'Blue Diamond' healing field is another such beneficial high-vibrational resource.

The alchemy of resonances and transformation

Before I came across energy psychotherapy, I spent many years using sound, chant, and mantra recitation to work with my emotions. In the chant of the *Vajrasattva* healing practice, each syllable of the 'One Hundred Syllable Mantra' represents one of the 'one hundred peaceful and wrathful deities' which are none other than the energies of our emotions. Chanting this deep earthy mantra with its rich resonance offers a powerful alchemical process for transforming energy.[10]

A friend of mine who had been advised to have a hysterectomy feels this practice helped heal her from cancer. She immersed herself in a daily routine of painting, chanting the mantra with its visualisation, and a detoxifying eating programme. When she went for a medical test, her tumour had gone, and she no longer needed surgery. I have included this mantra in the

---

[10] The mantra for the *Vajrasattva* practice for healing and purification is known as the 'One Hundred Syllable Mantra' which represents the '108 peaceful and wrathful deities'—i.e. our peaceful and conflicting emotions. This practice is referred to again in Chapter 6. The mantra and visualisation help purify and heal all the energies of the body emotions and spirit.

Appendix and people are welcome to download the chant as a gift from the Flame Centre website. www.theflamecentre.co.uk

The wisdom energy of emotions

Vajrayana Buddhism teaches the principle that emotional energies have purified and un-purified attributes. The five 'Buddha families' represent fundamental emotional energies which characterise us. They comprise five 'negative' emotions (the *Five Poisons*) which can be transformed into their wisdom counterparts, known as the *Five Wisdoms*. In this way:

> IGNORANCE becomes ALL ENCOMPASSING SPACE—the *wisdom of the Dharmadatu*
> ANGER/AGGRESSION becomes CLARITY—*mirror-like wisdom*
> PRIDE, ARROGANCE and MISERLINESS becomes GENEROSITY—*the wisdom of equality*
> NEGATIVE PASSION and GRASPING becomes DISCERNMENT—*discriminating wisdom*
> JEALOUSY AND ENVY becomes SKILLED ACTIVITY—*all accomplishing wisdom*

Understanding emotions as 'pure energy' helps to overcome dualistic perceptions of 'good' and 'bad' so they can be worked with in less judgemental ways. Therapeutically, the idea that troubling emotions can be transformed into wisdom can be inspiring for someone who feels plagued by—for example—anger. One of my clients found it very reassuring that instead of feeling bad about himself, he could work with his anger and see it emerging as clarity. Knowing that there is wisdom inherent in our emotions also provides a sense of purpose in how we work with and accept them. For instance, rather than just expressing and 'sounding off' about our jealousy, we work with it with positive intention in order to transform ourselves.

Soul-connecting and awakening consciousness

We have explored matter to light, energy, and frequency, but what of soul-connecting and awakening consciousness. How does this fit in? The following briefly lays out some questions we will explore as the book progresses.

Intention

When we become triggered and dysregulated, our emotions can feel so intense that it is easy to get lost. Energy therapy can bring relief and help us find balance, but more generally in therapy—and in life—what does 'working with emotions' involve? What can we fall back on to guide us when we want to lash out and blame others, stuck in ego and its reactions/ projections rather than owning our part and dealing with our own energies? We've been given an amazing palette of vibrations to play with—what vision of the world are we going to create? What pictures do we want to paint? How do we see ourselves? Who do we want to be?

A friend of mine, Benni, wrote a great song for Soulyard (a band we used to play in together), which had the catchy chorus:

Do as you would be done by
Woo as you would be won by
And only take what you can give
That's love's Demand

'Mrs Do-as-you-would -be-done-by' was a character from a childhood book, *The Water Babies*, which offered moral guidance (Kingsley, 1863). What type of moral choices do we want to make today?

Setting positive intentions creates a healing trajectory which informs the direction we wish to travel in and can make a significant difference as to how our life unfolds. The turmoil of emotions and life crises also provide circumstances where we can transform and grow. If we simply live in plodding ok-ness or complacency, such opportunities for choosing different directions, or waking up to new possibilities might not arise.

The life crisis in my life which led me to choose a significant fork in the road and take the 'Bodhisattva Vow' was when my sister was in tremendous pain, and I was lost, not knowing how to help. The Buddhist talk I attended explained so clearly the roots of suffering caused by our disconnection from our inherent true wisdom (our Buddha nature/our soul). A glimpse of awakening inspires the desire to help ourselves and others on the path of *dharma* (which means truth). I took this vow of love and compassion in France at a place called Joui, entirely unconscious of the synchronicity that Joui meant joy—it was only later that I connected the dots with my earlier decision to 'Choose the path of Joy'. Although I no longer formally follow Buddhism, this vow still guides me—perhaps choosing 'love and above' is an equivalent intention?

The lifting of the veils

In *A New Earth*, Eckhart Tolle expresses his concern that humanity is dangerously egocentric. Distinguishing between cleverness and intelligence, he declares that ego's qualities are not intelligent and moreover that the cleverness of ego divides, whereas intelligence includes. The Buddhist path is concerned with lifting the veils of ego, so we access heart-centred consciousness, wisdom, and compassion. Tolle celebrates that people are awakening from the deep sleep of ego to the state of awareness, the greatest agent for change. He summarises this awareness as: 'Conscious connection with universal intelligence. Another word for it is Presence: consciousness without thought' (Tolle, 2005). I use 'soul-connecting' to refer to the same thing, since my personal connection with universal intelligence is my soul.

Maya—the state of illusion

But what is the deep sleep of ego? Eastern and indigenous traditions have known for centuries that 'reality' is nothing but a construct of our mind. 'Maya' refers to the illusory nature of reality, described in the Buddhist prayer of compassion: 'mesmerised by the sheer variety of perceptions … beings wander endlessly astray in samsara's vicious cycle'.[11] The ignorance spoken of in 'samsara's vicious cycle' is equivalent to Freud's 'repetition compulsion'.[12] We go round and round in circles, stuck in a world where we can't seem to see what we are doing, and so we make the same mistakes again and again.

However, these 'veils' of ego and illusion are gradually lifting. The visionary Carl Jung speaks in *Dreams, Memories and Reflections* of his experiences beyond the ordinary cognitive mind, describing mystical states as being the 'real' reality: 'Our basis is ego-consciousness … our unconscious existence is the real one, and our conscious world, a kind of illusion … like a dream which seems a reality as long as we are in it' (Jung, 1973a, pp. 355–356).[13]

His writing prepares us for a different reality. The awakened state, formerly the preserve of mystics and visionaries throughout the ages is something which is accessible to us all, should people choose it. Within the therapy world and the public generally, many are interested in experiencing 'altered' states of consciousness. I remember avidly reading Carlos Castaneda's books in the seventies (Castaneda, 1968) which spoke about shamanic experience and the *dreamtime* of Shamanism's intuitive flow. As more train in shamanism these days, the increasing usage of psychedelics has significant implications for counselling and psychotherapy—there is a need for sufficient grounding to 'hold' such visionary states.

With spiritual epiphanies, and drug-induced transpersonal phenomena on the increase, people are beginning to wake up. Some, confused by their experience, seek psychotherapy to make sense of their 'altered states' of consciousness. As a therapist I feel our profession needs to consider the impact of such changes in consciousness, so we widen our clinical understanding. The new therapeutic methodologies such as energy psychotherapy, can be effective in assisting people as they go through such experiences.

The confusion about ego

In the territory of awakening consciousness, ego is quite confusing—people have so many different views of it. There is vast literature on the subject, and various terminologies are used

---

[11] The Prayer for generating *bodhicitta*—the awakened mind—is from a preliminary tantric practice, the *Longchen Nyingtik* 'Ngondro'.

[12] The concept of 'repetition compulsion' was noted formally by Sigmund Freud in his 1920 essay *Beyond the Pleasure Principle*, in which he observed a child throw his favourite toy from his crib, become upset at the loss, then reels the toy back in, only to repeat this action.

[13] The full quote is: 'Our basis is ego-consciousness, our whole world, the field of light centred upon the focal point of the ego. From that point we look out upon an enigmatic world of obscurity, never knowing to what extent the shadowy forms we see are caused by our consciousness, or possess a reality of their own … closer study shows that as a rule the images of the unconscious are not produced by consciousness, but have a reality and spontaneity of their own … the aim … is to effect a reversal of the relationship between ego-consciousness and the unconscious, and to represent the unconscious as the generator of the empirical personality. This reversal suggests that in the opinion of the "other side", our unconscious existence is the real one, and our conscious world a kind of illusion, an apparent reality constructed for a specific purpose, like a dream which seems a reality as long as we are in it' (Jung, 1973a, pp. 355–356).

within specific contexts, so here I present a range of views, which all seem to me to have validity. It does, however, depend on the perspective of reality from which we are viewing ego.

From a psychological perspective, energy psychotherapy, as with other forms of therapy, regards a functioning ego as a normal, necessary part of healthy human development. Broadly, I am referring here to the psychoanalytic definition of ego, the part of the mind that mediates between the conscious and the unconscious and is responsible for reality testing, providing us with a healthy sense of self and personal identity. It enables us to have a grounded capacity to negotiate reality: a biological, psychological, and social survival mechanism which helps us function in the world. We need our egos to live in this physical body.

3-D egoic consciousness

The third-dimensional physical world of Newtonian physics is governed by the laws of cause and effect. Our mental mind *separates* things through categorising into 'this' and 'that'. When we are in ego, we see ourselves as separate from—rather than interconnected with—others/the whole. The Buddha taught that our first dualistic experience of the world—the primary separation from unity consciousness—is the split between love and fear. One of the purposes of the 3-D dualistic world is to give us the experience of contrast in which we perceive others as separate, and through relationship, we bounce off them, which helps us to learn, grow, and expand.

When operating from the 3-D perspective there is a tendency to perceive our reality through the lens of 'victim consciousness'; we believe that 'things happen to us'; our narrative is one of circumstances assailing us from the outside world, causing us to feel the way we do, and we tend to blame the other and project out, finding it difficult to take responsibility for our part in creating situations. In the Piscean era, religion was largely characterised by the dualistic battle between 'good' and 'evil', and was concerned with themes of power, control, and authority, where the priest or 'Master' was placed above us. This perspective invited subservience, self-sacrifice, duty, and martyrdom. People tried to be 'holy' and 'righteous' in a world dominated by judgement. This is the era we are coming out of.

Self-esteem, self-inflation, and the 'not good enough' ego

When I was younger, to cope with my lack of self-esteem, I idealised others, putting them above me out of insecurity, and denying my own worth. Melanie Klein recognised the shadow of idealisation as envy, with its destructive backlash. Another aspect of low self-esteem concerns giving our power away to others, because we are frightened to own our light. Matt Kahn (2015) names the 'I am not good enough' position as the 'sacrificial ego' which he feels is just as 'big' and deluded as an arrogant, dominant, power-seeking ego. I lived out the inferior/superior axis in terror of becoming like my mother, who often came across as superior to others. While tending to inhabit my sacrificial supplicating ego, sometimes I unconsciously flipped into the shadow—like my mother, I too could be arrogant. The self-abasing judgement when I realised this was so unbearable that I would immediately revert in shame to my sacrificial ego.

I was initially confused after my first glimpses of awakening, trying to differentiate between expanded consciousness and egoic self-inflation. Ego self-consciously grasps on to experience, and easily misperceives the radiance of joyful expansion as an inflated sense of self. It is the after-thought which is the problem—not the experience itself. Once I had stabilised the experience of expanded consciousness, it gave me confidence, self-esteem, and security because I knew who I truly was. Experiencing pure awareness is quietening and strengthening. Knowing my Buddha nature and becoming familiar with a state of Presence gradually brought healing, and I became kinder to my confused ego.

Personal sovereignty and a sense of self

When I was part of the Buddhist community, the teacher with whom I took issue was intent on destroying or 'subjugating' our egos. It was completely accepted that 'ego was bad'. People were shamed and condemned if they were caught out for letting their egos 'show', though what I perceived the teacher doing was bullying those who spoke from a place of personal sovereignty, damaging their sense of confidence and self-worth. If someone is abusing us, it doesn't serve us to be doormats and accept this behaviour by thinking we can just float up and 'rise above it' into supposedly 'higher states' of consciousness—the MO for many in the community was spiritual bypassing. Ideally, we have self-respect and stand up against or walk away from abuse. It was my heart—my soul—and not my ego which guided me to walk away. It seemed to me there was considerable misunderstanding about ego. As Alan Watts said, 'Getting rid of ego is the last resort of invincible egoism' (Aletheia Luna, 2022, quoting Watts, 1989).

Dissolution of ego

From the third-dimensional perspective of everyday consciousness, ego is simply a story we tell about ourselves—of identifications, where I am a 'this', I am a 'that'—a musician, a therapist. We create a narrative where we identify with specific aspects of what we do in life, and our identities are fragile and changeable. While our souls are evolving, ego serves as a protective boundary. Perhaps it is not so much a question of *losing* our ego entirely, but rather, of no longer identifying with it.

'Awakening' does involve dissolution of the ego into the state of unity consciousness, so there is legitimate concern about what does or doesn't happen to ego. Ego is, however, also a vehicle we can use in the service of our spiritual evolution. According to William Linville in his 'Mastery of Creator Consciousness' series (2021), when we get beyond ego and become one with the wider reality, ego 'upgrades' to become our 'divine intellect'—a clarity which unites with wisdom and continues to serve the soul's higher purpose.

Transcendence of ego is a pathway into enlightenment, a pathway taken by many adepts. However, those who transcend the ego, transcend the aspect needed for action within physical incarnation. (There is an anecdote about this in Chapter 6 about the 'wearing out of phenomenal reality'.) The Dalai Lama has taught that we need our egos in life to get by in physical reality, so that we have sufficient desire to accomplish things, since it is the ego which drives us with forward-moving momentum. However, I also feel that Joy is a wonderful motivator, which doesn't feel at all egotistical.

It is also worth distinguishing between the transcendence of ego which occurs in total enlightenment as compared with 'Ascension'. People often speak about ascension and awakening in the same breath (though they are not the same thing) as part of the process of evolving consciousness. Petra Pixie usefully clarifies that 'Ascension is the taking of the body with you and one major aspect to this is harmonious integration with the ego … the steadfast commitment to integrate physical reality and enlightenment simultaneously' (Pixie, 2022)

The impermanence of ego compared with our everlasting soul consciousness

We are multidimensional beings, existing in several dimensions simultaneously, even if we are not aware of this. Negotiating reality can be very confusing and we need to do what is appropriate according to our evolving consciousness. This means that we flip in and out of different dimensions on our rollercoaster of awakening—the subject of my next book.

From a 'higher' dimensional perspective, ego is an illusion and isn't really 'You'. Buddhism speaks of its impermanent nature. In contrast to the truth of everlasting consciousness—what Christianity terms 'everlasting life'—ego has no real solidity or objectivity and is subject to birth change and decay. Ultimately, when we die, it all dissolves and we are nothing but consciousness. The aspect of us which has been there all along and is unchanging is our soul—our consciousness.

Duality—a state of separation

The *suffering* of ego is essentially about duality, torn between polarities, in a state of separation, a disconnection from 'Source' or Spirit, or from 'union with God' or however one wants to name this. Duality is the very nature of ego. Ego divides life into limiting ideas, beliefs, and concepts, makes judgements, and categorises experiences into 'good and bad', 'right and wrong' and so on. This creates suffering because it closes our perceptions. We get caught up in contracted states of criticism, fear, guilt, and negativity, feel separated from others, disconnected from our hearts, and stuck in judgement. Our ego feels hard done by, and from this place it is easy to slide into feelings of victimhood.

Rather than ego's judgement, we need discernment—the question is whether our capacity to discern is exercised by ego's harsh judgement or the soul's compassionate wisdom. The more we are caught in ego's judgement—which is ego's essential nature—the more we become distracted by negative responses to things—by resentment, bitterness, anger, fear, and so on. We not only become separated from others, but also dislike ourselves and feel disconnected. When we fall into these lower vibrations, we struggle with our shadow, and might prefer to avoid such a confrontation, finding it difficult to own and accept the part we play in creating our lives.

So getting beyond ego and duality is a challenge but it is also growthful, in the service of our evolution. When we remember to tap into our wisdom and ask, 'What does my soul say about this?', we can lift ourselves up. Our soul can then help us learn new ways and build positive habits such as developing gratitude by 'giving thanks for divine guidance'.

5-D heart and soul-centred consciousness

We emerge out of the dualistic world of separation, by opening our hearts, which is the gateway to our soul. This facilitates access to the multidimensional reality of the unified field of energy, where past present and future exist in the present moment of now. Awakening into the fifth dimension is characterised by breaking free of the restrictions of the cognitive mind, the ego, and its veil of separation from knowing our true nature. In 5-D we interpret all circumstances—everything that happens to us—as part of our soul's evolutionary journey, activating us to clear the blockages that each of us brought into this lifetime. We take every opportunity to resolve issues on our journey, and in the process contribute towards healing the collective consciousness. Few manage to live in 5-D—this requires a high level of mastery. When we see and embrace the essence of oneness, we have a taste of the first stage of enlightenment—a path which continues up to the twelve dimensions.

When client and therapist work from a soul-to-soul rather than an ego-to-ego state, we use the power of heart-based intention and let go, without clinging to a desired outcome, and let the energy do the work. This is Tiller's 'higher gauge' healing state, where the human aura and energy meridians contain intelligence as part of an information matrix, an 'intelligent data field'—or 'morphic field' (Sheldrake, 2023).

Connecting with our 'higher' levels—in whatever way is meaningful to each person—serves as a bridge to heal our ego states more easily. Finding our connection is uniquely personal. Some do so by being in nature, playing music, or through their spiritual faith, their trust in God, or using breath as a way of connecting with universal healing energy. If you are interested to explore this further, please use whatever is helpful, feels relevant, fits your understanding, or is inspiring to you. The most important point is to tune into your heart centre.

The unified field: zero point and non-dual consciousness

Unity consciousness takes us beyond ego, to non-dual consciousness within *The Divine Matrix* (Braden, 2007). The unified field is the infinite ocean of limitless possibilities where solutions can be found for everything. This field is characterised by unconditional love, wisdom, and interconnectedness. There is all the difference in the world between intellectual knowledge of it and a direct embodied cellular experience of non-dual consciousness—a state of peaceful as-it-isness.

We can only enter the state of unity consciousness by connecting through the portal of our open heart and soul. This opens into pure awareness of 'being one' with the unified quantum field. This field of fifth-dimensional consciousness is unaffected by time or space. It is the infinite repository of past, present, and future—of everything that has ever taken place and everything that has been or will be part of the universe.

Unity consciousness is an experience of spacious neutrality, compassion, intuitive intelligence, and non-judgement. We rest in our centre in a state of stillness—a state of equilibrium and coherence which is sometimes referred to as 'zero point field'.

The 'Shift'—the re-setting of planetary energy to the fifth dimension and the paradigm of 'new earth'—is bringing a circular rather than hierarchical operating system, which is of love, connection, and collaboration. It is a space of quantum coherence, balance, and community—of spaciousness, as-it-isness, and all-that-we-are.

Trinity—neutrality as the fulcrum between opposing poles

In this age of cosmic expansion, as we learn to find balance, it is helpful to recognise creation not just as a polarity but as a trinity. The nature of existence involves a trinity, with the balance point—or fulcrum in the still centre—being the third point. At this fulcrum of zero point we exist only in the moment of now. It is easier to deal with polarity from this place of as-it-isness, viewing different perspectives as they are. From the equilibrium of this neutrality, we can more easily choose without polarising and invalidating the position of the 'other'.

Raquel Spencer calls this the 'triwave':

> The triwave is the new magnetics that are anchoring onto the planet, taking us out of the binary and into Higher states of consciousness. It is the new platform that is superseding the old binary magnetics which we have been operating on for eons. It is the new blueprint, construct, platform that Creates the opportunity to move into higher states of consciousness. It is the new building block if you will … We cannot move into a higher state of consciousness within the old binary system. (Raquel Spencer, Facebook, 9 June 2022)

In a state of balance, we have greater freedom to choose. We can choose experiences which mitigate the effects of our limitations. Negativity can serve us in positive ways if we allow it to. For example, when we attract the opposite of our preferred experience, the comparison reminds us that this is what we *don't* want and helps us make a more positive choice. We can also use the exploration of shadow to accelerate the direction of our true self. In grappling with negativity, when we finally let it go, this experience can propel us further into the light.

Working with frequencies and vibrations offers the possibility of transformation and healing. When we release traumatic energy and blockages, we really can become free of the heavy vibrations of limiting thoughts and beliefs which makes it easier to experience love. Looked at from a vibrational perspective, one of the greatest services we can offer is to take responsibility for doing our own work and raise our own frequency. In so doing, our bodies hold more light which in turn contributes to the evolution of consciousness on our planet.

CHAPTER 3

The synergy of science in energy psychotherapy: neurobiology, cellular biology, and epigenetics

Mindbodyenergy and its interrelated systems[1]

Scientific disciplines used to exist within their separate realms, but today we think across different disciplines, working in the 'field' where every system is interconnected. The resulting synergy has profoundly affected our understanding of psychology and the ways we think about ourselves. This chapter outlines aspects of science which are relevant to energy psychotherapy, especially the neuroplasticity of the brain, the replication of cell patterns, molecules of emotion, epigenetics, mirror neurons, and a little about the quantum world.

The body and trauma

Historically, Freud's work with hysteria acknowledged the significance of neurology, the body, and libido. Wilhelm Reich recognised how trauma took on the form of 'muscular armour' as a defence against the patient's traumas, with his 'orgone' energy (similar to qi or prana), becoming the foundation for the body-based therapy, bioenergetics.[2] Generally, however, other than specifically body-based therapies, the body was largely omitted from therapy until we gained new understanding about trauma.

---

[1] See also, energy psychotherapy with *mindbodyenergy* and its many systems, Chapter 8.

[2] Wilhelm Reich believed that the loss of our 'orgone' energy, specifically measured through units called bions, which move between states in living and inanimate matter, could result in various ailments. Basically, this energy was the life force that traverses through all things, which others refer to as qi (chi) or prana. Reich thus theorised that if one could harvest this energy and recharge the body with it, it could be beneficial to our health, so to this end he went on to invent the Orgone Box.

The 'one-person psyche' approach prevailed in analysis for many years, focusing largely on talking, analysing, and thinking. References to the body concerned countertransference, particularly projective identification (Klein, 1946), and somatisation. A move from a one-person to a two-person psychology approach (Greenberg & Mitchell, 1984) led to interpersonal and relational schools. Intersubjective therapy had a sense of the energetic transmission occurring between two people, and attachment theory recognised that regulation of affect can occur when two attuned bodies are together in a room.

Talking therapy and the difficulties of re-traumatisation

Phil Mollon spoke of the hazards of trying to resolve trauma by simply talking, which can potentially make things worse without bringing relief:

> I became aware of how extensive the experience of trauma had been in the childhood … and how unhelpful conventional talking therapy, of whatever kind, often was in relation to trauma. Although …we might achieve some understanding of their development and of the dynamics of their mind, this did not seem to help. Sometimes it would make people worse; self-harm would be a common outcome. Talking of trauma … may leave a person *re-traumatised* … the affect simply cycling around the psychosomatic system. This presented an agonising clinical dilemma: many people who have suffered traumas need help in processing their traumatic memories, but accessing the memories leads to a worsening in their mental and behavioural state. (Mollon, 2008, p. 4)

These days many analysts and psychotherapists recognise the need for nonverbal processes with traumatised clients. Bion's thinking posits that difficult nonverbal emotions and states of mind can be taken in and contained by the therapist (Bion, 1967). A 'generative split' within the therapist's psyche then enables her to reflect on, process, and detoxify the intolerable feeling states for as long as it takes to render them more bearable to the client (Bollas, 1987). This process in itself is therapeutic work and perhaps nothing further need be said in the therapy—though the client may wish to communicate something about their experience verbally once the feelings have been rendered more bearable through this process. Or, as Anne Alvarez very movingly writes, sometimes there is the need for the sexually abused client *not* to talk about their experience at all (Alvarez, 1992)—perhaps she came to the same realisation as Phil Mollon.

Metabolisation of the client's processes by the therapist is, however, potentially hazardous. In Chapter 8 I talk about energy boundaries and the dangers of the therapist taking in too much toxic energy and becoming ill; the advent of energy methods provides a very helpful way of overcoming this problem.

Greater emphasis on working with the body occurred with eye movement desensitisation and reprocessing (EMDR) brain reprocessing, and sensorimotor therapy (Ogden, Minton, &

Pain 2006), and it became apparent that including the body and its sensory components made the work more effective. Then, largely through the pioneering work of Allan Schore and others, the relevance of neurobiology became globally integrated within psychotherapy, and with it, an increasing awareness of the body.

When our therapeutic focus includes the body, clients become more present and aware of their bodily sensations and what they are experiencing, which highlights just how much emotions are bodily events. However, when emotions remain unexpressed—which is often the case with trauma—blocked or repressed emotions are channelled into the body via the pathways of energy meridians where they are felt as bodily sensations, pain, and illness. This phenomenon can be likened to Bion's protomental system, where the energy has neither progressed to the mental nor the physical realms. Potential emotions can be blocked from entering the mind, denied access to language and/or are simply foreclosed, going down into the body. Bringing energy into the equation helps us get above the level of these difficulties. Energy brings more leverage and power to effect change, releasing the stuck energy and freeing up the *mindbodyenergy*, which brings relief without re-traumatisation.

Neurobiology and the brain

The rapid technological advances in neuroscience that began in the 90s have changed our perceptions about emotional, psychological, and physiological stress. Neurobiology, rooted in a multidisciplinary background including biology, chemistry, biochemistry, physics, and computer science, is particularly relevant to energy psychotherapy.

Brain development is an experience-dependent social process that can override genetics. Neurobiology involves the nervous system, its functions and structures. This includes the cells and tissues of the nervous system, ways they form structures and pathways in the body, and how these processes inform and mediate behaviour. Neurobiology also includes the brain, spinal cord, nerves, and neurons and the billions of nerve cells—or neurons—that receive and send electrical impulses throughout the body.

There is much lively research in neuroscience and its literature about the inextricable links between mind and body. Here, I mention a few key contributors: Allan Schore (2003, 2019a, 2019b) and Cozolino (2006) brought to psychotherapy an understanding about attachment and the regulation of affect; Dan Siegel's *Mindsight* (2010) taught us about the brain's capacity for both insight and empathy; the popularisation of Anthony Bateman and Peter Fonagy's work on mentalization (2004) changed the shape of therapy in the NHS; and a number of books have made information about neuroscience widely accessible to the public, including Sue Gerhardt's *Why Love Matters*, (2004) which explains the traumatic impact of a lack of a loving connection on the baby's developing brain, and Norman Doidge, who popularised the idea of *The Brain that Changes Itself* (2007).

The plasticity of the brain—re-sculpting neural pathways

The plasticity of the brain is highly relevant to energy psychotherapy, which works with neural pathways and aspects of the brain all the time. 'Experience-dependent neuroplasticity' demonstrates how the brain is not a fully formed structure, but rather, a dynamic process undergoing constant development and reconstruction across the lifespan (Cozolino, 2006). Day after day, our mind is building our brain, as neural patterns develop out of experiences and patterns of activity which become 'hard wired'. New experiences create neurological connections which arise directly from the electrochemical conversions which take place between them, and new synaptic connections are made. Thus, the process of change in the brain occurs when the activity of neurons creates new patterns in the mind-brain. Dan Siegel, a pioneer of interpersonal biology shows how in using 'Mindsight' (2010), we can transform reactive impulsiveness to receptive awareness, enabling us to make intelligent choices instead of blindly repeating maladaptive behaviours. In so doing, we re-sculpt the neural pathways and break free from the mental patterns that hold us back.

So how do our neural pathways and patterns develop? The saying that 'neurons wire together if they fire together' (Hebb, 1949) speaks of the close interconnection of neural networks. The more often the respective neurons 'talk' to each other, the more the synapses (unions between neurons) become solidified. So, when we think about something, the neural networks fire up and when we return to thinking about the same subject or similar, the neurons connect together again. In this way, through making repeated connections, mental states become neural traits.

The problem comes when our networks keep connecting to and returning to unhappy memories. Repeatedly going back to the same old negative experience doesn't help us at all— its like beating a bruise, as if this will make the bruise better. A well-known quote, supposedly attributed to Jung—'what you resist, persists'—has profound implications for our daily lives and for psychotherapy. It seems that to really change—i.e. change our brains—we need to dampen down those old connections and allow ourselves to be fired up by positive experiences, which then build new beneficial networks. Synchronously, while neuroscience was making these discoveries about the importance of creating new neural networks, Steve de Shazer brought solution-focused therapy with its focus on positive intentions, into the domain of therapy with his book *Words Were Originally Magic* (1994).

One of the amazing aspects of energy psychotherapy is that it can quite rapidly facilitate changing patterns in the brain. It accesses the neural pathways via the subtle energy system and clears out the old patterns of trauma and negative beliefs, replacing them with words and/or phrases which state positive new intentions. Since energy work is self-applied, anyone can use these methods, as evidenced by the increasing use of tapping with EFT (Emotional Freedom Techniques) by the general public (see Chapter 7).

Mirror neurons

Seeing and doing are the same thing

The discovery of mirror neurons was another major discovery. In the early 1990s, Giacomo Rizzolatti (Rizzolatti & Sinnigagli, 2008) experimented, recording the activities of neurons in the brain of macaque monkeys before, during, and after the monkey picked up a peanut. Then, upon seeing an experimenter pick up the peanut, the monkey's neurons fired according to the same pattern as when the monkey had picked up the peanut itself. Later research using brain imaging from UCLA demonstrated that specialised brain cells, known as mirror neurons, activate when we observe the actions of others; similarly when we simply read sentences describing that same action (or see others on film). Mirror neurons, found in Broca's area and in the premotor cortex of the brain, 'mirror' the behaviour of another person, as though the observer was performing the action, first-hand. They replicate the electrical signals and brain chemistry of the person we are observing (or reading about or watching). For mirror neurons, seeing and doing are the same thing.

Cozolino (2006) argued that mirror neurons were at the crossroads of the processing of inner and outer experience and are most likely involved in the evolution of gestural communication and empathy. When we interact with someone, our mirror neurons enable us to create within our minds, representations of their actions, sensations, and emotions. Without any conscious effort, our brain instantly mirrors theirs, allowing us to have a level of understanding of what they feel. This gives us the capacity to see things from the other's perspective and attune to the person we are observing or thinking about.

Our brain encodes sensory experiences within the neuronal pathways via neurotransmitter connections. In infancy, these brain connections are made by human interaction, so a deficit in human contact can result in failure for the brain to connect at different levels.

The following example illustrates how we can work with such ideas in practice.

EXAMPLE

Anna came for therapy, desperate to have a relationship but 'whenever I try to meet men, no one shows any interest in me, I start having a conversation and they switch off after thirty seconds'. Anna had always felt rather disconnected from her mother, whom, it also transpired, was on the autistic spectrum. I had just been to a training by Allan Schore on mirror neurons, so I decided to introduce the idea of mirror neurons into the energy work and attempt to treat Anna's connection patterns.

Anna and I co-created the following phrases to describe exactly what happened to her during this infant attachment trauma, where Anna's attempts to relate with her mum were met with her mother's disconnection from her. She then cleared this traumatised energy, including the pattern of her mirror neurons, through her chakras. She repeated the following phrases to inform the neural pathways which energy and information needed to be transformed:

> *All my distress at all the times and ways mum disconnected from me when I was trying to get her attention when I was a baby.*

Repetition compulsion is astonishing—time and time again we notice in energy therapy how traumatic patterns repeat exactly:

> *Because mum switched off from me after thirty seconds of connection when I was a baby, I resonate with the pattern of her disconnected mirror neurons, so men also disconnect from me after a similar length of time, and I can't get their attention.*

While doing the energy clearing, we also worked with a 'Post-it' note with the words 'mirror neurons' written on it to carry the energetic frequency of the relevant part of the *mindbody-energy* in the field. This was based on work I had learned on the principle of treating allergies from seminars undertaken with Sandi Radomski, ('Allergy Antidotes'), Tony Roffers, ('Sensitivities'), and Asha Clinton ('Presence and Dissociation'). It is also possible to include other aspects of the body, brain, or nervous system in the field when doing trauma clearing, which helps strengthen their functioning.[3]

After clearing those phrases, we positively reframed this trauma using energy methods to create new neural pathways. The phrase Anna chose was: 'I attract men who stay present, interested and connected with me'. It is worth noting here that energy methods are more powerful than affirmations, since they work beyond the cognitive level, at the 'higher gauge' with the entire *mindbodyenergy*.

I think I was as amazed as Anna when, the following week, she reported she had been on a date and managed to make a good connection with the man. She subsequently went on to have a relationship with him, get married and she came to visit me in my consulting room a year later to show me their beautiful baby. It was wonderful to see how happy she was. It would be wrong to imply that all energy therapy is as easy as this—but it is heartening to see how much it can help people.

Implicit motion, the mirror neuron system, and regulation of affect

Schore (2003) stresses that attachment communications of trauma patients are implicit, affective, nonverbal 'states'. The unconscious affect regulation expressed in rapid nonverbal communications at levels beneath conscious awareness within the dynamic intersubjective field, play a critical psycho-biological role within the psychotherapy relationship. The mirror neurons system, the insula, and amygdala are active during emotional expressions, and correlate with

---

[3] Nambudripad's Allergy Elimination Techniques (NAET®) was discovered by Dr Devi S. Nambudripad in November of 1983. This work offers a non-invasive, drug-free, natural solution to alleviate allergies of all types and intensities using a blend of selective energy balancing, testing, and treatment procedures from acupuncture/acupressure, allopathy, chiropractic, nutritional, and kinesiological disciplines of medicine. Dr Devi's work has informed other energy practitioners.

maternal reflective functioning and empathy. Because mirror neurons are crucial to empathy and the neurological substrates of attunement, the presence of the therapist is important in noticing and naming what is happening.

Energy psychotherapy amplifies this effect; the neuroplasticity of the brain can be beneficially affected by trauma clearing, and then working with positive intention helps to build links and connectivity that were previously missing.

The brain and stress

Chapter 7 describes methods for releasing stress and balancing exercises to clear 'neurological dis-organisation' for therapist and client.

Chapters 7 and 8 explore methods for clearing PTSD, aspects of fight, flight, freeze, flop and, early developmental trauma.

Trauma, attachment, and stress disorders

The neuroscience concerning the emotional attachment bond formed between an infant and its primary caretaker is well known, with love playing a central role in shaping and influencing the developing baby's brain (Gerhardt, 2004). Infant and caretaker both need to connect calmly for positive attachment to occur, so if either parent or child is unable to maintain a balanced nervous state, the attachment bond may be compromised. Lack of love is very stressful—a traumatic attachment, whether caused by abuse, neglect, or emotional unavailability on the part of the caretaker, negatively impacts brain structure and function. Treating such developmental trauma is a core area of work in energy psychotherapy

Neurons in the cortex of a developing foetus are already firing in response to events at twenty weeks (Music, 2013) so neurological dysregulation which occurs on account of stressful prenatal experiences in the womb and at birth can interfere with the attachment bond. Women who were pregnant and happened to be present at the World Trade Centre on 9/11, and who subsequently developed post-traumatic stress symptoms, had children with altered stress responses and cortisol levels (Yehuda et al., 2005, quoted in Music, 2013). As Sandi Radomski says, 'It is all in the first trauma' which creates a 'blueprint' which affects the trajectory of our lives.[4]

Brain technology recognises the difference between normal stress responses that return to a state of regulation, and traumatic stress responses that do not normalise. According to Dr Connie Lillas (Lillas & Turnbull, 2011), when someone is stressed, the stress responses (at any age) can go into one of three primary directions: 'too hot' a stress response, where there is an acceleration of the nervous system resulting from frustration or anger; 'too cold' a stress

---

[4] Sandi Radomski was discussing that 'It's all in the first trauma' in a supervision/development group I attended with her, working with *Ask and Receive*. She emphasised the crucial work which needs to be done with infant trauma, since it creates profound 'blueprints' which affect the trajectory of our lives. This is explored more in Chapter 8.

response, when there are shutting-down and tuning-out behaviours; and a 'mix' of hot and cold stress responses, where there is a blend of out-of-balance behaviour, including anxious withdrawal, anxious clinging, or hypervigilance (NICABM, www.nicabm.com offer useful training programmes for therapists which explore the stress responses in detail).

Preverbal trauma and stress

Adverse childhood experiences (ACEs) are well documented. Less so is the significant correlation between in-utero, prenatal and preverbal trauma in infancy, and vulnerability to being adversely impacted by stressful experiences in later in life. This can include a range of conditions such as PTSD, depression, anxiety, ADHD, chronic physical health problems, and difficulties with managing feelings, thoughts, and emotions.

If a baby/young child has not been soothed by their carer, they have not learned how to self-soothe. Without containment, the child lacks safety and struggles to regulate emotions or even tolerate having feelings at all. In adulthood, people become hypervigilant, extremely sensitive, and easily triggered into volatile mood swings. Alternatively, they might have difficulties thinking, 'mentalizing', or putting experiences into words. Not least are difficulties in learning—many so-called 'learning disabilities' are simply the result of traumatised stuck brains, which makes it hard to take things in.

All this undermines the development of a healthy sense of self. In energy psychotherapy, we work with the above traumas and conditions, clearing foetal distress and bringing in positive new neural connections and patterns. Our clients regularly report feelings of significant change and greater ease in their lives.

When, through post-partum depression, premature birth, or ongoing neglect or brutality, there has been severe attachment trauma and a failure of the maternal–infant bond, the oxytocin system—which optimises love, well-being, and health—is disrupted. Deprivation in the maternal environment can affect brain chemistry to such an extent that it may cause endogenous depression in adults, which can become very stuck and engrained. However, when people are motivated to get better, longer-term energy psychotherapy can help somewhat with deep depression, though this requires the clearing of considerable amounts of trauma and the installation of positive intentions to create positive new neural pathways.

Freeing trauma through relationship and movement

Cozolino's work (2006) showed the potential healing impact relationships have on the brain. When the traumatised brain feels stuck and 'fixed', it is the connection with self and other which opens opportunities to make changes. The brain also benefits when we focus on positive information rather than using its energy to fight its limitations. Van der Kolk (2015) spoke of the importance of movement when trauma is frozen in the body. The groundbreaking work of Anat Baniel in *Kids Beyond Limits* (2012) offers an interesting example. A clinical psychologist, dancer, and leader in the field of movement/brain relationship, Baniel helped children who had started out in life with severe disability and brain trauma, which affected all levels of their functioning, to overcome astonishing limitations.

Baniel felt that at the core of change is movement, which is energy: movement was the most powerful way to communicate with the brain, since movement *is* change. She also emphasised thinking as movement, since this creates something new in the neural pathways which wasn't there before. Emotions—'energy in motion'—which were previously stuck, can also begin to flow and be freely expressed.

This understanding is just as relevant for energy psychotherapy. First, we need to fight the automatic habit of repeating what we did before. Going over old ground only deepens existing dysfunctional patterns and loses the opportunity for making other free-floating neurological connections which are 'waiting to be'. This idea emphasises how important it is to find new ways to address pain and trauma in psychotherapy.

The second is recognising the significance of our human need for safety. Neurosciences tell us that body and brain are constantly responding to perceived threats from our environment, deciding—at a cellular level—whether we are safe. How secure we feel profoundly affects not only our physical and immune health, but our brain's health, which, in turn, determines our mental well-being. We often avoid change because it disturbs what is familiar, and instead fixate on an experience or get stuck in a rut. Sandler spoke of how familiarity provides our sense of safety—'better the devil you know' (Sandler, 2003). As people seek safety above all other considerations, anxiety and fear can sabotage our need for change.

Third, to be healthy, the brain needs to make new connections and new patterns throughout life. Without this increased complexity we remain stuck and can't develop and evolve. Sometimes in energy psychotherapy when we work with transforming limiting core beliefs, people viscerally feel the effort their brain is making, 'working' to try and formulate new alternatives as new neural pathways open up.

Nonverbal cues

The brain is very attuned socially. The infant's brain is shaped to a large degree by the right-brain-to-right-brain process of unspoken nonverbal communications, which set blueprints for subsequent thoughts, feelings, and behaviours. Nonverbal cues are estimated to be responsible for eighty per cent of what helps clients feel safe in therapy so to create reparatory change for clients who have been traumatised during this nonverbal phase, as well as consciously reflecting (left-brain function), therapists need to follow the physical and emotional experiences of their clients moment by moment. Allan Schore talks about the vital role of such nonverbal communications when working with suicidal patients.[5] Consequently, nonverbal forms of

---

[5] Dr Allan Schore, a YouTube talk on 'The Role of Non-verbal Communication in Treating Suicidal Patients'.

communication, including eye contact, facial expression, tone of voice, posture, intensity, and timing or pace are very important. Subtle cues are picked up from the clients' body language, tone of voice, etc., and transmitted back as nonverbal understanding that the therapist knows of the client's deepest experiences.

Energy work fits well and easily into this arena. When the therapist shares the client's sensate experience by feeling it to some degree within their own *mindbodyenergy* this helps to regulate the client's feeling states. (Chapter 8 speaks of the difference between 'Presence' and empathy, and how not to 'take on' the client's energy.) The therapist mirrors the client during energy clearings; the client repeats a clearing phrase and works with their meridians (tapping), chakras, or using intention methods such as *Ask and Receive* to release stress through their subtle energy system. As they do so, the therapist also holds or taps their own meridians or chakras in the same places.

This mirroring serves two functions. It heightens the psycho-biological attunement between therapist and client while protecting the therapist from picking up too much bodily counter-transference (i.e. protecting the therapist's energy centres from 'taking in' the client's trauma). Mirroring the client's movements—such as the energetic releases of breathing, and yawning— also develops an increased space of intimacy, affect regulation, and intuitive connection between therapist and client, very similar to mother/baby attunement.

I and my clients yawn quite a lot during the process of energy releases so I was interested to see a scientific explanation of this in *How God Changes your Brain* (Newberg & Waldman, 2009). Yawning positively influences many functions of the brain, evoking neural activity in areas associated with creating feelings of empathy. The precuneus—a tiny structure hidden within the folds of the parietal lobe—plays a central role in consciousness, self-reflection, and memory retrieval. The precuneus is stimulated by yogic breathing, which helps explain why different forms of meditation contribute to an increased sense of self-awareness. Newberg explains how yawning helps us maintain an optimally healthy brain; 'although your eyes may start watering and your nose may begin to run, you'll also feel utterly present, incredibly relaxed and highly alert'. These symptoms are frequently present during energy therapy releases

Traumatisation—stress frozen in place

In normal responses to stress, hormones release, our heartbeat speeds up, and blood pressure increases. We breath quicker, move faster, hit harder, see better, and hear more accurately. These neurological and physiological changes help protect us in the moment. Once the danger has passed, our nervous systems calm down and we return to a state of equilibrium or neurological balance. However, when someone becomes traumatised, the stress becomes frozen in place—locked into a pattern of neurological distress that doesn't return to a state of equilibrium.

The triune brain

Energy psychotherapy works with all aspects of the brain and nervous system. (The vagus nerve will be discussed in Chapter 8.) A serviceable model of the brain emerged in the 1960s when Paul MacLean (1990) grouped brain neurons by function into three areas. This hierarchy, known as the triune brain, developed in a particular order through evolution.

MacLean's triune brain model is oversimplified and a little out of date now. Contemporary advances in brain-imaging show there is no such neat division, since primal, emotional, and rational experiences are the product of neural activity in more than one of the three regions addressed and it is their *collective* energy which creates human experience. However, Shadid (2021) argues that MacLean's brain model provides revolutionary insights in thinking about different levels of consciousness, so these divisions—describing the structure and function of specific brain regions—are nonetheless helpful.

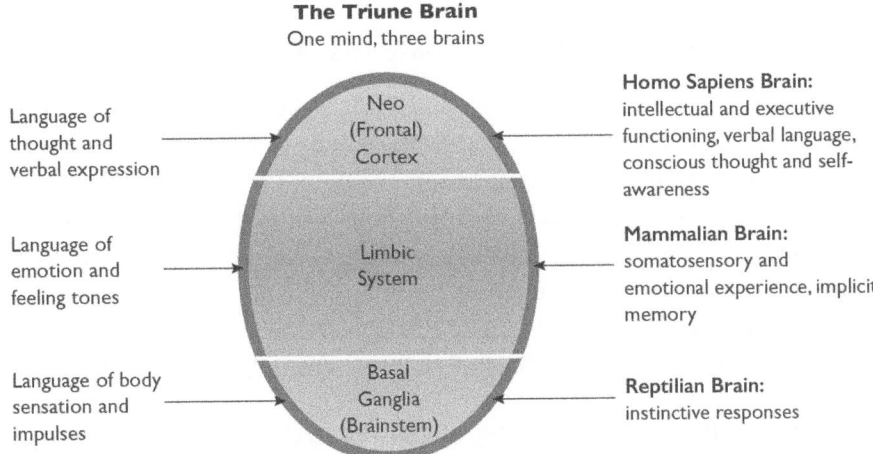

The Triune Brain
One mind, three brains

Language of thought and verbal expression → Neo (Frontal) Cortex

Language of emotion and feeling tones → Limbic System

Language of body sensation and impulses → Basal Ganglia (Brainstem)

Homo Sapiens Brain: intellectual and executive functioning, verbal language, conscious thought and self-awareness

Mammalian Brain: somatosensory and emotional experience, implicit memory

Reptilian Brain: instinctive responses

Figure 5 Maclean's model of the triune brain in evolution: role in paleocerebral functions

The *reptilian brain* (the basal ganglia/brainstem) concerns our basic need for safety and survival. It is responsible for our automatic instinctive responses and bodily reflexes, and regulates our core physiological functions—our heartbeat, breathing, and other vital organs—as well as our habitual unconscious social behaviour patterns like handshakes and head nods. When we feel safe, we are peaceful and calm—when unsafe, we live in fear, and our nervous system is in 'survival' mode.

The *mammalian mid-brain*—our emotional brain—is responsible for feelings, emotions, our implicit memory, and our need to feel satisfied. It contains the limbic system comprising the hippocampus and amygdala—our somatosensory system. The amygdala 'decides' whether our environment is safe or threatening, triggering the fight/flight/freeze survival response based on perceived emotional tone. It perceives danger ahead of the neocortex (our conscious brain), so we often feel fear before we are consciously aware of its cause.

Finally, the *human* (*Homo sapiens*) *brain* comprises the neocortex and frontal lobes. This primate brain governs higher mental functions including regulating attention, complex reasoning, abstract and rational thought, imagination, language (our capacity to put things into words), and empathy. It is the seat of our conscious awareness and is also concerned with our basic human need for attachment/connection with others.

While subsequent researchers have presented considerably more interconnected models of the brain, MacLean's model claims that functions in the three brain regions are largely distinct. For example, out of self-preservation, the reptilian brain prepares us for action when we are in danger by initiating the release of chemicals throughout the body. The limbic system—our emotional brain—is stimulated to release chemicals which create our experience of emotions when we watch shocking news or receive an upsetting message. Finally, we engage our human brain—the neocortex—when making decisions, solving problems, or reasoning.

Cellular science—thoughts, feelings, and emotions

The replication of cellular patterns—Deepak Chopra[6]

Deepak Chopra a renowned endocrinologist and leader in the field of quantum physics and mind–body healing, was an early advocate of the mind–body connection. He held that thoughts, feelings, and emotions have physical consequences (Chopra, 1989). Every thought, feeling, and emotion creates a molecule known as a neuropeptide. Neuropeptides travel throughout our body and hook onto receptor sites of cells and neurons. Our brain takes in the information, converts it into chemicals, and lets the whole body know if there is trouble in the world, or cause for celebration. These molecules course through the bloodstream, directly influencing our bodies by delivering the energetic effect of whatever our brain is thinking and feeling.

Replication of traumatic memory in degenerative (traumatised) cell patterns

Chopra established that cells inside the body regenerate at different speeds—for instance, liver cells regenerate in six weeks. One might ask why someone with liver cancer in January would still be riddled with cancer in June? Dr Chopra explains this by 'phantom memories' stored inside our cells. Inside the degenerative cancer cell lies a traumatic memory which it passes on to the next cell generation being born. So, the new cell is born as an exact replica of the previous cell. Thus, the cells keep replicating themselves, passing on the degenerative memory from one generation to the next and so on. What is being replicated is the degenerative (traumatised) cell pattern stored inside. Simply put, cell memory retains 'ill-causing' information. Chopra discovered through studying thousands of case studies, that the successful survivors of serious diseases had two things in common:

- First, those who got well were able to get in touch with their body's wisdom—what Chopra referred to as its infinite intelligence, or 'Source'. In energy psychotherapy we can access

---

[6] Since writing this, it has been discovered that Chopra was caught up in the Epstein scandal. Nonetheless, his clinical research is still valid.

this intelligence through energy/muscle testing which guides us as to which trauma needs to be released, and also through connecting with our souls or 'higher levels'.

- Second, they were able to get access to, resolve and let go of the traumatic memory residing in the cells. When the person released this trauma, the degenerative memory was not passed on to the next cell generation, so the next cell was born as a new regenerative organically healthy cell, thereby putting an end to the degenerative cycle.

This is precisely the work we do in energy therapy, releasing 'ill-causing' trauma from the cells. The free association of memories that emerge provides us with a 'flow' of information, which brings out what needs to be cleared and also helps guide the direction of the work.

Molecules of emotion—Candace Pert

'The molecules of emotion run every system in the body' (Pert, 1999).

Dr Candace Pert, an award-winning cellular biologist and biophysicist unequivocally established that emotions and the body are neurologically linked. Pert was among the earliest contributors to 'psycho-neuro-immunology', and her work in the 1980s led to her theory of how the 'bodymind' functions as a single psychosomatic network of information molecules which control our health and physiology.

In *Molecules of Emotion* Pert revealed how her study of information-processing receptors on nerve cell membranes led her to discover that the same 'neural' receptors were present on most, if not all, of the body's cells. Bruce Lipton, who drew on her work said:

> Her elegant experiments established that the 'mind' was not focussed in the head but was distributed via signal molecules to the whole body. As importantly, her work emphasised that emotions were not only derived through a feedback of the body's environmental information. Through self-consciousness, the mind can use the brain to generate 'molecules of emotion' and override the system. While proper use of consciousness can bring health to an ailing body, inappropriate unconscious control of emotions can easily make a healthy body diseased. (Lipton, 2010)

Neuronal plasticity—healing and renewal at a cellular level

We have previously mentioned neuronal plasticity, the capacity for healing and renewal by replacing old neuronal connections with new ones, and how repeated experiences change the neural pathways. This is healing at a cellular level. What is interesting is that the production of a single thought requires a complex system of interactions amongst all three levels of the brain—the reptilian brain, the limbic system, and the neo-cortex. When we formulate a 'clearing' phrase and repeat it during energy clearings, we are communicating this information throughout the neuronal pathways to every cell of our being on all levels, telling the body what it is that needs to be cleared from the *mindbodyenergy* or the positive energy which needs to be 'installed'.

Neuropeptides—the molecules of emotion

In the field of psychosomatic medicine, it is recognised that some people have difficulties discriminating between physical and mental pain. When we become 'stuck' in an unpleasant emotional event—a trauma from the past—this is stored at every level of our nervous system including at the cellular level. Pert uses the word 'trauma' to describe both physical and mental damage. This has been a key part of her theory of how the molecules of emotion integrate what we feel at every level of *mindbodyenergy*. The memories in these cells are constantly replicating, renewing the old traumatic patterns. Pert's laboratory research has suggested that all the senses—sight, sound, smell, touch, and taste—are filtered, and these sensate memories are stored through the molecules of emotions, mostly the neuropeptides and their receptors, at every level.

Repressing emotions—blocked energy

Chemistry is associated with every emotion that we have. At a purely chemical level, consciousness and emotions are affecting our cells. When we repress an emotion, it releases a chemical into the blood stream, which will go to certain cell receptors and block them, leaving them incapable of communicating with the rest of the cells in the body. If those cell receptors remain blocked over a long period of time, this creates a propensity for disease to occur in the area which is blocked, referred to in *The Power of Now* as the 'pain body'.

> The remnants of pain left behind by every strong negative emotion that is not fully faced, accepted and let go of join together to form an energy field that lives in the very cells of your body. (Tolle, 1999)

Expressing emotions—flowing energy and open cell receptors

Conversely Dr Pert also found that when we *express* an emotion wholesomely i.e. it is fully expressed and we are open to that emotion (not avoiding, hiding from it, repressing it, or pushing it away), then the cell receptors remain open. This scientific theory highlights the benefits of energy psychotherapy, which facilitates unblocking repressed emotions and the free-flowing expression of emotion, so that we remain 'open' rather than closed.

Emotions, feelings, and cognitions—Antonio Damasio

Damasio's neuroscientific discoveries show that our rationality is built on the building blocks of emotion. In developmental terms, feelings come first—cognitive processes elaborate on emotional processes but could not exist without them (Damasio, 2003, 2010). However, rationality does not exist merely 'on top of' the apparatus of biological regulation but comes from it and with it. Damasio considered that emotions belong to the body, triggering a series of specific chemicals and organic alterations; then after emotions come feelings, which have a deeper relationship with our thoughts.

The 'biology of belief'

Epigenetics

Dr Bruce Lipton's groundbreaking research where he cloned stem cells in petri dishes, established the role of epigenetics and the *Biology of Belief* (2010). His work synthesised the latest and best research in cell biology and quantum physics, demonstrating that our bodies change because of the change in our thinking. He showed us how 'the biology of belief' works.

In Lipton's experiments, in environment A, the cells differentiated and formed muscle; in environment B the cells differentiated and formed bone; in environment C the cells differentiated and formed fat. Since the cells were genetically identical, this experiment proved that it was the environment that influenced the behaviour and genetic activity of the cells. Termed epigenetics in 1990, 'epi' means above, and so 'epigenetic control' literally means 'control above the genes'. Lipton's experiments demonstrated the powerful role of perceptions in this process.

Signal transduction and gene switching

In Lipton's explanation of quantum bio-physics (2016) he describes how certain proteins work as on–off switches to DNA. Amazingly, environmental factors—including our own beliefs—can create such switches. When such an environmental signal is picked up by the skin of the cell, the signal is relayed inside the cell and goes into the nucleus to activate the genes. Termed 'signal transduction', this is a leading edge of science. The skin of the cell is not just skin, but it is also the brain. The cell's brain is the mem-'brain' of the cell. The cell membrane senses the signals and responds to them. It is empowering when we realise that we can control our genes by our thoughts and emotions. This means that we can change our environment, by choosing how we perceive that environment—positively or negatively.

Rather than modifying the genes themselves, our thoughts and feelings modify gene *expression*. The cell's operations are primarily moulded by its interaction with the environment, not with its genetic code. In effect, our biological (cellular) behaviour can be influenced by *physical forces* (such as chemical signals from food, and medications) and by *consciousness*—vibrational signals from our thoughts and emotions. In the *Biology of Belief* Lipton provided the scientific underpinning for pharmaceutical-free energy medicine. His work also reminds us that chemistry is based on physics, and that the new cell biology cannot be adequately explained by Newtonian physics which has no 'field' effect.

CHAPTER 4

The quantum field: energy, information, frequency, and consciousness

From a quantum mechanics perspective, energy is information, resonance, and consciousness. Our mind controls our body through electromagnetic fields. Our cells respond to all forms of electromagnetic fields, energetic fields, and quantum mechanical properties as well. Life in the cells expresses itself in the changing shape of protein which is controlled by signalling. Matter is formed from specific energy frequencies and change is brought about by specific frequencies activating different functions in the cells. We have approximately 50 trillion cells in the body and the brain is the mechanism of perception, like a chemist that translates the signals into chemistry. In summary, our biology is controlled by both the environment around us and our perceptions and beliefs. It is the electromagnetic translation of our perception or beliefs of that environment that controls our biology.

We can use the power of *intention* to connect with the vast data of 'the field' through the quantum waves that it emits and receive information via a quantum frequency wave. As Einstein said, 'The mind is the sole generating agency of the particle called the body' (quoted by Lipton, 2016).

In relating this to energy psychotherapy, we therefore interact with energy which influences and organises the factors that regulate life. How does this work? The subatomic particles (information) are like powerful miniature force fields or nano tornadoes. As there is no physicality to an atom, the atom is generating waves—and thus broadcasting energy through the field. Every atom or molecule emits and absorbs light of characteristic wavelengths. Since we're made out of atoms and molecules, our bodies are emitting and absorbing light.

Dr Peter Gariaev (1942–2020): language, the wave genome, and its positive implications for self-healing

The primary signals which control life are not chemicals, but energetic signals, the vital life force (*prana* or *qi*). Dr Peter Gariaev (1942–2020), a Russian quantum scientist, contributed to the quantum paradigm shift and our new understanding of the biosphere with his work on linguistics and the wave genome. He found a direct link between our genetic code and the structure and construction of language, which was backed up by others, including Nobel Prize winner Luc Montagnier (Jacobi, 2022).

Lipton's work on epigenetics showed us that our beliefs are 'encoded' in our DNA. Gariaev's work on linguistic wave genetics demonstrates the power of language—how word and sound activate these 'codes' and 'recodes' them, enabling us to switch our genetic codes on or off, which changes and restructures our DNA/genome. This is the very essence of energy psychotherapy with tremendously positive implications for self-healing. It all comes down to resonance/ frequency. In life generally, our sonic expression/vibration—that is to say, whatever we think or express—becomes a hologram contributing to the creation of our reality. When we set positive intentions, the unified field matches the (high) frequency we put out. By consistently taking action to stay in this frequency and maintain its potency—physically, emotionally, mentally, and spiritually—we gradually evolve, supporting our ascension to *Homo luminous*.

In 'Choosing the path of joy' I mentioned how 'ascension' involves lighting up the vestigial strands of DNA which transforms our genetic code. Humanity is also being assisted by the high frequency plasma light pouring onto earth, which is accelerating the massive planetary changes and 'decoding' everyone's dormant DNA. As this light is absorbed into our bodies, its 'light codes' activate our cells, awaken new DNA strands—alongside our consciousness—and bring corresponding gifts such as enhanced intuition. All this occurs via our crystalline light body—or *Merkabah*—our personal quantum energy field or biosphere. The blueprint of our life force is constituted by the sum of the molecules of our DNA/RNA, which together are entangled at a biological level, creating a lattice of pure crystalline liquid—'aether' or 'plasma light'. Our high vibrational light body is an ideal transmitter and receiver of energetic resonance and intercommunication, which interfaces with our ordinary consciousness. Soul-connecting creates a bridge between our spiritual and physical body thereby raising our vibration and facilitating our personal evolution.

Quantum coherence and interpersonal neurobiology—Daniel Siegel

The influence of quantum theory is also found in Daniel Siegel's work on interpersonal neurobiology. Contributing to the synthesis of advances across a range of disciplines—including brain science, psychiatry, attachment theory, quantum physics, and spirituality—Siegel expanded our understanding of consciousness, and what this means for the practice of psychotherapy. Siegel is especially interested in the idea that the universe is chaotic and dynamic, but 'the field' can be brought to order and quantum coherence by *relationship*. Scientifically speaking, this coherence—or essential order—lends itself to the logical transference of data through its emissions and transmissions.

Siegel defines a core aspect of the mind as an embodied, relational process that regulates the flow of energy and information through the mind's *interpretation* of events. The mind interprets the signals from the environment and generates its own signal and electromagnetic field. The electromagnetic signalling of the neurons in the brain shapes which chemistry is released by the brain. If you change the vibration of the cell, you change the response of the cell, which then changes the response of the body and there is an energetic movement.

We know that this science is actual, rather than merely theoretical, because many people do energy work at a distance using zoom and things still shift in our field. Despite being online, client and therapist have visceral interpersonal experiences of working together—for instance, yawning together during the release of traumatised energy. Such direct experience of 'quantum entanglement', and the 'spooky actions at a distance' which Einstein spoke of, shows the unified field in action.

Siegel felt his concept of interpersonal neurobiology provided a new basis for psychotherapy. His hypotheses are that first, a healthy mind is at the root of self-regulation, utilising an integrated system which has adaptability and flexibility in responding to external stimuli. Second, he considers that all self-regulation emerges through the process of integration (he defined integration as the linkage of differentiated parts). When this integration is impaired, chaos and rigidity (in the nervous system's response to external stimuli) lead to dysregulation and ultimately to psychopathology.

Siegel considered that psychotherapists can specifically aid integration at psychological and neurological levels by identifying the areas of chaos and rigidity (i.e. the traumatic roots) in their clients' lives and promote self-regulating interventions (energy treatments) which bring about coherence. Finally, he considers that effective psychotherapy improves the integrative growth of fibres in the brain (long-term neuroplasticity). In energy psychotherapy we offer a range of mind/body ways of working which seek to do precisely all that Siegel describes.

Concerning the quantum world

I was listening to a webinar by Dr Richard Alan Miller, a renowned quantum physicist, polymath, and spiritual practitioner who has written countless books, including on quantum physics. Miller, with the highest possible level of clearance in military intelligence, is regularly called into the secret space programme (SSP) to sort out 'difficult problems'. He was commenting that developments in quantum physics are advancing so rapidly that the Marvel movie *Doctor Strange in the Multiverse of Madness*, with its extraordinary multidimensionality, is truer than we might wish to believe. Miller recognises that few scientists can keep up with the emerging new discoveries, so he is writing another book about deeper layers and levels of quantum science, in the hope that someone will be able to understand it. Such knowledge is very humbling and gives us a perspective on the vastness of multiverses.

***

Bringing us back to something we can aspire to understand, I have been having a more ordinary conversation with Phil Mollon about the nature of science in energy psychotherapy. It is difficult to know precisely which scientific territory we enter when we think about this, particularly if one is not a quantum scientist, so the following explorations seek to reach some kind of understanding. Phil's books (2005, 2008, 2022) explore scientific aspects of energy psychotherapy in more detail, for those who are interested.

In Chapter 2, 'From matter to light', I discuss how in the vibrational universe, mind is no longer separate from body. In the multidimensional quantum world, everything is fundamentally interrelated, and moreover, there is not one truth but several possible truths. The quantum model is concerned with field effects and entanglement. One event impacts another, and that event influences the original one in a fractal process. Cause and effect depend on the vantage point, on where you are starting in the loop of a cycle that is infinite.

The term 'quantum' originally relates to the way electrons were discovered to shift their position not in gradual ways but in quantum leaps. Later, the term quantum physics/mechanics was used to refer to the whole realm of the very tiny—the subatomic realm. It was found that small particles, such as photons or electrons, would behave as waves, but, puzzlingly, as soon as a human observer enters the picture, they become particles. The distributed probability wave becomes fixed by the act of human observation—thus human consciousness somehow alters how subatomic particles behave. McTaggart and many others have drawn on this basic and well-established phenomenon, to explore the effects of human intention.

In quantum physics, atoms interact, not as physical interactions, but as the interaction of waves given off by the atoms. If you bring these energy sources close together, then the ripples interact in very specific ways, known as 'interference' or 'super position'. Essentially, every particle or quantum entity or 'packet'—described as either a wave or a particle—is held in a field of infinite possibility ('the unified field') until something—perhaps a thought or intention—creatively brings it into form. This is relevant to our understanding about 'thought fields' and why the creativity of our thoughts, feelings, and intentions is so important in energy psychotherapy.

Intention—a 'higher gauge' realm

Aspects of the brain are known through esoteric yogic traditions to relate to the spiritual aspects of a person's development and can lead to greater intuitive awareness beyond the cognitive mind. For instance, the pineal/pituitary axis—the 'third eye', the area of the brain largely concerned with spiritual and transpersonal dimensions of experience—serves as a gateway to what William Tiller termed 'higher gauge' realms. I am grateful to Phil Mollon for introducing me to the work of Tiller (Emeritus Professor of Material Science at Stamford University) and his ideas about intention.

There have been many successful intention experiments using meditation: Hagelin (1993) focused on reducing crime in Washington DC (quoted in Chapter 1); many other experiments are quoted in *Mind to Matter* (Church, 2018); and McTaggart (2001). All these relate their research to hypotheses concerning the quantum level of reality.

Lynne McTaggart's experiments on the power of intention discovered that:

> Human intention could be used as an extraordinarily potent healing force. It appeared that we could order the random fluctuations in the Zero Point Field and use this to establish greater 'order' in another person. With this type of capability, one person should be able to act as a healing conduit, allowing The Field to realign another person's structure. (McTaggart, 2001, p. 235)

William Tiller's intention experiments

Tiller's intention experiments at Walnut Creek resulted in a 'psychoenergetic science' (Tiller, 2007). He had meditators imprint intention into a simple 'Intention Imprinted Electrical Device' and these experiments revealed the existence of 'two unique levels of physical reality'. These are:

1. our conventional, particulate, electrical, atom/molecular level and
2. a new, magnetic, information wave level that has much in common with the old 'ether' concept of the 1800s.[1]

He found that the second level of physical reality operated quite differently 'from our normal electric atom/molecule level … The 'stuff' of this physical vacuum level consists of magnetic information waves … [and] the physics of this new level is modulatable by the human mind, human intentions, and human consciousness in general' (p. 13).

Tiller's research provides an alternative theory for intention, not based on quantum physics. Most crucially for energy psychology, Tiller finds that the human subtle energy system is the portal, or 'coupler system', to this Level-2 reality that is at a higher dimensional level ('higher gauge') than Level-1 physical reality (Tiller, 1993, pp. 293–304).

Tiller then posed the question:

> Is it possible that … there exists a … body system … at the higher electromagnetic symmetry state (higher thermodynamic free energy per unit volume state)? If so, then this could drive all the processes (mechanical, chemical, electrical, and optical) of the rest of the body and would look like a *source* of life? (p. 88)

His results demonstrated that this was so: 'our acupuncture meridian/chakra system is the human body system that is at this higher thermodynamic free energy per unit volume state' (p. 8) and that 'the behaviour of the physical world alters in the presence of subtle energy'.

---

[1] Ronald Beesley's *The Creative Ethers* (1978) concerns the basic functions and order by which the universe keeps in motion. There are seven wavelength circuits and Part 1 deals with the Creative Ethers. Ethers are also understood with Tibetan Buddhism to relate to the fifth element, the dimension of 'space'.

Tiller therefore does not believe that the theories of quantum physics are adequate to explain his findings about intention. As a result of his experiments, Tiller revised Einstein's principle of *mass–energy* to that of *mass–energy–information–consciousness* and his model was elaborated on by Debra Greene (2021) to explain energy psychology.

However, Chris Essonne's brief video (2022) further expands the 'old ether concept of the 1800s' mentioned by Tiller, offering an explanation of the physics of the aethers which *does* allow us to unify quantum physics, gravity, and electromagnetism.

Phil Mollon feels that Tiller's theory of a 'higher gauge' realm may provide a better explanation than quantum physics for intention effects. In some correspondence with Phil about the applications of this to energy psychotherapy, he said:

> Regarding Tiller, it is not so much that he argues the solution to our problems lies at a higher gauge—but that he identified a higher gauge, a realm where the laws of physics are subtly different, and which is responsive to our intention. This higher gauge seems to be the realm in which the subtle energy systems of the body and mind operate. Actually, I suppose the argument that the solution to our problems lies in working at a higher dimensional level is one that I have made—inspired by Tiller's findings. Thus, we can say that energy psychotherapy is more effective than conventional psychotherapy because it draws upon higher dimensional levels—a higher gauge, if you like—and thereby exerts more power over the lower levels. (Phil Mollon, email 4 June 2022)

Unity consciousness, higher dimensional trance states, and the brain

So how do we deal with the paradox of creating positive outcomes that unfold in 3-D time and space out of 5-D states of non-dual consciousness? Tom Kenyan, a sound healer who works with the Hathors (Kenyan, 2012, online reference), explains that in 'higher dimensional trance states', we are led to expanded states of being that, by their very nature, transcend both time and space. It is in the expanded non-localised sense of ourselves that the magic of manifesting enters the 'higher gauge' order of expression. If we expand on Tiller's idea that 'the human subtle energy system is the portal, or "coupler system" to this Level 2 reality', Kenyan's reference to a 'conduit' seems to be saying something remarkably similar:

> Non-dual states of consciousness, which we call the 'Mother of All Things' (i.e. the Void), are the wellspring and the source of manifest reality. We have found that using non-dual states of consciousness as a springboard to create positive outcomes generates more masterful creations. One of the paradoxes involved in the perception of non-dual states is the fact that you perceive these states via your nervous system, which is firmly rooted in duality. Indeed, as you read these words, or hear them spoken, the bioelectric fluctuations in your brain and nervous system operate from a dualistic template. As nerve impulses pass through your neurons, the minute biochemical and electrical events responsible for thought and mental/emotional impressions co-exist in a dynamic dualistic matrix. Yet non-duality, itself, exists outside the dualistic reality of your nervous

system. In functional terms you enter into an awareness of non-duality when your brain/ mind enters a higher dimensional trance state of consciousness. In this unique trance state, there is a *conduit*, or shift in awareness, through which you can experience your own non-dual nature. In more advanced states of consciousness, you can operate in both relative sensory experience and non-dual experience simultaneously. In other words, you can experience the sensory world with its multiple complex duality at the same time you experience the deep calmness and centeredness of your non-dual nature. (2012)

Straddling the two worlds of duality and non-duality (non-local awareness) is quite advanced. For most of us, the task of creating positive outcomes

involves stepping outside the box of perception, the limitations of belief that led you to conclude you are trapped in a linear flow of time. This perception of time may be true for your physical body at your current level of evolution, but it is not true for your consciousness. All that needs to take place is for you to find the conduit, or the channel, that leads to an expanded state of awareness and being. For us, not all trance states of consciousness are the same. *Higher dimensional trance states* are not simply expressions of brain function; they are an inherent human ability that allows you to enter a conduit that connects you to other aspects of your being, which are outside the constraints of perceived time and space. In other words, when you enter a *higher dimensional trance state*, you functionally transcend aspects of neurological activity within your nervous system. While your brain/mind is still bound by the neurological realities of your nervous system, an aspect of your consciousness is no longer bound by these limitations. We call this *the conduit*, and in some ways, it is a metaphor while in other ways it is an apt description, because it is much like a wormhole that connects you to vaster aspects of your nature.' (2012)

It seems to me that Kenyon's 'conduit' of a 'higher dimensional trance state' is similar to Tiller's 'higher gauge state'. Whatever scientific understanding we have, on an experiential level I feel this conduit can be found through connecting with our souls—our 'divine consciousness'. To my mind, this 'higher gauge' level is equivalent to 'soul-connecting'.

The healing and learning state of quantum 'flow'

Chapter 2 outlined the dualistic nature of ego's perception and how fifth-dimensional 'quantum' consciousness is available to all who open their hearts to it. This idea is percolating into the mainstream, where businesses are creating models based on quantum 'flow':

We are entering into an unprecedented time in human history, whereby we are undergoing a shift in consciousness that will change everything … All systems and industries will evolve and elevate to new levels, such that coherence, integrity, transparency, and responsibility, along with working knowledge of the Unified Field, become the vital components of a successful business model. (Heflin, 2017)

Heart- and soul-based states resonate at 500 and above and as we move into these higher frequencies we begin to go beyond the time/space dimensions of the 'ordinary' world and experience 'spooky' effects which defy third-dimensional 'rules'. The entanglement of consciousness and quantum level of phenomena is widely discussed where there appear to be magical causalities and instances of synchronicity increase. See also: Zukav (1979), Bentov (1977), Radin (2006), Church (2018), Lanza and Berman (2008), Levy (2018), Currivan (2017), and many more.

Gene Ang, with a doctorate in neurobiology at Yale, works full time with quantum energy healing methods. Quoting Bache (2008), Ang suggests that accessing the quantum field of unity consciousness facilitates healing by bringing us into the higher vibrational states of 'wave-like' energy, characterised by ease and being 'in the flow'. According to Ang, this quantum 'flow' state creates a vortex which amplifies intelligence and 'super-learning' and enables us to access and receive patterns of energy and information from the wider field—or 'collective consciousness'. Being in a state of 'quantum healing hypnosis' (very similar, surely, to Kenyon's 'higher-dimensional trance states' or Tiller's 'higher-gauge' realm), facilitates access to our guides and 'higher teachers', including our own soul or higher self, so we can 'download' wisdom and information which isn't otherwise readily available to us. Consequently, we can have direct access to the akashic records, which hold the memories of all the soul's lifetimes.

Quantum 'flow' is amplified in group healing or learning situations. When we are in resonance with one another, this flow state is relaxing and enables us to receive the exchange of energy and information with 'ease and grace'. Phil Mollon's 'Blue Diamond' is one such healing field, a 'flow' state which makes learning easy and harmonious.

Work with the quantum field is burgeoning. According to Dr David Clements (https://isee-infynergy.com/about-us.htm), one of the beautiful aspects of this 'creator field' of pure potential is that it is benevolent and always operates in life-expressive and expansive ways. Clements developed a system called INFYNERGY based on the interconnectedness of all things where 'intent codes' are absorbed and transmitted. Clements holds that the quantum field is key in moving into a world of heart centeredness. New life-assisting applications are being developed that naturally operate in synergy with life and the expansion of divine consciousness. His research has led to a concept he calls infinity, synergy, energy, and evolution (ISEE). Using attributes of the quantum field to help humanity, he has created products which draw on three principles:

- to repurpose degenerative energy structures into generative ones
- to assist and strengthen the connection to the living Earth fields
- to assist people in expanding and moving beyond the level where degenerative energy structures have a harmful effect, into a deeper state of living connectedness.

This is remarkably similar to the purpose of energy psychotherapy.

CHAPTER 5

Energy psychotherapy: a new therapeutic focus

*T*his chapter offers an outline of the therapeutic process, with more detailed explanations in Part II.

The heart-centred work of energy psychotherapy draws on the core therapeutic approaches, relational skills, and theoretical resources of each therapist's training in counselling or psychotherapy. In this therapeutic paradigm we bring in the dimensions of working with the body, vibrations, and frequencies. This experiential work is easy to learn. Co-created between client and therapist, the energy work itself is done by the client on and for themselves using straightforward self-help methods working with subtle energy, facilitated by the therapist.

Beyond analysis

There are many contradictory perspectives in energy psychotherapy—one size does not fit all and there is no inherent fixed view about this work, which can be couched in a variety of ways. Analysis and understanding—which is of course valuable in bringing insight—expands to a holistic psychotherapy which focuses on releasing the 'dense' stressed energy of trauma from the body.

The approach is relational and client led, involving all the usual tenets of safe, grounded work in therapy. It includes curiosity, exploration and playfulness, knowing and not knowing, and finding a balance between the needs of body, mind, and soul. As with any psychotherapy, sometimes people may simply wish to talk, explore and feel their feelings, and there may be no energy work to do in some sessions. Above all, I cannot emphasise enough that energy psychotherapy is an *integration* of energy methods within the therapeutic relationship.

A wide remit

Energy psychotherapy has a wide remit, working comprehensively with the physical, emotional, mental, spiritual, and energetic dimensions of experience. It can be used across most therapeutic disciplines, and with most forms of psychological disturbance and symptomatology. The methods work effectively with psychodynamic formulations, the treatment of phobias, attachment trauma, anxiety, depression, panic disorders, and so-called 'personality disorders', limiting core beliefs (somewhat like an energy therapy form of CBT), the treatment of PTSD, complex trauma, and dissociative disorders including dissociative identity disorder (DID). If a client is in an *actively* psychotic or bipolar state however, energy methods are not generally recommended, though we can undertake useful trauma work when a person comes back into balance. As with other psychotherapies, the client's motivation to be well makes a significant difference.

The self-application of energy methods clears disturbances or 'perturbations' in the energy field, using chakras, meridians, thought fields, and the solution-focused energy of intention. This work can bring people to a state of balance by clearing energetically a range of issues including: clearing trauma and PTSD; overcoming developmental blocks; integrating splits and fragments of the psyche; and building a healthier more resilient ego/sense of self. A special feature of energy psychotherapy, when people are motivated to do the work, is that it can help overcome what are termed energetic 'reversals' or 'massive reversals', including complex self-sabotaging tendencies. We can also work with complex trauma and integrate archetypal shadow energies and inner attacking parts.

All aspects of the life cycle can be worked with. This includes trauma around conception, in-utero, birth, and infancy, and troubling relational patterns that we form, based on attachment traumas, abandonments, and insecurity in our upbringing. In the process of developing a sense of self, people experience various wounds and employ defence mechanisms and unconscious processes to survive which can also be addressed by energy psychotherapy; for instance, releasing child parts who are stuck in arrested development, where a trauma has held the person frozen in time at a young age, even when other aspects of their life may have progressed. Other depth work includes clearing cultural, transgenerational, transpersonal, and spiritual trauma.

A particularly useful feature of energy psychotherapy is that it can work without language. This enables us to work across cultures—for example, with traumatised refugees where there has been sudden uprooting from one culture into another—and with people who are unable to put their experiences into words.

We can also use energy work with couples and in groups. For example, Asha Clinton and others undertook a project in Guatemala for women who had experienced rape and extreme loss. They did group energy clearings of trauma, which was greatly restorative, both individually and for the community.

Experiential work with the body

Focus on the body is not new, but its importance is gaining wider recognition. Since our ego is 'first and foremost a bodily ego' (Freud, 1923b), to work effectively with trauma we need to include the body. With his background as a neurologist, Freud's early work with hysteria was a precursor to PTSD. When treating his patients, he sometimes touched them at specific centres—such as the forehead—bringing about abreactions which brought relief. Freud's concept of libido is similar to that of energy, *qi*, or *prana*, so these abreactions are like the energetic releases which occur when clearing trauma through the subtle energy system.

Well-known trauma specialists speak of the vital role the body plays. In *The Body Remembers* Rothschild emphasises how our body remembers everything that has happened to us throughout our life and knows information of which we may not be conscious or have recollection (Rothschild, 2000). Pert (1999)—see Chapter 3—speaks about cellular memory. This is also held in our DNA, so our bodies can access transpersonal information including intergenerational trauma and memories held in the akashic records which hold records throughout time and space of the entirety of our soul's journey. The free associations of the body are another way we receive information. Memories emerge naturally when we do energy work, and as this happens, the trauma is gently released from the cells

Van der Kolk's idea that 'the body keeps the score' (2015) can be applied quite literally in energy psychotherapy. Our bodies are very precise, enabling us to energy test exactly how much trauma is in the body using subjective units of distress (SUDs). These measure from 0–10 how much energetic 'charge' is present, either as perturbation in the subtle energy system and energy field, or—looked at another way—the amount of distress and triggering the person is experiencing.

A wide definition of trauma—'difficult emotions and/or physical symptoms'

Energy psychotherapy views trauma—which is very much held in the body—as the cause of most psychological disturbances. Asha Clinton, who developed Advanced Integrative Therapy (AIT) offers a broad definition of trauma to include developmental, relational, and situational trauma as well as well as catastrophic and life-threatening events:

> Trauma can be viewed as being any occurrence which, when we think of it, or when it is triggered by some present event, evokes difficult emotions and/or physical symptoms. In this way, all psychological imbalances can be viewed as being caused by trauma of one form or another. (Clinton, *AIT BASICS manual*, https://ait.institute)

Once therapists and clients experience for themselves the psychobiological/sensate aspects and the relief that energy therapy brings, it is easier to recognise the centrality of this focus on trauma.

Co creation—the playful exchange between client and therapist

One aspect of the therapeutic process involves formulating phrases which sum up the essence of the client's distress. These phrases can be written on a tablet or laptop, so the client can read them easily without having to remember all the words. Energy work is also equally effective when the client simply thinks of, or pictures, their issues, where spoken words are not required. If a client is distressed during clearings, it is also possible for the therapist to speak the words on behalf of the client, since the information is shared in the energy field. This is especially useful when working with small-baby or extremely traumatised parts who have no voice.

The client may have been wounded at different ages, so we bring these parts into the energy clearings into a 'healing circle', which acknowledges the multiplicity of wounded parts and archetypal energies of the complex. The healing circle helps to integrate these parts, while resourcing them at the same time.

Following the flow of the process

Energy psychotherapy may feel uncomfortably new to many therapists, though its process—in its use of free association and following the flow of the unconscious—has a surprising amount in common with psychoanalytic therapy. Jung said that the unconscious guides us in purposeful ways, and this is very much the case in energy psychotherapy. The client is invited to free-associate while they do energy work and as we follow the flow, the wisdom of the unconscious brings things to light, intelligently leading us to issues which need our attention. For instance, when someone is triggered, this energetic 'charge' indicates there is something to clear. We then co-create trauma-clearing phrases which 'tell the story of 'what happened' and the client repeats while tapping on meridians or moving down the chakras. Repeating the clearing phrase indicates to the body and its neural pathways the precise stresses to be released.

Identifying links between the underlying historical trauma and the presenting issue generally makes the work more effective. For instance, if someone is habitually hypervigilant because they were abandoned in infancy, a phrase like 'Mum left me, so I am hypervigilant, and always expect my partner to leave me' will bring about increasing embodiment and emotional resilience. Clearing trauma enables clients to tolerate and integrate previously avoided feelings and emotions. This brings coherence to the ego (both psychologically and bodily), effecting change at structural levels relatively quickly, including changes in the brain; calming stress, the nervous system and PTSD; reducing and in some cases eliminating triggering altogether.

We honour the truth of our bodily responses, so if we suddenly feel nauseous, have a strong body memory, or become neurologically imbalanced, this is a sign that the energy system has been activated. 'Following the energy' also involves trusting dreams and what comes up in the moment as being acutely relevant. We ask for and trust the soul's guidance—of both client and therapist—and follow the promptings of the quiet inner voice.

The timing of when to clear using energy methods may be indicated by a perturbation in the field, such as feelings of overwhelm, shortness of breath, or racing heartbeat and we may wish to clear the issue there and then. Alternatively, after talking and reflecting we might do energy clearings towards the end of the sessions.

The energy psychotherapist takes an active role: as well as noticing the energetic charge and flow of energy, we need to act in the moment. For instance, if a client describes a difficult experience using 'charged' words like 'I felt flayed alive', such language often indicates there is a significant underlying traumatic component. We might stop and say something like 'let's see if we need to clear that now', using muscle/energy testing to check 'it is in my best interest to clear this trauma now'. If the client's energy system tests strong to that, they will then use self-energy clearing methods, with the therapist mirroring this alongside them.

The balance of time spent talking and clearing varies from person to person. The relational aspects of energy psychotherapy may take up a significant proportion of the sessions. I work with attachment-based principles in the therapeutic alliance, where there is a sense of 'play', of discovery, a relaxed exploration—we don't have to get it right, we are working together, finding out what is going on. It is a very intimate way of working, with many of what Daniel Stern (Stern et al., 1998) calls 'now' moments.

Although transference and countertransference still occur, the therapeutic alliance tends to reduce these elements. However, when powerful dynamics occur, these can be worked with energetically. If an unconscious re-enactment is occurring, we explore it and if it is blocking the work, this can be cleared energetically so the flow can continue. One client felt that, like her mother, I was mis-attuning to her, which caused her distress and distrust. First, I acknowledged the rupture, and the reality that she was right and that I had mis-attuned to her. Then we went on to do an energy clearing, linking the past with the present trauma with a phrase *Mum mis-attuned to me, so I felt hurt that Ruthie did the same, and I am not sure if I can trust her anymore.* Clearing this through the chakras brought us back into relationship again, and the rupture was repaired while at the same time bringing insight about her relationship with her mother. Transference can also be discussed in supervision; for instance, around a deadening feeling, or a feeling of enmeshment, where the therapist can't think. Clearing such dynamics energetically in supervision with a phrase such as *all this enmeshment and confusion* brings coherence and clarity back into the field. The attention to free association and flow involves us being connected with our bodies. There may be less emphasis on analysing and thinking, and instead, we work energetically, tending to clear stress in the moment it arises.

Beyond belief

Although part of this book focuses on soul-connecting and awakening consciousness, energy psychotherapy does not require a person to have faith for it to work. Its methods are effective regardless of belief—this applies to both therapists and clients.

Atheistic views have been put forward by many, including Richard Dawkins (2006) and Stephen Hawking (2018) who felt that one can't prove that God doesn't exist, but science makes God unnecessary. The controversial views of Yuval Harari (2011, 2017) are also widely held, so ideas about awakening and evolving consciousness may not feel relevant for some and might even be off putting. Taking a broad and perhaps over-generalised view, we could say that for many left-leaning Europeans, non-religious, non-spiritual rationalist ideologies are seen as essential. If spiritual concerns feel irrelevant, energy psychotherapy can perfectly well be practised without any consideration of 'souls' or 'awakening'.

A significant part of American culture on the other hand tends to embrace spiritual or religious outlooks, while the 'New Age' is generically 'spiritual', with aspiration to connect with universal consciousness, or the life force of 'universal prana'.

As with any therapy, naturally we respect intercultural perspectives, so whatever belief is held, an open, non-judgemental attitude towards all is desirable. Intercultural therapy training can help therapists who do not have any beliefs to work effectively with clients who hold religious, non-dualistic, or transpersonal beliefs.

Heart-and soul-based work

Energy psychotherapy is nonetheless essentially heart- and soul-based work. Although analysis is often involved in the formulation of the problems, there is less focus on thinking and more on experiential work clearing trauma. Energy work also raises people's frequency which supports the evolution of consciousness for those who are interested. One of the by-products of connecting directly with the wisdom of the *mindbodyenergy* at a soul level, is the natural development of intuitive flow in both client and therapist. The experiential states we arrive at, which Kenyon (2012) described as 'higher dimensional trance states' (see Chapter 4) are 'beyond analysis'—beyond thought and cognition—operating in the 'higher gauge' quantum realm which may perhaps be linked in some way with Bion's concept of 'O' (Grotstein, 2007).

Working safely with energy

Since this book outlines energy practices for you to try out for yourself and with clients, considerations of safety are important. From the outset we follow practices of safety, grounding, and embodiment. Sessions generally start with energy balancing, and we pay attention to states of emotional and physiological regulation throughout the work. Energy Balancing is described in Chapter 7.

Caution with complex trauma (explored in Chapters 8 and 9)

Although energy work is essentially gentle, as a cautionary note, when therapists first train in energy therapy, working with complex trauma is not advised—without experience, one can destabilise the person or their survival defences. In *Trauma and Recovery* (1992, p. 155) Judith Herman outlines basic tenets for safe, contained practice, and the need for a staged treatment plan as a general framework for working with PTSD and complex trauma. Establishing a safe therapeutic relationship is naturally important to start with. Since trauma dysregulates people both emotionally and physically, working within Dan Siegel's 'window of tolerance' (1999) is another useful concept. Energy work helps establish that window through energy balancing and clearing small pieces of trauma.

Using kinesiology to guide the work safely

Energy testing/kinesiology, described in Chapter 7, is a key method for guiding the work and establishing that it is safe to clear specific pieces of trauma. Linking with the client's body and energy field, it acts like a 'sat nav' to determine a safe way forward. First discovered in the 1930s, kinesiology still feels quite revolutionary and is something both therapists and clients can learn to use. The therapist can self-energy test on behalf of the client, (this also works on Zoom) or alternatively, test the client's arm directly, if the client gives their consent. When working together, therapist and client share the same 'field' which connects the subtle energy system and thought fields (see Figure 6). The information to be tested for is therefore readily available.

We can use energy testing to ascertain the roots of trauma including when it first occurred. Binary statements are presented to the client's energy system via this method, and the Yes/No responses often bring forward information of which the client is not consciously aware.

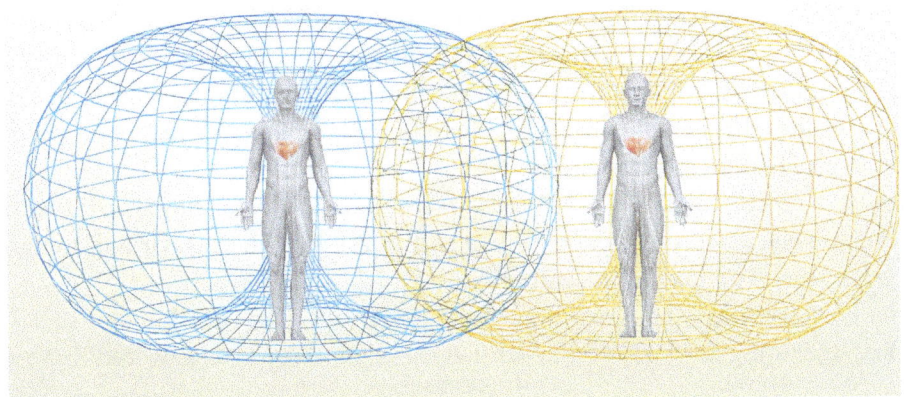

Figure 6 Shared energy field between client and therapist

The state of 'Presence' of both therapist and client in energy testing is important, akin to Bion's concept of reverie. It helps to harmonise the field. Figure 6 shows a coherent regulated energy flow which becomes scrambled if a person becomes dysregulated. This is why it is essential to make sure that both therapist and client are balanced before they energy test.

The profound empowering tool of energy testing helps many have a deeper trust in their bodies and connection with their spirit.

Understanding the roots of trauma

Energy psychotherapy involves getting to the roots of issues. We need to know if there is unresolved early trauma precipitating the client's presenting issues which requires knowledge of the personal history. I generally ask clients to fill in a form before they start therapy to provide a comprehensive history, including traumas, patterns, and themes, and clients sometimes comment that this process is in itself quite therapeutic. Naturally everyone has their own way of taking a history, but essentially the information we gather might include:

- *Indicators of patterns of repeated trauma* in earlier life which link with the present.
- *Areas of vulnerability*, including 'small child' parts, triggering and potential PTSD, and propensities to fragment or dissociate.
- *How do the defences and resistances operate?* What coping mechanisms and survival defences are part of the picture?—for example, addictions, fragmentation, dissociation, disconnection, self-harm, potential areas of risk and so on. Are there specific resistances or self-sabotage to consider?
- *Developmental stuckness*—areas and ages of unresolved early developmental trauma from which they have been unable to progress.
- *Core themes*: if the work is time limited, it can be helpful to work with themes such as being silenced; sense of identity; repeated experiences/patterns of abandonment; co-dependence; being victimised; traumatic loss—and so on.
- *Risk, resources, resilience, and safety*: what protective factors and resources does the client have to support them? Are there ongoing concerns regarding self-harm or risk? What strengths does this person have? What helpful coping strategies do they use? What have they survived/come through and how?
- *Substance 'misuse' and/or addictions*: if there is a history of ongoing difficulties with recovery, is the person ready and motivated to start with energy work or do they need— for example—to go to a detox centre first?
- *Social circumstance*: a consideration of the practical living situation and social circumstances, including any kind of support that the client does or doesn't have.

'Coming down to earth'

People who have experienced complex trauma are often unable to remember their history, in which case we focus on what the client brings in the moment. The example which follows is work with someone who was going in and out of an 'altered state' of consciousness. The therapeutic approach focuses on grounding the client.

EXAMPLE

Neville had an out-of-body experience after a trauma at a spiritual retreat centre and someone paid for him to have ten therapy sessions to help. His spiritual experience had gone to his head, and he was somewhat borderline and grandiose, feeling he was a 'superior being'. He held confused views about compassion, selflessness, and his 'mission to help humanity' and was quite ungrounded, split off from reality, unable to function in the world. Neville hinted that the spiritual experience had activated unworked-through childhood trauma.

To establish safety, the primary therapeutic task was to stabilise Neville, get him back into his body and integrate his fragmented ego. We started with energy balancing and focused on ordinary worldly tasks and basic self-care such as ensuring that he ate regularly, washed, and had a routine. Eventually we considered ways he might start earning his living and he got a part-time job packing vegetables. Energy clearing helps to stabilise the ego, so working on 'small' issues to start with, Neville gradually became accustomed to energy work and its benefits. The karate-chop (KC) technique which deals with reversed energy was very useful, enabling him to verbalise his conflict and distress while tapping in the KC point on the side of the hand. As an example, we used phrases such as:

> *Even though I feel ungrounded by my spiritual experience and struggle to be in my body, I completely accept myself.*

Once stabilised, the next stage was to approach clearing the underlying early trauma which had caused his fragmentation. Neville's 'spiritual' experience could neither be approached nor integrated until this fundamental embodied work was undertaken. Through free association, memories arose that he had been abused by a priest in childhood. We cleared this trauma and distress, using methods described in Chapters 7 and 8 which helped to integrate fragmented parts. Consequently, Neville became more centred and grounded in his body, and had establishing a safe-enough, secure-enough base to come down to earth. At the end of the sessions, Neville reported feeling much better. He could offer a coherent narrative of what had happened, a sign that trauma has been resolved. He recognised that his wounded abused child-self had avoided pain by spiritual bypassing, to hide from the terrible shame of his early trauma. He was also able to value and integrate aspects of his spiritual experience.

CHAPTER 6

Psychotherapy in the quantum era: 'maps' for working with energy and evolving consciousness

This chapter explores various 'maps' which identify therapeutic need and developmental focus according to emotional, psychological, spiritual, and transpersonal experience, to situate the work of energy psychotherapy. Overviews help us think and formulate. As well as 'following the flow', we need to ground the work with clinical understanding. What work will be beneficial? Is it to strengthen the fragile ego and build a sense of self, where we honour ego's way of perceiving and negotiating reality? Or if someone feels firmly on their soul's path, the focus will be different. Or a mixture. There is no judgement about 'higher' or 'lower'. What is important is that therapy is congruent, meeting each person where they are.

Orientation

'I don't know what to do or how to be if I let go of my old patterns'

People can benefit from having a map when navigating new territory. 'Janine' felt rather lost trying to negotiate a new family situation. A bright, warm-hearted soul, and the 'feral' (her words) child of an alcoholic mother, Janine survived this neglect and fought all the way to the top of the corporate world. After an extremely traumatic incident of family betrayal, she was struggling with feeling 'hard-hearted', locked in an angry battle without any internal guidance other than catholic guilt. Operating from her customary 'winners and losers' mindset, she felt she could either lock her heart down and become embittered, or open to a wider perspective. The issue was less about her family—she could do civil and polite—but how could she care for her heart, so she did not shut down? Janine connected deeply with her grief and vulnerability. She was pleased at this breakthrough but wondered—'I don't know what to do, or how to be if I let go of my old patterns'—how should she move forward without a spiritual/ethical background to guide her?

Soul-searching questions from clients such as these led me to include this chapter. How do people orient themselves when they are lost, since there is not one 'truth' nor neat guidelines for life's situations? Setting intentions for life is helpful, but what guides those intentions?

'Road maps' provide signposts for stages in a person's journey. Here I offer two developmental overviews from psychological and spiritual perspectives, and two frameworks concerned with different levels of 'truth'/emerging consciousness—one, an energetic map of the chakras and the other, an evolutionary spiritual framework. Such maps can help orient the work by assessing and clarifying areas which might need further attention.

Developmental perspectives and the sense of self

Psychological perspectives

Psychological theories help us understand what might lie at the roots of underlying difficulties. It is assumed that the reader is familiar with basic psychological concepts and theories about the psyche and human development. Here, I highlight a few perspectives I have found relevant in energy psychotherapy, focusing mainly on attachment-based, psychoanalytic, and Jungian theory. Naturally, those with different clinical orientations will also have their own models to draw on and I hope that for those readers who have no background in theories, this will nonetheless be helpful for you.

Daniel Stern, (1985) a key figure in attachment theory, brought the interpersonal world of the infant, with its sensory experiences of light, colour, and sound, to our awareness. The carer intersubjectively and intuitively attunes, connects with, and responds to the energy of the baby, laughing or sighing in resonance, naturally mirroring and matching baby's 'vitality of affect'. The 'language' of energy therapy is similarly one of resonance, vibration, and energetic 'charge'. Like the infant–parent dyad, working with energy involves intimate psycho-biological attunement between client and therapist. This work facilitates the regulation of affect, even on-line or on the telephone, (where such ways of working became a necessity during the early 2020s, though many prefer an 'in-person' connection).

From Stern's work we understand that the baby's sense of self exists before language—by 'sense' I mean simple (non self-reflexive) awareness. *We are speaking at the level of direct experience not concept.* This language is also very much in tune with Dzogchen.

In Chapter 3 we explored how infant developmental research recognises how our minds emerge, and our emotions become organised through engagement with other minds. The interdependence and interconnectedness in early relational experiences form the blueprint of the ways we relate to others. These energetic and relational patterns are embodied in our energy bodies and affect not only psychological predilections but also physiological patterns, energetically woven into our body and brain from babyhood.

Energy psychotherapy can access and work relatively easily with the sensory 'field' of in-utero, neonatal, and preverbal trauma. Although the foetus or baby would not have had language at the time of the trauma, the subtle energy system nonetheless understands words that we use to describe the circumstances of the trauma. In this instance, the clearing phrases focus straight-forwardly on 'what happened' to him.

EXAMPLE

Jonathon presented with an immobilising depression precipitated by a relationship breakup. He was also dissociated. He was unable to function in his life and was in danger of losing his hard-won career as a solicitor. His early history was one of considerable neglect. He had detailed memories of early, abandonment traumas, and long periods of isolation. During our work, trauma emerged largely through free association and his visceral body memories. Some of his history was from stories recounted to him, such as suffering a near-death experience aged three months old when he was admitted to hospital unable to breathe. We cleared each trauma as it arose, using either tapping or chakra work. Here I include a few key traumas including traumatic patterns

CLEARING PHRASE
Because of all the times and ways mum was disconnected and not 'present' I never felt properly attached, so I feel constantly abandoned, and separation is very painful and difficult for me.

HEALING/RESOURCE CIRCLE
Dissociated self, child self, baby self, The Absent Mother, The Abandoned child, Guardian angel, Mother Mary

A few months into the therapy, Jonathon cleared a sequence of trauma concerning his near-death experience. This helped him become more grounded, back in his body, and mobilised again.

CLEARING PHRASE
All my shame when no one recognised my beseeching eyes and my desperate need *for help when I was dying, so it's very difficult to ask for help now.*

HEALING CIRCLE
Baby self, dissociated self, 'floating-off' soul, Mother Mary, Guardian Angel

CLEARING PHRASES
All my terror when I nearly died, confined in an incubator where I had no control, so I floated off to survive. Because of this, when I am confined and have no control or choice to go at my own pace, I become highly anxious and dissociate to cope.

All my trauma when I was ignored and nearly died as a baby. Then too many doctors examined me insensitively on the table. I was squirming, exposed, and shamed and had to shut down and hide to survive. My soul fragmented, and I didn't want to come back, so part of my soul was left behind and I am not really here.

It was extraordinary how viscerally Jonathon's three-month-old body-memories came back to him through free association. His abreactions showed him to be totally immersed in these early baby experiences. He felt considerable relief after the clearings, though he also needed time to rest and recover.

Jonathon did about a year of energy therapy and cleared extensive amounts of trauma. During this time, his depression lifted, his PTSD was considerably reduced, and he became more connected with his body. His self- care improved considerably, such that he was able to move home and start a new job. Although Jonathon made a good recovery, I feel it is possible at some point he may need further therapy.

Ego strengthening: working with trauma and defence mechanisms

Freud felt a key aim in psychoanalysis was 'to strengthen the Ego, to make it more independent of the Superego, to widen its field of vision, and so to extend its organization that it can take over new portions of the Id. Where Id was, there shall Ego be' (Freud, 1933a).

When the ego becomes split and fragmented by early developmental neglect and/or other life-shattering events, clearing trauma helps strengthen it. Energy work with the subtle energy system stabilises people, so they no longer fall into 'shattered states' or feel overwhelmed by impinging traumatic thoughts. Since defences such as splitting, projection, fragmentation and so on play such a key role in developmental trauma, and in the functioning of ego/sense of self, working directly with the defences fruitfully brings about structural change. The examples I give are quite basic defences.

EXAMPLE

Neil's infant bonding with a terrifying mother had resulted in persecuting anxiety (Klein, 1946, paranoid–schizoid position) where he was habitually caught between extremes of 'good' and 'bad'. Such polarised states manifested throughout his life.

Unable to feel wholehearted about any relationships, Neil suffered a lot from anger and disappointment, and presented in therapy in tortuous ambivalence. Over a period of a few months, we cleared extensive traumas, concerning his early life which had been chaotic and 'unheld'. We undertook trauma-clearing about his unstable mother, his frantic early preoedipal anxieties, and his overly responsible child-self. Each clearing brought new insight as to why he felt the way he did, while he simultaneously experienced beneficial changes.

We finally came to work energetically with his habitual ambivalence, expressed by Neil flip-flopping back and forth with extremes of judgement about himself and his partner, not being able to decide whether to stay with her or leave.

CLEARING PHRASE
When I was a baby, I was torn between my polarised parents, completely overwhelmed by traumatic extremes and couldn't find anywhere safe to be, so I am habitually ambivalent, and in my relationship I lurch between being supercritical and judgemental and then contrite and loving, and I can't find balance or a place to settle.

This clearing finally helped Neil to settle. The following week he was astonished to report that he had completely calmed down. The pendulum had stopped swinging back and forth, to such an extent that he stopped criticising his partner, felt more spaciousness, and had finally decided to commit to her and accept her as she was. He was surprised to feel this new centredness—it was quite foreign for him to feel at peace with himself. Clearing the associated traumas which linked this early infant trauma with his presenting difficulties had helped to bring stabilisation and integration.

Another commonly occurring defence concerns difficulties with being authentic. Winnicott's classic paper, 'Ego distortion in terms of true and false self' (1960) highlights the defence of adapting and hiding true feelings. Clearing specific trauma concerned with not being able to be/express/or having to hide one's true self, makes it safer for the person to be themselves.

EXAMPLE

Rose had been a 'parentified child' from a very young age and had spent her life 'people-pleasing'. The first thing she said when she came to therapy was 'I can't put myself first—I just can't do it'. Rose had cared for and was extremely attached to her volatile, dismissing narcissistic mother, who punished Rose if she expressed her true feelings—most notably her anger—by neglecting and abandoning her. The ultimate abandonment had been when she died, leaving Rose bereft. In adult life, Rose found herself in similar relationships where she was again 'treated badly'. While finding it impossible to be herself and express what she truly felt, Rose was frustrated that people 'expected her to put up with this bad treatment of her'. She was so terrified of being abandoned; she unconsciously repressed her feelings and her 'child self' felt that her very survival was at stake. As she became more conscious during therapy, this became suppression. We did extensive trauma-clearing which gradually strengthened her sense of self but a particular trauma, which made a great deal of difference was:

CLEARING PHRASE
It's not safe to be me, or to express my anger in case I am abandoned, so I am compliant, and suppress my feelings to survive because I don't feel worthy of being loved.

HEALING CIRCLE OF PARTS
The parentified child, baby self, the compliant one, the abandoning mother, the abandoned child, True Self, Soul, The Universe

Over time and extensive trauma clearing, Rose was able to tolerate her absolute terror of abandonment and come to terms with the loss of her mother. Much of our work involved connecting with her abandoned child self and working with the specific traumas of this part of her who had come to 'take over her life'. Rose has done a lot of work to move beyond her co-dependent attachments. She managed to separate from a damaging partner, has developed a greater sense of herself, and now dares to speak her mind.

Dissociation and 'energy boundaries'

We can also work with dissociation and, over time, someone can learn to be safely in their body.

EXAMPLE

Rachel had a mentally ill, violent mother who had been inconsistent, abandoning, and terrifying. All her life, almost any feeling triggered Rachel into dissociated states, and she struggled to be in her body. She operated largely from an adaptive 'false self'. Clearing her terrifyingly traumatic and disconnected experiences in infancy and early childhood helped her to feel safe enough to be more connected and remain present in her body. Over a period of long-term energy psychotherapy, she gradually learned to stay with and tolerate her feelings instead of immediately leaving her body. Eventually she was able to evolve from passive aggression to the capacity to own her angry feelings. In this way, clearing trauma facilitated the emergence of a stronger more resilient self, who was able to bear and cope with reality, experience her feelings, and express herself.

Energy boundaries

The subtle layers in the energy field around a person are often compromised by severe trauma. Esther Bick wrote papers on 'the petrified self' (Willoughby, 2006), and 'second skin formation' (Bick, 1968) pertaining to this delicate area of the psychic skin. When people have been invaded—psychically, physically, or emotionally—they develop 'holes' in their aura and the 'energy boundaries'—our sense of personal coherence and integrity is compromised. Sensitive people can be particularly vulnerable to intrusions from others. Bion's concept of the 'contact barrier' is relevant here: the severely traumatised person cannot process her feelings sufficiently using 'alpha function' or the different stages of symbolisation to create a contact barrier that protects her from the projective intrusions of others (White, 2006, p. 70). Energy psycho-therapy offers simple ways of strengthening energy boundaries providing invaluable self-care for therapists and clients alike, in not 'taking on' the traumatised energy of others, so they can establish greater resilience (see Chapter 8).

'Resistance' and 'energetic reversals'

Getting stuck is one of the banes of psychotherapy. 'Resistance' (Freud, 1920g, 1926d), or 'avoidance' in attachment terms, are known in energy therapy as 'psycho-energetic reversals'. When reversals occur

> It is not a matter of slowing the work down, but of a complete block on any energetic movement. (Mollon, 2008, p. 141)

When the forward-flowing process of life energy is blocked, this is quite literally, a 'reversal' in the flow of energy. The blockage itself can be taken as the focus for energy clearings, and once this is released, the work can move forward again in a life-affirming way.

Commonly occurring reversals are often based in limiting core beliefs such as a lack of self-love, feelings of lack of worth and lack of deservedness. Methods for clearing these will be discussed more fully in Chapter 7, but simply for now, by tapping on the karate-chop point (KC) on the side of the hand with fingertips from the other hand, repeating a reversals correction statement, facilitates change, clearing the blocked energy so the person's psychological mindset and physical body becomes available for continuing work. An example of clearing a reversal is to say something like the following: (the essential parts of the phrase being those in italic bold) while tapping on the side of the hand:

REVERSAL CORRECTION PHRASE

Even though … e.g. I feel terrible shame about my issue (or whatever the conflict is) ***I love and accept myself***

Lack of healthy self-love lies at the heart of many mental health conditions so saying this statement may bring a protest—'but I *don't* love myself'—in which case the phrase can be modified to something which feels more possible such as 'I aspire to love myself'. 'I accept myself' or 'I'm OK'. The very process of confronting lack of love often results in tears, and a sense of relief at unblocking the resistance. Psychophysical biological bonding strengthens the therapeutic alliance during such clearings and makes it possible to continue. This simple process is incredibly useful and provides a valuable self-help resource which can be used by both clients and therapists.

Repetition compulsion

Clearing repeating patterns is key in energy work. Psychoanalyst Paul Russell (Russell, 1973, 1998) considered repetition compulsion to be one of Freud's greatest legacies, where the cost of an un-mourned loss is like an addiction 'as if drawn to some fatal flame'. The re-creation of the same old traumatic patterns in life can be hard to shift, though in energy psychotherapy, once recognised and cleared energetically, the traumatic pattern can be stopped. These repetitions occur when what cannot be remembered, felt in the body, or resolved, is repeated, and so the past is transferred onto the present.

In depth work, recognising the original causes of trauma and connecting them with the present issue is a central focus for energy clearings. The scientific discoveries of Chopra, Pert, and others, discussed in Chapter 3, show how trauma is transmitted at a cellular level, going back through generations of cells via the DNA. One of the wonderful aspects of energy psychotherapy is that it can clear and put an end to such traumatised transgenerational and transpersonal traumatic patterns.

EXAMPLE

A pregnant client, Annabel, was terrified she would be unable to bond with her infant, not least because there was a significant transgenerational history of mental illness in her family. She cleared the following traumatic pattern:

CLEARING PHRASE
Because of all the times and ways and lifetimes (ATTAWAL) women in my family throughout many generations suffered post-natal depression and struggled to bond with their infants, I am terrified I might repeat this pattern and not be able to connect with my baby.

Annabel cleared this and other aspects of her fears around being a mother and experienced a significant shift after this trauma clearing. She went on to deliver a healthy baby with whom she has a close healthy attachment bond.

The space between ego and soul

A key focus for this book is the idea of moving from ego-based to heart-based consciousness—or 'soul-connecting'. The path of discovering the differences between the two has, for me, been very interesting. Therapy undertaken in the first half of life is often spent coming to terms with developmental issues, family dynamics and surviving trauma from early life and clearing trauma. As a child, we are somewhat victims of circumstances, but when mid-life crises dawn, a certain dissatisfaction looms—perhaps the 'dukka' Buddha spoke of. There is more recognition of choice and freewill, and a greater sense of responsibility in exercising this—a search for something more. The phenomena of the 'dark night of the soul' can be a time when people have a longing which awakens different aspirations. Does one choose ego's path of 'service to self', or the soul's path of 'service to the whole'?

Spiritual and heart- and soul-based approaches

These days the general public listen to literally hundreds of podcasts and spiritual 'webinars', such as Transformation into the New Paradigm, New Earth One Network, Beyond the Ordinary, and so on, which often start with a meditation connecting with the heart centre, the portal to the soul. It is also not uncommon for people to experience transformational epiphanies as part of everyday life when their heart opens—for instance, listening to beautiful music or during a spectacular sunset—and they experience their awakened state. This comes full circle to the 'direct experience' Stern spoke about in infants—though in adulthood, this is at a conscious level, where ego's filter falls away.

However, within psychotherapy, apart from approaches specifically designated as spiritual, most trainings omit a spiritual or transpersonal perspective.

I mentioned the dichotomy between rational and spiritual approaches in 'Choosing the path of joy' and in subsequent chapters explore how the vibrational nature of energy psychotherapy helps to integrate 'higher gauge' levels, where the spiritual/soul-level brings assistance in working with ego's problems. The ideas of 'soul-connecting' and awakening consciousness are not new. Various psychotherapists, psychologists and analysts have been interested in the expansion of consciousness, including notions of truth and ethics, so I wish to mention a few who bring the soul into psychotherapy, as a reminder of their enriching contribution. There is not space to do justice to the depth and breadth of their work, and I have had to leave out many. I have not approached these in chronological order.

Narcissism and 'the life-giver'

Neville Symington (1994) was an analyst concerned with the adoption of an overtly ethical and spiritual stance. Noting the collapse of core values central to 'mature religion' and the importance of integrating Shadow, Symington suggests (1994): 'If the goal of psychoanalysis is the transformation of bad actions into good, is it not right to call this a spiritual aim?' He felt therapy needed to foster a healthy sense of self—the 'Life-giver'– to counter the destructive 'service-to-self' narcissism which so plagues this era. (Interestingly, some Buddhist teachers say that narcissism is an emanation of a haughty spirit of this age named Gyalpo.) Influenced by core Buddhist teachings, Symington argued that humanity was self-absorbedly wrapped up in narcissism, taking its own ego as the 'love object'. He suggested psychotherapy needed to transcend egoic 'self-clinging' by fostering an understanding of the interdependence of our shared human condition, thereby facilitating the evolution from a selfish egotistical position to a life-affirming one of healthy love of self and others. Symington was criticised for his evangelism in arguing that psychoanalysis served as a 'secular form of religion', where analysts assume the role formerly taken by that of priests:

> the struggle with the Shadow is against those dark forces which try to prevent us saying 'Yes' to the Life-giver within us. It is this struggle with which psychoanalysis is concerned. As a spiritual method relevant to the modern world … its spiritual nature must be recognised. (Symington, 1994, p. 137)

There are interesting similarities between Symington's life-giver vs narcissism, Freud's Eros and Thanatos (life drive vs death drive), and the concept of positive forward-flowing energy vs 'massive reversals' in energy psychotherapy, explored in Chapter 9.

Growth trajectories, post-Kleinians, and beyond

Jean White in her account of contemporary analysis speaks of signifiers of psychic growth and development, and specifically, the growth trajectories of 'Openness, desirousness, aliveness and flexibility' (White, 2006, p. 181), qualities which resonate at high frequencies. The late works of Bion (his concepts of transformation) and Lacan (his continual reaching out towards 'the beyond' and the jouissance of the drive) also resonate powerfully with the concept of the fifth dimension.[1] Bion's highly original work with his interest in the unconscious as the seat of infinite, ineffable uncertainty and the 'absolute truth' about ultimate reality, was reaching for something more. This culminated in his discovery of 'O' and the 'deep and formless infinite' (Grotstein, 2007).

The truth of the body

In promoting self-actualisation, William James (1902) recognised that what is true is experienced in the body, so we can only be self-realised from within the body. In energy psychotherapy we often refer to this as 'the wisdom of the body' and the truth of its messages to us. James also acknowledged the existence of a wider 'field'. Mystical states were seen as states of knowledge where we can experience union with something larger than ourselves and in that union find our greatest peace.

Jung's concept of the 'Self'

The application of Jung's ideas in energy psychotherapy has added considerable depth. Quite differently from Freud's understanding, Jung viewed the 'encounter with the unconscious' as a rich force, the source of all, and full of creative potential. This was central to his writing and the process of individuation. Jung recognised the need to transcend human suffering, so rather than focusing on neurosis and the territory of ego, he emphasised the individual's lived experiences of 'inner life'. He also explored Eastern mystical chakra meditations as powerful methods for arriving at transpersonal states of consciousness. Moacanin (1986) describes how Jung's approach aims at the 'cure of souls', the approach to the numinous where the goal is not only the healing of pathology, but above all, the fulfilment of individual wholeness or self-realisation.

Jung's analytical psychology values personal mystical experience, the creative process, and, like Buddhism, our subjective experience—the perceptions of mind and how we see things. He saw the constant dynamic interplay between conscious and unconscious experience as providing the impetus for growth and change. Through his journey of visionary experiences and dreams, Jung experienced the distinction between self (the ego or little 'I') and the 'Self' which transcends this level of experience and enters another reality altogether. Like Assagioli's concept of the 'superconscious', and Buddhism's 'Rigpa' (pure awareness), Jung's notion of 'Self', (Jung, 1973a, b; Miller, 2024) brought expanded states of consciousness into wider recognition. When we dissolve our perceptions into the pure energetic reality beyond ego-consciousness, an intuitive wisdom state arises which opens the door to a significant perceptual shift.

---

[1] Regarding this, the discussion of Bion's and Lacan's late works in *Generation: Preoccupations and Conflicts in Contemporary Psychoanalysis* is very helpful (White, 2006, pp. 187–196).

The collective unconscious and archetypes

Jung also understood that the realisation of the 'Self' involved integrating the wholeness of the human spirit. Observing the human tendency to ignore 'shadow', he emphasised the importance of embracing multifaceted aspects of the psyche—light and dark. Recognising the universality of the human condition, and our deep interconnectedness with one another, his concept of the collective unconscious contains the huge range of qualities and characteristics of archetypal energies within it. A significant aspect of energy psychotherapy concerns the integration of these, using mandala-like healing circles (explained in Chapter 9).

Duality, the Transcendent Function—the alchemical unions of opposites

Jung's concept of the Transcendent Function plays an important role in the alchemical process of energy psychotherapy. In considering a wounded bird, Jung noticed that the healing impulse was balanced by an impulse to crush and destroy. We generally prefer to think of ourselves as healers rather than own our sadistic urges and Jung regarded this tension—the polarity of opposing forces—as a dynamic energy which helps us evolve and progress on our path. Integrating these polarised energies is an important aspect of the 'alchemical union of opposites'; it helps us become whole and complete. In energy psychotherapy, we use the Transcendent Function in the healing of complexes, where polarised or disharmonious energies in a situation are brought together to be accepted and integrated (see also Chapter 9).

Jung's *Memories, Dreams and Reflections* (1973a), and *The Red Book,* offer vivid accounts of the journey of the human soul to 'Self'-realisation. For those who follow the path to individuation, each has their own unique potential to evolve and gain spiritual realisation.

Assagioli's 'Self-actualisation'

Assagioli, (1961, 1988) who developed psychosynthesis, was another pioneer in transpersonal therapy. He agreed with Freud that healing childhood trauma and developing a healthy ego were necessary aims of psychotherapy and one aspect of his contribution to energy psychotherapy was his emphasis on working with 'parts'. He also held that human growth could not be limited to ego development. A student of philosophical and spiritual traditions of both East and West, Assagioli supported the blossoming of human potential into *self-actualisation,* arguing that transpersonal development is possible for everybody. He mapped out the spiritual dimensions of human experience and the 'superconscious' (another term for awakening, like Jung's notion of 'Self').

The Soul as the central, organising construct for psychotherapy

The sixties saw a movement away from materialism, and Jung's views gained more credence. James Hillman (1967, 1996, 2010) developed Jung's ideas on spirituality, focusing on the soul as the central, organising construct for psychotherapy, and arguing that psychology needs to return to its roots as 'the study of the soul'. Several Jungians, and in particular Nathan Schwartz-Salant (1989) and Donald Kalsched (1996, 2013) applied Jung's archetypal understanding in their creative work with trauma. Donald Kalsched in *Trauma and the Soul* (2013) speaks of the mystical or spiritual moments that often occur around the intimacies of psychoanalytic work, demonstrating that

> depth psychotherapy with trauma's survivors can open both analytic partners to 'another world' of non-ordinary reality in which daimonic powers reside, both light and dark. This mytho-poetic work, he suggests, is not simply … defensive … but a mystery that is often at the very centre of the healing process—and yet at other times, strangely resists it. (From the front matter of Trauma and the Soul)

Elkins (1995) amplified Hillman's ideas by mapping a theory of the soul. He argued that psychopathology is really (or at least includes) the suffering of the soul, and that psychotherapy is the process by which therapists touch, nurture, and heal the client's soul. Also in the nineties, Yeomans (1994) noted a gathering momentum during the seventies to the nineties at the fringes of the profession, where psychotherapists were exploring, experimenting, and expanding their thinking to include the spiritual dimension and its relationship to human suffering.

Psycho-spiritual traditions

Psycho-spiritual therapy has long been part of the mystical Sufi tradition. Almaas (2004), well known for *The Diamond Approach*, was concerned with the transformation of narcissistic self-preoccupation. He quotes Idries Shah (1978, pp. 51–52) describing the Sufi 'seven stages' developmental view of 'Self' as 'a *consciousness* that can experience itself within different planes of existence and can evolve towards wholeness and spiritual realisation'. Shah goes on to say that

> The Self … goes through certain stages in Sufi development, first existing as a mixture of physical reactions, conditioned behaviour, and various subjective aspirations. The seven stages of the Self constitute the transformation process, ending with the stage of perfection and clarification. Some have called this process the 'refinement of ego'. (Shah, 1978, p. 82)

Various organisations offer spiritual forms of therapy such as core process psychotherapy (a Buddhist approach of The Karuna Institute), and a Sufi approach to transpersonal counselling and psychotherapy (Centre for Counselling and Psychotherapy Education (CCPE)).

Evolving models of consciousness

Ken Wilbur's models of human consciousness (1993, 2000) provided a groundbreaking synthesis of religion, philosophy, physics, and psychology helping us recognise different 'levels' of the spiritual evolution of consciousness on 'the journey back 'home'. His integration of the psychological systems of the West with the contemplative traditions of the East in his *The Spectrum of Consciousness* (1977) and *Integral Psychology: Consciousness, Spirit, Psychology* (2000) provide significant reference points for integrating psychology and spirituality.

Maps for our soul's evolution

Energetic maps of the chakras

Methods for clearing trauma through the chakras will be discussed in Chapter 7.

Different models of the chakras

Psychotherapeutically, the chakra map helps us assess areas of development which need attention and provides a way of understanding stages of evolving consciousness. As previously stated, our energy reflects our truth, so refining our energy forms the basis for self-realisation— as our consciousness evolves, our energy or 'light bodies' can carry more light.

There is not 'one truth' about the chakras. Some say there are hundreds of chakras all over the body. In recent years, a twelve-chakra systems model has become prevalent with numerous variations, some with chakras within and some outside the body. The most referenced have two or three additional chakras above the crown, and the Earth chakra, which is located below the root chakra and the surface of the earth. Raquel Spencer notes a newly configured twelve-chakra system centred in the heart which enables us to experience a higher level of direct connection, and more easily become one with the unified field. A full explanation is offered in the Appendix, but briefly:

> A new chakra system is evolving which takes us out of the current program and the collective matrix and establishes a new way of processing Light with the core functionality fuelled and powered by the Heart. The heart is the 'Zero Point' access to Source energy allowing a self-rejuvenating and infinitely expansive field of life force energy to flow into our personal energy matrix. (Raquel Spencer, Facebook, 9 June 2022)

Dr Suzanne Lie (2015) speaks of the chakras as our 'light body systems', a method for communicating with our higher dimensional self. Each chakra represents a certain area of our nervous system (spine and brain), our endocrine system, and a major nerve plexus.

> When we come into alignment with our chakra systems, our consciousness instantly expands into higher frequency brainwaves … you simply plug into it, let go of your ego self, and 'allow' the inter-dimensional information to come into you.

The degree to which the chakras are balanced and in alignment enhances our consciousness and allows us to connect with higher and higher frequencies/dimensions. According to Dr Lie, we receive light messages many times throughout the day but when lost in our '3-D life', we become unconscious to these amazing messages.

The seven main energy centres/chakras

In energy psychotherapy, we predominantly work with the seven main energy centres which are like mini 'brains' located along the spine/nervous system. These act somewhat like energy junction boxes, connecting also with the meridians. Just as in Erikson's (1950) stages of psychological development, all the chakras—lower or higher—have useful evolutionary functions and lessons to teach us, and they work together holistically as a system. We can only perceive through the lens of development that we have ourselves realised. Just as a dog hears the high frequency of a whistle where humans cannot, so, too, we cannot fully perceive someone who is operating from a higher frequency and level of chakric development than our own.

The chakras have positive and negative qualities (refined and unrefined aspects), and their energetic condition—their distortions, blockages, and biases—provide indicators of our motives, desires, and intentions and the issues we need to deal with. As a personal example, when I first started working with energy, nearly all my issues were focused on my throat chakra. Quite apart from constantly having throat infections, my traumas were broadly concerned with finding my voice and struggling to speak my truth. Since clearing these issues, I am grateful that I now have remarkably few throat problems.

As energetic blockages in the chakras manifest, and we work to clear them, we learn the developmental lessons related to each centre. Once cleared, we can then utilise the best qualities offered by each chakra and bring them into alignment in the 'line of the light'.

The 'fight/flight' axis and 'service-to-self' mentality of the first three chakras

Developmentally, the first three chakras, are concerned with our basic survival as human beings. They are dominated by competition and the fight/flight responses of the instinctual realms of the reptilian brain and motivated by our desire for possession. To arrive at the wisdom offered by the higher chakras, we need first to gain clarity in the ways our vision is biased, and our perception distorted at the lower three chakras. It's helpful to clear issues held at these lower chakras first, since these form the foundation for holding the more spiritual perspectives, and without this developmental work, spiritual experiences can become ungrounded. However, there are no hard and fast rules, not least because our development does not necessarily progress in linear order, and we need to focus on specific chakras at different times as issues arise in our lives.

The overall level of consciousness of the first three chakras is a 'service-to-self' mentality. There is no real ability to stand in the shoes of the other and there is a somewhat selfish, self-absorbed notion of existence. Concern is largely for ourselves and our family (1st chakra), or for 'our group/gang' (2nd chakra), or for our nation (3rd chakra). There is little room for the wider understanding of the whole, of co-operation, growing together and interdependence. This is brought when the heart chakra opens, offering a wider, more connected perspective.

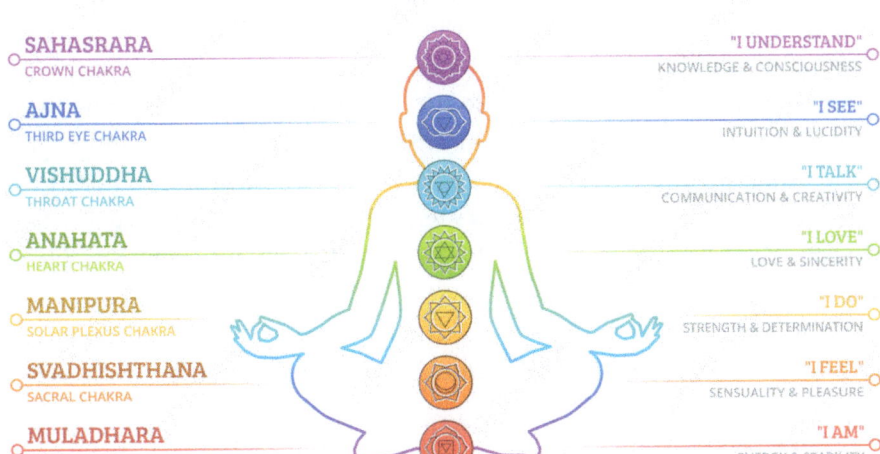

Figure 7 The seven chakras and their key issues

1st CHAKRA RED—ROOT (BASE): *mother, basic trust, fundamental security, and survival*
The root chakra, located at the base of the spine between the perineum and the anus, is concerned with fundamental security and survival. It is like Bowlby's 'secure base' (1988) where we work through issues relating to our early upbringing, relationship with parents, and the ways we were cared for in infancy. The state of our root chakra has far-reaching consequences for how secure or insecure we are as people, how much we trust, and our sense of dependence or independence. It often pertains to abandonment issues and our connection with the 'divine feminine'. If we have a weak base chakra, there is often a lack of grounding and dependence on others.

2nd CHAKRA ORANGE—SACRAL: *consumption, sex, food, money, addictions,*
meeting needs and appetites
Located at the lower abdomen, this chakra concerns issues of creativity and consumption, of meeting our needs and appetites for sex, food, and money. When the second chakra is out of balance, gratification, greed, and excess (such as addictions) are used as ways of avoiding coping with the pain of feelings. In evolutionary terms, the second chakra is like the evolution from a small family to a group of early settlers. In developmental terms, the 2nd chakra represents the teenage phase where gangs, peer groups, passions, extremes, and self-interest are prevalent. There is a concern about scarcity, and competition for money or resources at the 2nd chakra, so the person may find it hard to share, or may have a 'winners-and-losers' mentality. Other issues may concern aspects of sexuality—reproduction, trauma, and development.

3rd CHAKRA YELLOW—SOLAR PLEXUS: *wisdom, power, personal responsibility, and sovereignty*

The solar plexus is a complex system of radiating nerves and ganglia found in the pit of the stomach between the navel and lower part of the chest. It is concerned with developing a sense of self, the onset of adulthood, and issues to do with power, control, authority (and abuses of these functions), and autonomy issues. It also relates to the fiery emotions such as anger and rage. A well-functioning 3rd chakra can digest and deal with ideas and cognitive issues effectively and brings the ability for a person to hold responsible adult positions in society and stand in their own sovereignty. In evolutionary terms the 3rd chakra relates to the nation-states. In physical terms it governs digestion (the stomach, internal organs, pancreas, spleen, kidneys, liver and gallbladder, and the intestines).

The upper chakras—the spiritual axis, and service to the whole

The flowering of spirituality starts at the awakened heart chakra. We cannot evolve very far if we remain on ego's path of 'service to self'. Developmentally, the upper chakras are concerned with the awakening state of consciousness where we recognise our interconnectedness with 'the-all'. At this stage of our human evolution, living from the heart, we naturally adopt an outlook of co-operation, compassion, harmony, non-judgement and 'service to others' (which also includes appropriate love and care for the self.)

4th CHAKRA GREEN—THE AWAKENED HEART *of love, healing, interconnectedness, and co-operation*

When fully open, the loving heart is generous and giving and has the capacity to stand in another's shoes and feel the wider (transpersonal) connection with the greater whole. This is a non-judgemental place of peacefulness, neutrality, and balance, sometimes referred to as 'Zero Point'. Having an open heart requires grounding, so the three lower chakras need to be balanced and cleared of blockages to create a firm foundation. When the heart centre comes up in energy clearings, it covers a wide range of issues including love, grief, compassion, sadness, fear, shock, betrayal, resentment, and spiritual issues. 'Service to others' involves genuine giving without comparing oneself with others or martyring or sacrificing oneself. Some speak of two heart chakras—a lower and a higher heart chakra. The lower heart chakra may be more inclined to sentimentality, whereas the 'higher' heart, located at the thymus point and where Phil Mollon's Blue Diamond point is located, is able to take a broader compassionate overview and hence can take more mature and difficult decisions.

5th CHAKRA BLUE—THROAT: *communication, and 'speaking your truth'*
The 5th throat chakra is concerned with truth. It is also about the expression of thoughts and feelings and 'finding your voice'. The physical aspects of the throat chakra are the throat and mouth. The thyroid, throat, and neck are vulnerable to a variety of ailments connected with

communications or self-expression. When listening to the sound of the voice it gives a great deal of information through the quality, tone, and timbre.

6th CHAKRA INDIGO—FOREHEAD (AJNA CENTRE/'THIRD EYE'): *awareness, vision, intuition, trauma*

The 6th chakra is physically connected with all the organs of perception associated with the senses of sight, smell, hearing, taste, and the brain and the pineal pituitary glands. Some people's perceptions are more sensitive to sound and speech, others have more visual or sensory tendencies. When the 6th chakra is open, intuition and psychic abilities relate to the third eye, bringing insight, wisdom, vision, and clarity of thought. Intuition manifests naturally within an ethical framework as part of the evolution of the heart and the capacity to stand in others' shoes. Without an open heart it is dangerous to force the development of the third eye and its psychic abilities. When the frontal lobe is overloaded by trauma, this results in stuckness, difficulties thinking, isolation, and a lack of integration.

7th CROWN CHAKRA VIOLET (The thousand-petalled lotus): *'Father' energy, spiritual energy*

The 7th chakra brings the finest spiritual energy into the body. While having an open crown chakra is a blessing, it is necessary for all the chakras to be properly functioning and in balance to live well in the world. If the lower chakras are unstable, an open crown chakra can lead to ungrounded behaviour and unrealistic attitudes. The colour violet is integrating and helps to overcome disconnection and isolation. I see the violet flame during my meditations, and include a meditation of this in the Appendix.

The chakras as vehicles for awakening consciousness

When the chakras are clear, in alignment, and open out into the 'unified field', 'kundalini arising' may occur, facilitating access to multidimensional experiences and dimensions. This can be a powerful and confusing experience, and some have challenges in grounding the energy. Meditations on the chakras also provide methods for arriving at higher states of consciousness. According to Paramahansa Yogananda (1946), 'Christ Consciousness' resides at the 'third eye'. Our perception is key: 'The eye is the lamp of the body. If your eyes are healthy, your whole body will be full of light' (Matthew 6: 22–23). The cosmic consciousness centre is at the top of the crown. By a series of meditation exercises called Kriya Yoga, it is possible to speed up the evolution of human consciousness to realise cosmic consciousness.

Grounding the journey of awakening

Just as a child goes through a developmental process to arrive at maturity and adulthood, so too, the journey of awakening needs to be properly grounded. Spiritual problems arise when people open the upper chakras without having proper balance and grounding in the lower chakras, so the developmental framework of the chakras can be helpful. Blockages at specific chakras provide useful 'diagnostic' information. For example, imbalances at the base chakra concern basic survival and development of the 'secure base' (Bowlby, 1988); at the 2nd chakra they concern needs, desires, and consumption; and at the 3rd chakra, the development of a sense of personal power and responsibility—and so on. Using chakras as a diagnostic tool increases our discernment so we can distinguish (for instance) between a genuine spiritual state of ecstasy as compared with mania, where spiritual bypassing involves the deployment of manic defences to avoid dealing with unbearable grief and pain (Klein, 1940). It is not until we have worked through developmental issues and arrived at psychological maturation that we have sufficient grounding to open the spiritual centre at the heart chakra and the chakras above, leading to the spiritual realisation of 'unity consciousness' or 'the awakened state'.

Although it might appear that there is a 'hierarchy' of chakras, this would be a mistake. No one chakra is better than another. All the chakras need to function well together in harmony as a unified system, so the energy can flow in balance and alignment along the 'line of the light'.

A map of evolving consciousness

People approach life in many ways. Some follow particular religions or spiritual 'paths to enlightenment', some, who are interested in 'awakening' are spiritual but not religious, and others are explicitly atheist though they may have humanitarian and heart-based values. I wish to honour whichever path you follow or values you hold. Please feel free to skip this section if it does not interest you. None of the following is necessary for practising energy psychotherapy.

Having meditated since the late 1970s, I have a long-standing passion for the integration of awakening consciousness in psychotherapy and am happy that more people are interested in meditation, mindfulness, and going on retreats. I am grateful to Tibetan Buddhism, which gave me grounding and a taste of the expanded consciousness of my true awakened essence—or soul consciousness if you like. (There are many levels of realisation, glimpses of awakening being entirely different from a fully enlightened state.) Buddhism provided a spiritual education—a staged path for spiritual transformation.

In response to clients asking questions about 3-D and 5-D, I felt it might be helpful to outline the evolutionary frame of 'The Nine Yanas' (vehicles) of Tibetan Buddhism, with its understandings about truth and ethics at different levels of consciousness leading to Dzgochen. Other traditions have equally valid approaches—for instance, to my mind, Dzogchen is also the same as what others term 'Christ Consciousness'. The Dzogchen approach is just the one with which I am familiar, and I feel is very relevant during this time of planetary awakening.

Dzogchen and quantum flow—the 'king of medicines'

Dzogchen, soul-connecting, and energy therapy have in common that they tune into the quantum flow. If the conditions are right, we can access states of consciousness beyond thought and concept in the heart-centred space of the unified (quantum) field. Everything falls away in the simplicity of pure awareness. In Dzogchen, this flow state is known as the 'King of Medicines', where healing occurs effortlessly, 'like the snake unwinding its knots' (a phrase from a key Dzogchen text called *Hitting the Essence in Three Words*).[2]

In moments of 'flow' people may experience their spiritual nature—a sense of relaxation, joy, and lightness. A client with a background of severe complex trauma slipped into such a state and decided to lie down and 'just be'. About twenty minutes later he uttered a phrase from the Bible: 'The peace of God which passeth all understanding'. Arriving quite naturally at this state of peace and healing, he was profoundly moved by this experience, as was I. Such embodied states operate in the realm of energy[3]—they are experiential rather than cognitive, characterised by naturalness, purity, and effortless simplicity.

Outline of The Nine Yanas of the Nyingma tradition of Tibetan Buddhism

[For a table outlining details of The Nine Yanas, please see the Appendix.]

Dharma—the path of truth and discernment

The Nine Yanas is a progressive path helping us to arrive at wisdom and maturity. '*Dharma*' means truth. We have free will and the path of *dharma* presents us with choices for which we are responsible. We often get lost on the journey as we learn how to discern—which forks in the road should we take and which to leave behind? Hopefully, through our experiences we come to trust that life itself is our greatest teacher.

Just as the energetic development of the chakras hold different realisations about truth at each 'level', so too, The Nine Yanas shows that truths or 'realisations' are built upon sequentially. 'Truth' is, of course, a vast subject. Ethical and moral principles are inherent to any spiritual path as we find authenticity and balance. We develop the capacity to discern the changing nature of truths which provides a basis for making decisions about what to do, or not to do, in life's complex situations. Through this process we become sovereign. Rather than being lost in relativist positions, not knowing where to stand, or seeking others to tell us what or how to think, we go within, connecting with our higher guidance, listening to and trusting our own senses and 'knowing'.

---

[2] *Hitting the Essence in Three Words* is a key Dzogchen text: it is the final testament of Garab Dorje, the first Dzogchen Master and the Root Text and Commentary is by the nineteenth-century Dzogchen Master Patrul Rinpoche. Known as *The Special Teaching of the Wise and Glorious King,* these teachings used to be secret but are now more widely available. The *Three Words* has been translated variously by others as *The Three Golden Letters* and *The Three Statements*.

[3] 'Energy' and consciousness are here used as a loose equivalence with the three qualities in Dzogchen: *tukje* (compassion) is the indivisibility of *ngowo* (essence) and *rangshyi*n (nature/clarity/luminosity/cognisance). The fuller description of this is:

Ngowo tongpa: the essence of mind is empty

Rangshyin salwa: its nature is cognisant

Tukje gakme/tukje kun khyap: its compassionate energy is unconfined and all pervasive.

Broadly, the first eight yanas operate in the realm of ordinary 'mind'. (In Buddhism 'mind' includes emotions as well as thoughts). These subdivide into three yanas, which encapsulate Buddha's essential teachings:

- *'To do no harm'*—the *Hinayana* path or 'lesser vehicle' establishes basic principles of self-discipline, morality, and ethics.
- *'To do good to perfection'*—the *Mahayana* path or 'greater vehicle', brings the realisation of 'emptiness' of the Heart Sutra, with compassion as life's guiding principle.
- *'To tame this mind, again and again'*—the transformative path of *Vajrayana* and the tantras works to purify the energy of our perceptions and emotions and arrive at the non-dual state of 'pure perception'—of not judging others.

'Heaven on Earth'—a universal consciousness, 'blazing like the sun'

Dzogchen, the ninth yana, is the apex of the path, the state of pure awareness which takes us beyond mind altogether. This 'direct path' works with the *wisdom mind* rather than with the ego's manifestations (our thoughts and projections). We awaken into ultimate reality, an enlightened 'view' of non-dual wisdom, otherwise known as 'the nature of mind'. The great Dzogchen Yogi, Padmasambhava (sixth century BC) prophesised that in this age, Dzogchen—a *universal* state of consciousness beyond religious doctrine—would spread far and wide and 'blaze like the sun'.[4] Otherwise known as the fifth dimension, or 'Christ Consciousness', this is the prophesised 'heaven on earth'. It brings us directly to Source—or 'soul connecting'. No 'belief' is required, so it is relevant even to those who consider themselves atheists.

Stages of the path

As the path progresses, the 'truth' of the view of the previous perspective provides the foundation for higher realisations. In reality, 'higher' or 'lower' are not the correct words, since all are essential and co-exist at the same time. Just as establishing a 'secure base' is important in human development, so too with 'The Nine Yanas', the 'higher' the 'view', the deeper and more grounded the spiritual foundations need to be.

Each yana holds a different understanding and 'realisation' with respective 'laws'. His Holiness Dudjom Rinpoche illustrated these with a traditional teaching about a poisonous plant, symbolising various ways of working with our emotional blockages and negativity. According to each yana/level, different antidotes are applied to render the plant harmless.

---

[4] I know several Christian monks and nuns who have studied Dzogchen and found its meditation adds meaning and depth to their faith.

Hinayana (Sutrayana): the path of renunciation

Sometimes termed 'the lesser vehicle', Hinayana is known as the foundational path of renunciation. Hinayana practice is focused inwards to develop the experience of egolessness in meditation with the simple practice of *Shamatha*—'peacefully remaining'. (The practice of mindfulness and awareness originated from this.) *Shamatha* cultivates awareness by working with ordinary mind, letting the busyness of thoughts and emotions settle like sediment sinking to the bottom of a glass of water, until we gain increasing clarity. There is a sense of 'minding your own business'—dealing with one's own issues, and not comparing oneself with others. We simplify and focus. Desire is given up in favour of the simple path of meditation, self-reflection, and abstinence.

Study in Hinayana is cognitive, and concerns analysis
We study 'the aggregates of ego' and how the 'ordinary' logical mind is constructed. *Sutras* are taught, including 'The Four Noble Truths' which outlines the causes of suffering or 'dukka'. The remedy for this suffering—our profound dissatisfaction with life—is to realise the 'awakened state'.

The 'view' of enlightenment in Hinayana is egolessness, an aspect of 'absolute truth'
The path takes an ethical stance of acknowledging good and bad, with the desire to 'to do no harm and to cultivate good'. This is achieved by cultivating the moral values of the 'The Eightfold Path'. Time, effort, patience, and self-discipline are required to establish this sound spiritual foundation. Without this base, the rest of spiritual development cannot follow. So, although Hinayana is called the 'lesser' vehicle, it forms a vital underpinning for all further work.

The poisonous plant analogy at the Hinayana level

> A group of people discover a poisonous plant growing in the garden. They panic, as they recognise that this is very dangerous, so they try to cut down the plant. This is the approach of *renunciation,* the Hinayana method for overcoming the ego and the negative emotions.

Mahayana view—the awakened mind of 'emptiness'

The realisation of the Heart Sutra is the gateway to the 'greater vehicle' of the Mahayana. When we awaken to the 'view' of 'emptiness'—true reality—our heart opens and 'absolute *bodhicitta*'—or compassion—naturally arises. In Tibetan, the word for mind and heart are one, so '*citta*' is translated as mind/heart, and '*bodhi*' means our inherent Buddha nature, our seed of 'awakening'.

The profound 'glimpse' of 'emptiness' is a 'view' of a sacred reality which shines the light on our deluded so-called 'normal' egoic reality. We recognise how confused we have been on account of our ignorance and our suffering ceases in that moment—we realise that enlightenment is possible. We also experience oneness—our interdependence and interconnectedness with the greater whole—and that we can no longer gain at another's expense. This is the union of wisdom and compassion.

The view of Mahayana awakens us to another dimension—the enlightened view of *absolute* truth. The absolute unchanging truths are very few—one is all-encompassing love and compassion; another, eternal consciousness. Awakening inspires us to renounces egoic selfishness and take the *bodhicitta* vow as a way of life, living from the heart until enlightenment. The service-to-other *Bodhisattva path* is one of compassion and generosity where activities of our body, mind, and spirit are dedicated for the benefit of all.[5]

We also learn that *relative* truths are illusory and change all the time. We live predominantly within the relative egoic world until—eventually—we can stabilise the 'absolute' state of awakened consciousness. To help us evolve, we cultivate the 'Four Immeasurables' (mentioned previously) of Love, Compassion, Joy, and Equanimity of the awakened mind of *bodhicitta*, guided by the 'Six Paramitas'—the qualities of generosity, discipline/morality, patience, enthusiasm, meditation, and wisdom. This heart-centred focus refines our energy on the journey to enlightenment.

Despite 'wandering endlessly astray in samsara's vicious cycle' we do our best, following our sense of what feels right at the time, with less chance of getting lost when we live led by our hearts. We aspire to integrate all our experiences, and compassion helps us to forgive ourselves and others when we make mistakes or get out of balance. It is not so much a question of 'getting it right' as of developing the ability to move and change through circumstances, and to not judge self or others. In this way we evolve spiritually as we progress through life.

The poisonous plant analogy at the Mahayana 'level'

> People realise that the poisonous plant is dangerous, and that simply cutting it will not suffice, since its roots remain to sprout anew. They therefore throw hot ash or boiling water over the roots to prevent the plant from growing again. The Mahayana approach applies the 'realisation of emptiness' as the antidote to *ignorance* (ignorance being the root of ego and negativity).

---

[5] Bodhicitta: Buddha Maitreya in the *Abhisamayalankara* (Ngön Tok Gyen):
> Arousing the bodhicitta is:
> For the sake of others,
> Longing to attain complete enlightenment.

We focus on compassion, reflecting on how all sentient beings have the capacity to overcome the causes and results of suffering by developing wisdom and attaining enlightenment. Everyone can arrive at the precious level of complete Buddhahood, attaining complete liberation from suffering.

Vajrayana/tantra: 'sacred outlook'/'pure perception'—the path of transformation

The lotus—a symbol in Vajrayana—represents the power of the human family to transform its energy into enlightenment. Just as the lotus rises out of muddy swamps, so too, the pure energy of our enlightened awareness arises out of the mud of distorted, confused emotions, projections, and perceptions. The essence of this path is to transmute the Five Poisons—pride/arrogance; jealousy/envy; greed; desire/attachment and anger—into their wisdom counterparts, the Five Buddha Families (as described in Chapter 2). Tantra is also known as the path of joy because we enjoy our experiences on the path. Rather than renouncing our emotions, perceptions, and desires, we refine and transmute them through visualisation practices, until we arrive at clear seeing. Regardless as to whether circumstances appear as good or bad, we completely trust life as the path, and that we will benefit in some way from each experience. The high vibrational view of 'pure perception' sees life through the guaranteed lens of The Five Perfections. This is very relevant in our lives today. Though it is a challenging path, if we can learn to trust the sacred outlook of the Five Perfections where everything that occurs is regarded as 'perfect', it can cut through much confusion and 'victim consciousness':

- *The perfect teacher*—the 'teacher' is not necessarily a person and can arise as life's circumstances manifesting to teach us on our path.
- *The perfect teaching*—this is the knowledge and wisdom to be learned from whatever situation arises.
- The *perfect place*—we can guarantee that whatever we learn always happens at the right place.
- *The perfect assembly*—this is the appropriate constellation of people who manifest to teach us through life's experiences and relationships.
- *The perfect time*—the circumstances of teaching and learning always occur at the perfect time.

Sacred outlook involves seeing things directly and simply in 'as-it-isness'—recognising the pure, sacred divine nature in all things. This clear sight is non-dual 5-D perception. We see all people as Buddhas—or divine beings—and all realms as the Buddha fields—'heaven on earth'. In everyday life we can practise this by observing the ideas, thoughts, and emotions which arise in our interactions and relations with other people. When we encounter difficulties, we might be tempted to project out by judging or blaming others saying, 'he said/she said' and so on. Instead of worrying about what anybody else is doing, we reflect—'what did *I* do?' By taking responsibility for our own thoughts and actions, we aspire to develop clear sight.

The outer and inner tantras
The outer and inner tantras are not the scope of this book so I will only mention them briefly.

Visualisation (*Kyerim*) and dissolution practices (*Dzogrim*) are key in Vajrayana, providing methods for purifying our perception. Elaborate visualisations facilitate the integration or our peaceful or wrathful energies/emotions—termed 'deities'. We project out the energy to be worked with in the form of the visualisation, and then re-integrate it by dissolving the visualisation. For instance, in the healing practice of *Vajrasattva* we visualise a peaceful waterfall of light nectar, whereas its wrathful counterpart, *Vajrakilaya*, purifies by destroying with fire. Ultimately, both practices are healing and transformative. Our qualities are not judged dualistically as being either good or bad but viewed with compassion from the pure state of energy—of 'as-it-isness'. This is very similar to working with Jung's archetypal energies.

In the dissolution phase (*Dzogrim*), all is dissolved into the simplicity of the pure natural state. There is no further need to 'fabricate' or create visualisation, but simply to 'be', relaxed and open, resting in the uncontrived, *unaltered* state of non-duality. Visualisation practices share similarities with the classical psychoanalytic process—of projecting issues and emotions onto the (blank-screen) analyst to see them, through having them reflected back. In this way we learn to recognise who we are, and to own previously unknown or unconscious qualities and emotions. This expands our sense of who we are and helps us become more complete.

The poisonous plant analogy at the Vajrayana 'level'

> A group of doctors are delighted to find the poisonous plant with its valuable medicinal properties which they transform into medicine. This is the tantric approach of the Vajrayana, which does not abandon the negative emotions, but through the power of purification and transformation, uses their energy as a vehicle to bring realisation.

The 'higher tantras'—Anuyoga and Atiyoga

Anuyoga and Atiyoga, the 'completion stages' of the path, both have things in common with energy psychotherapy.

- Anuyoga works with the inner mandala, specifically purifying the energy of the subtle 'channels, inner air and energy', including chakras, the inner air of prana, our psychic force, and sexual energy.
- Atiyoga or Dzogchen is the 'direct path' of our consciousness—an experiential wisdom path of liberation which connects us directly with the unified field.

Dzogchen: the non-conceptual path of liberation

After the intense visualisations in Vajrayana, everything falls away into total purity and simplicity. Known as the 'Great Completeness', the essence of Dzogchen practice is 'Taking perceptual experience and [*Rigpa*] as the path ...'.[6] An alternative translation is to 'make projections and mind the path'.[7]

Dzogchen has two principal practice pathways which suit different people's dispositions and lead to liberation: these are *Trekchö* and *Tögal*. Dilgo Khyentse Rinpoche offered a succinct summary at a retreat I attended in France in 1984:

> The practice of Dzogchen or Atiyoga, is to realise... buddha nature which has been present in our nature since the very beginning ... to recognise this Nature, the practice should be utterly beyond fabrication. The practice is simply to realise the radiance, the natural expression of wisdom, which is beyond all intellectual concepts. It is the true realisation of the Absolute Nature just as it is, the ultimate fruition. At the present moment, our awareness is entangled within our mind, completely enveloped and obscured by mental activity. Through the practice of Trekchö, or 'cutting through all attachment', and the 'direct realization' of Tögal, one can unmask this awareness and let its radiance arise. (Dilgo Khyentse Rinpoche, Khyentse 2011)[8]

Trekchö 'cuts through' the egoic mind, bringing the practitioner to the state of pure awareness or *Rigpa* (non-dual consciousness): 'Since pure awareness of nowness is the real Buddha, in openness and contentment we find the Buddha in our heart'.[9] Pure awareness operates in the stillness of 'zero point' of the quantum/'unified field', which is the vibration of love. Dudjom Rinpoche describes the realisation of emptiness thus:[10]

> No words can describe it.
> No example can point to it
> Samsara does not make it worse
> Nirvana does not make it better
> It has never been born
> It has never ceased
> It has never been liberated
> It has never been deluded
> It has never existed

---

[6] From the bardo teachings of *The Tibetan Book of the Dead*.

[7] 'Make projections and mind the path': This is a quote from the 'Main (or Root) Verses of the Six Bardos', a terma (mind treasure) revealed by Karma Lingpa of the Dzogchen tantras of Padmasambhava. In Tibetan this text is called Bardo Thödol, ('Liberation in the Intermediate State Through Hearing' or 'The Great Liberation by Hearing in the Intermediate States').

- Francesca Fremantle and Chogyam Trungpa use the translation 'making projections and mind the path' in *The Tibetan Book of the Dead, translation and commentary* (Shambhala, 1975, pp. 98–99).
- Gyurme Dorje translates it as: 'Taking perceptual experience and [the nature of] mind as the path...' in *The Tibetan Book of the Dead* (Penguin Books, 2005, pp. 32–34).

[8] Dilgo Khyentse Rinpoche outlined the whole path of Dzogchen in Dordogne France in 1984 in a teaching on the Longchen Nyingtik Guru Yoga. The full version can be found on Rigpa Wiki.

[9] From H. H. Dudjom Rinpoche's prayer, 'Calling the Lama from Afar'.

[10] Quoted in *The Tibetan Book of Living and Dying* (Rinpoche, Gaffney & Harvey 2002).

It has never been non-existent
It has no limits at all
It does not fall into any kind of category

Tögal, translated as 'leap over' or 'direct approach', is a rapid path to enlightenment which works with the inner clear light 'spontaneously present' within all phenomena. In the different levels of enlightenment, the fourth stage of *Tögal* leads to a total transcendence of egoic senses known as the 'wearing out of phenomenal reality'.[11] Masters who have realised this stage are unable to function in the everyday world, because if sitting in meditation in the freezing cold, or in boiling hot sun, they wouldn't register their physical needs.

An anecdote about H. H. Dilgo Khyentse Rinpoche describes this: on a plane, Dilgo Khyentse's attendant handed him a drink which he drank with total equanimity. His attendant became very anxious because he suddenly realised he had put an entire packet of extremely hot English mustard into the tea, mistaking it for honey. Most people if they had just one sip of such a burning drink would cough and splutter. Dilgo Khyentse, who was always in a non-dual state of consciousness, remained totally calm and unperturbed. At this level of realisation, experience is neither good nor bad, and all is accepted as 'one-taste'.

H. H. Dudjom Rinpoche's poisonous plant analogy at the level of Dzogchen

A peacock lands, and dances with joy when it sees the poison. It immediately consumes the poisonous plant, and it turns, miraculously, into beauty. The peacock represents Dzogchen, the direct path of self-liberation, the fruition of all the nine yanas, where 'liberation from suffering happens instantaneously'.

Dzogchen—taking us beyond, to the 'peak experience'

I find Dzogchen very inspiring because it instantly cuts through the ordinary rational mind bringing us to a completely different state of consciousness. It is not, however, a question of attaining something—at this level we transcend the concept of evolving consciousness altogether, because we arrive at an unchanging state which has always been with us since the very beginning, 'It has never been born, It has never ceased' (Dudjom Rinpoche). This 'innermost secret teaching' is an energy state which raises our vibration, a 'short cut' like a rocket which takes us beyond, to the 'peak experience'.

---

[11] The Four Visions of Tögal are:
  1. Direct realisation of reality itself
  2. Increasing experience
  3. Awareness reaching full maturity
  4. Dissolution of experience into the nature of reality (also translated as 'the wearing out of phenomenal reality').

We can only arrive at this consciousness through the heart, in a state of openness and humility. As it says in Matthew 19.24, 'It is easier for a camel to pass through the eye of a needle than for a rich man to enter the kingdom of God.' If we are inflated by ego or pride, we cannot get through the gap. This vast, unobstructed wisdom is all encompassing, a naked non-dual consciousness which perceives directly. It is said that having a glimpse of enlightenment and resting in this natural state can cut through aeons of suffering, and our negativity can be purified in an instant. This is why Dzogchen is known as 'the king of all medicines'.

How do we know if we truly find liberation?

> The real, true sign of whether you can liberate or not is when you actually meet, face to face, negative circumstances and thoughts, which arise blazing like a raging fire or bubbling like boiling water. If at that very moment you are able to liberate them, then that is really the same as a true miracle. (Terton Sogyal, Dzogchen Master (translation 2019))

Or as Mooji says: 'We can only find [this heartfelt state of consciousness] by coming to a true and profound experiential understanding of what I am, what you are' (Sri Mooji, 2022).

Part II

The practice of energy psychotherapy

Introduction to Part II

During an era of tremendous change, new quantum healing techniques and processes are finding their way into therapists' consulting rooms. Energy psychology and its methods have long been established in the USA with the Association for Comprehensive Energy Psychology (ACEP) spearheading the way generously and creatively. In the UK, which has a different training model for its therapists, we too have been evolving our own forms of this work which we term energy psychotherapy.

The second section—Chapters 7 to 10—is concerned with the actual practices of energy psychotherapy and describes various methods you can try out for yourself. My focus is on practical application—how this embodied way of working can easily and naturally be integrated within the normal frame of talking therapy, the 'felt sense' and the psychotherapeutic relationship. These methods are 'self-applied' and easy to use, which is empowering for the client, and I offer some vignettes to illustrate. Since working with energy can be quite powerful there is an emphasis on safety and grounding as core fundamentals of the work.

Chapter 7 provides the energy psychotherapy toolkit itemised on the contents page. It includes learning how to balance the system, which is very useful for self-regulation of clients and therapists and explains how to self-energy test to guide the work. A number of methods are described for clearing traumatised energy from the body and reprogramming neural pathways working with meridians, energy centres/chakras, 'thought fields', and intention.

Chapter 8 focuses on integrating *mindbodyenergy* and its many systems and includes an exploration of the subtle energy systems. It considers trauma and its impact on the body, touches on polyvagal theory and the parasympathetic/sympathetic nervous systems, hyper- and hypo-arousal, and offers energy methods to balance and regulate the nervous system. In considering the needs for self-care for therapists and clients, the differences between presence and empathy are explored and the need to retain healthy 'energy boundaries'.

Chapter 9 explores the multidimensional clinical terrain of the work to clear trauma at all levels. This includes preverbal and transpersonal trauma where energy is a 'language beyond words', working with early attachment trauma and the importance of establishing safety. There are considerations of PTSD, and the use of gentle non-traumatising methods to bring about wholeness and integration using healing circles (resource circles). In addition there is a focus on working with parts and integrating archetypal 'shadow' work including deep resistance or massive 'energetic reversals' where people are sometimes blocked from moving forward.

Chapter 10 considers some transpersonal issues and their implications for training therapists in working with the new clinical terrain, and concludes with some personal reflections.

I hope you enjoy this introduction to working with energy and how it can bring us to states of wholeness, integration, peace, and well-being.

CHAPTER 7

Energy psychotherapy 'toolkit'

This chapter introduces components of the practice of energy psychotherapy. It outlines various methods which you can try out with vignettes illustrating their benefits. I refer to Asha Clinton's broad definition of 'trauma' mentioned in Chapter 5.

Feel free to try these methods out for yourself as self-help techniques. If you are a therapist, you may like to start by introducing energy balancing and karate-chop to your clients. If you wish to work in more depth, it is advisable to do a training in energy psychotherapy and ensure you are in supervision with an energy psychotherapist.

Preliminaries: energy balancing, hydration, and regulation

When we work with energy, we start with preliminary exercises to ensure we are energetically balanced and well hydrated. If you are a therapist or client doing energy work together, this applies to you both. So, at the start of and throughout energy work make sure you are:

- well hydrated
- energetically balanced with the correct electromagnetic polarity
- homolaterally balanced horizontally, across the body from left to right

Hydration

The electromagnetic flow of working with energy requires that we are well hydrated. We are made up of 60–80 per cent water and many are dehydrated, so you may be surprised by how much water you need to drink. Energy work can make people thirsty, and signs of dehydration include exhaustion, an inability to think clearly, and getting muddled—so when you work with clients make sure that you provide—and both drink—plenty of water. It is not uncommon for people to drink a litre of water in a session. It is also beneficial to drink water from as pure a source as you can find. Adding electrolytes to the water will replenish your energy.

Energy balancing

Any of us can easily go out of balance, so having balanced and correctly polarised energy systems is important. The following energy balancing methods calm down and self-regulate the energy system, which is especially useful for traumatised clients in hypervigilant states of PTSD. Becoming dysregulated takes various forms—the electromagnetic polarity can become disorganised (vertical, from the crown to the root), or the homolateral balance (from left to right across the body) can go out of alignment.

Signs of energy imbalance

- when the person is triggered
- general confusion and brain fog (also applies to dehydration)
- getting muddled up, stumbling over, and struggling to find words
- being clumsy

Methods for balancing the subtle energy system

There are many effective methods for regulating emotional distress, triggered states, and putting the subtle energy system into balance The following are a small selection. They are useful for all of us—please feel free to try them out straightaway.

MEDULLA UNDER-THE-NOSE HOLD

1. Make sure your legs are uncrossed.
2. Place two fingers in the little hollow under the nose and press firmly.
3. Gently cup the bottom of the skull at the back of your head in your other palm.
4. Sit like this for 60–90 seconds (eyes open or closed) whilst breathing normally.

COOK'S HOOK-UP (a version of the Wayne Cook posture)

1. Cross your left ankle over your right ankle.
2. Place your right arm over your left arm with your hands resting on the thighs.
3. Place the tongue against the roof of the mouth behind your upper teeth.
4. Sit and breathe naturally for a minute or so (5–6 deep silent breaths).

SIMPLIFIED COLLAR-BONE BREATHING

A simplified collar-bone breathing is demonstrated by Phil Mollon on video, which has multi-purpose beneficial effects (www.philmollon.co.uk/BREATHING-EXERCISE.html).

HOMOLATERAL BALANCING (to balance left and right sides of body)

1. Tap your knees with your fingertips and then cross your hands to tap the opposite knees.
2. When crossing-over, do so with vigour, tapping for longer in the crossed position.
3. Repeat a few times, ending in the crossed position.

Grounding energy

Lots of people are not fully in their bodies, so the following exercises can help people to become more grounded.

NAVEL BREATHING

Breathe slowly in and out through the navel, considering that your breath enters and leaves your body through your navel. This practice supports the heart and is beneficial for people in states of anxiety and fear, or who tend to leave their bodies and dissociate. Navel breathing brings a sense of personal coherence, centring, and grounding. It is also useful for bringing the energy down into the centre of the body (the hara) for those who tend to get stuck in their heads.

FEET ON THE GROUND

Place your feet on the ground (bare feet on grass or earth is ideal on occasions when it is possible) and experience the connection with the ground/earth, allowing the energy to flow down through your body, your feet, and into the ground. Some people find it helpful to visualise roots growing from their feet anchoring them deep in the earth.

Calming the nervous/energy system

Stress and PTSD are debilitating, so simple self-care methods can calm down the nervous system, helping people enter the 'rest digest', relaxed, and peaceful states. This is discussed further in Chapter 8.

TAPPING JUST ABOVE THE NAVEL

If you are triggered, or in a state of hyper-arousal, tap above the navel about fifteen times or simply rub the area gently. This is also useful for balancing the energy system.

LUNG MERIDIAN BREATHING

This is simple and soothing, and very useful for states of shock.
1. Cross your hands over your chest and heart centre, with the fingertips tucked in to the hollows of the shoulder—under the collar bone.
2. To find the place, move your fingers along from the edge of the shoulder, under the collar bone—there is a 'hollow' or indented area, quite large (linked to the lung meridian).
3. Breathe naturally in whatever way feels comfortable to you as you press into these points and allow stress to be released gently through the calm rhythmic process of breathing.

'TRIPLE WARMER' OR 'BIRD BEAK'

This pose is comforting and calming
1. Use thumb, index, and middle fingers of your right hand to make a 'bird beak'.
2. Place this 'bird beak' into the V of your throat, the little hollow just above the collarbones.
3. Rest your cheek into the flat of your left hand (head tilted to the side) and fingertips coming up over the gall bladder point (side of eye, at the end of the eyebrow).
4. Rest for a while.
5. If you wish you can repeat on the other side.

The triple warmer is a natural pose—people often cup their chin in their hand and rest on the side of the cheek like this. It is good for calming down stress and is particularly helpful with PTSD, hyper-arousal, and traumatised 'child-states'.

Energy testing—otherwise known as kinesiology/muscle testing

> For the most part we are not measuring the gross muscle strength of the muscle, but we are monitoring the muscle response as an indicator of the energy system. (Dr John F. Thie, the founder of *Touch for Health*)

Energy testing, otherwise known as muscle testing or kinesiology, is used for guiding the work of energy psychotherapy safely. Anyone can learn to self-energy test themselves, and it is an invaluable skill. Self-energy testing can also be done on behalf of others, with their consent. When we energy test directly in-person, we generally test the arm of the other person if they are happy to be tested in this way. This is a collaborative process where we get our minds out of the way and connect in a state of 'Presence' (with soul, or 'Source'). We follow the 'flow' of energy which bridges and integrates the physical, the psychological, and consciousness itself, a process which brings a deeper connection with self and other. Direct in-person energy testing can feel empowering for the client, connecting as it does directly with the wisdom of their own body's responses.

Adopting the optimum ethical stance as a practitioner involves boundaries and seeking permission; respect for the vulnerability of the client and potential power imbalance; and an open attitude. When we first start energy testing with a client, we might say something like: 'I don't presume any knowledge, I only know what your energy system tells me'. Our task is to facilitate the client's system's communication and to be guided by the client's whole system—their conscious thoughts and words, and their deeper wisdom. In terms of the ethics of energy testing, according to Phil Mollon, the energy system can't be misused and will only co-operate if we are sincere, respectful, and humble—if we try to misuse energy testing for personal power it won't co-operate.

Accessing information through energy testing

Through energy testing we can access the origins of trauma which may not otherwise be consciously known. This means we can quite easily work with preverbal and deeper layers of trauma in the system. Statements are addressed to the person's subtle energy system which, when tested, provide Yes/No answers. For instance:

- *This trauma occurred between the ages of 0–5.*
- *There is a transgenerational component to this trauma.*

Energy testing is a living resource of enormous potential, and its implications are profound. While the technique is simple, our relationship with the experience is interesting and complex. There is an immense amount to be learnt and explored. This is particularly true about energy testing oneself ('self-energy testing') as we learn how to access our own personal 'satnav'— our guidance system—and use this method for ourselves. As you hone your skills, you find that energy testing is nuanced, distinguishing the subtle differences between 'I want to be over this problem', where the result may be strong, whereas testing 'I want to be *completely* over this problem' might test weak, indicating a slight ambivalence.

There are many ways to energy test, including sway tests and testing various parts of the body. Here I focus on self-energy testing. This skill involves testing statements for Yes/No answers which provide us with information. We can self-energy test for ourselves, and test on behalf of others, so since many therapists work on Zoom these days, this is phenomenally useful.

Self-energy testing methods include using the index and third finger; the O ring test; the 'sway test'; and the sticky thumb nail test and many others. Try out different ones to see what works for you. It is helpful if you entrain your body to 'know' how to do this by repeatedly practising. Here are a couple for you to try out.

How to self-muscle/energy test by entraining the body

- Make sure that your system is in alignment and balanced before you start by doing the preliminary energy balancing.
- Drink water before you start.
- When you test simple binary statements, these statements will register as YES, 'true' or NO, 'false'.
- A response that is STRONG/firm is taken as YES.

- A response that is WEAK/slack is taken as NO.
- Some people 'get' how to energy test straightway—others may need a period of entraining the body's responses.

USING INDEX AND THIRD FINGER (ONE-HANDED METHOD)

- Use the index finger as the muscle to be tested.
- Use your third finger to push down on the index finger. (In so doing it is as if the index finger serves as the 'arm' and the third finger is like another 'arm' pushing down on it.)
- Test a statement—e.g. 'My name is ...' by pushing down on your index finger with your third finger.
  - If the index finger holds strong, this is YES; the statement tested as TRUE.
  - If the index finger is unable to resist the pressure and is WEAK, this is NO; the statement tested as FALSE.

'O' RING (TWO-HANDED) ENERGY TEST

Make a circle of your forefinger and thumb and try to prise the 'O' apart with the fingers and thumb of the other hand.

- When the ring is strong and difficult to prise apart, this tests as STRONG and means YES or that the statement tested is TRUE.
- When the ring is WEAK and breaks, it is easy to prise apart and that means NO or that the statement tested is FALSE.

We can entrain the body as it likes. The main thing is to find a consistent response.

Once you have found a method you like, you can experiment and 'play' with energy testing. Examples of simple Yes/No *statements* (presenting statements *not* questions):

My name is (true name) should be STRONG
My name is (made up name) should be WEAK

Today is ... (incorrect) should be WEAK
Today is ... (correct) should be STRONG

You can also explore what strengthens or weakens your energy system. So, if you imagine someone who engenders positive feelings, the energy test is likely to be strong, whereas for someone who brings up negative feelings, the response is likely to be weak. You can also energy test when shopping for food as to which foods best suit your body.

The technique of energy testing is relatively simple; some take to it like a duck to water, whereas others struggle. I remember being astonished when Sandi Radomski (known as 'the Queen of muscle testing', who does this effortlessly) told us in a workshop that she had difficulties in the beginning—so it is well worth persevering. The main thing is not to be put off by initial blips such as doubting the results, or letting your head get in the way of what is essentially an energetic process. It takes practice to develop confidence. If you find yourself being sceptical, this is something that many others have also felt. You can work through your scepticism using energy methods such as acupoint tapping or chakra clearing, to overcome your difficulties and anxieties about it.

As you become more confident, self-energy testing is very useful for:

- Checking your own energy system to make sure you are balanced.
- Checking for guidance about the energy work which needs doing.
- Checking the timing and when it is safe—or not—to do specific pieces of energy work.
- Using energy testing whilst working online or on the phone.

Energy testing—key points

Energy testing is an art, not a science. It accesses the information in the 'field' between client and therapist, which is why the therapist can test on behalf of the client and use it on Zoom.

Energy testing overrides the cognitive mind, directly accessing the body and soul's wisdom—it is the body and energy which does the 'work'; we get our minds out of the way and energy test with an attitude of not knowing the outcome. This is a mysterious and sometimes playful process which we undertake with wonder. The yes/no answers give us information, but this is not 'the truth', since there are variables to consider which need to be interpreted and understood.

The energy system needs to be in balance for testing to be accurate, which is why it is important for both client and therapist to do energy balancing and drink water first. We test clear binary *statements* to produce direct yes/no answers (rather than test questions). Since the body/energy system is very literal and can be a bit pedantic, we make sure the wording of a statements is precise. For example:

- 'It's in my highest interest to work with this', e.g. energy tests, YES
- 'It's in my highest interest to work with this NOW', e.g. energy tests, NO

Energy testing follows the client's healing process to 'guide' the therapy, informing us what to clear, when, and whether it is safe to do so. Energy testing is also used to measure SUDs (subjective units of distress measure the energetic 'charge' or level of stress in the body) by testing, e.g. 'The SUDs for this are 6 out of 10'.

We can use the process of energy testing to explore and ascertain information about the origins of trauma, including preverbal and transpersonal experiences, body memories, and depth psychology. To do this we use energy testing phrases like:

- 'This trauma occurred when I was in-utero'.
- 'It is safe for me to clear this trauma now'.
- 'The root of this trauma is in my maternal line'.

The numinous 'presence' of energy testing helps us become more sensitive to energy, connecting us with the guidance of our soul and Source energy.

Clearing resistance (psycho-energetic reversals) using karate-chop (KC) tapping

Energy 'flowing the wrong way'

A special feature of energy therapy is its capacity to identify internal objections to therapeutic work. It is often these resistances and blockages, usually unconscious, which prevent us from getting better. Psycho-energetic 'reversals' are quite literally a reversed flow of energy which gets in the way of a person being well. Roger Callaghan, developer of Thought Field Therapy (TFT), discovered psychological reversals by muscle testing his patients, where the muscles—or energy—tests strong if the statement is true, or weak if it is false. 'I found to my chagrin that a large number of my clients got weak when they thought of getting better and stronger when they thought of getting worse' (The Five-Minute Phobia Cure, 1985, p. 49). In such instances the subtle energy or 'chi' in the body is flowing 'the wrong way', quite literally reversed, akin to Freud's 'Death Instinct'.

An unconscious block to 'clearing' an issue

Hover-Kramer coined the term 'psycho-energetic' reversals:

> A reversal is the energetic equivalent of an unconsciously held belief that influences the energy system and interferes with the conscious changes that the client wishes to make. (Hover-Kramer, 2002)

Working with psychological reversal is crucial. When there is a blockage to 'clearing' a trauma, unless such reversals are addressed in the energy system, energy techniques will have little effect.

Common, universal themes for psycho-energetic reversals

1. **Core beliefs** about recovery and healing overall:
   'I'll never recover'—'I'm too bad to be helped'
   'It's not possible for me to get over this problem'
2. **Underlying conflicts**—the psychodynamics, internal conflicts, and psychological motivations behind reversals. We can energy test for:
   SAFETY (or lack of it)—'It's not safe to get over this problem'
   DESERVEDNESS (lack of it)—'I don't deserve to …'
   IDENTITY (and threats to it)—'I won't be me if …'
3. **Resistances** to getting completely over a problem, where we hang on to part of it (self-sabotage) or are in two minds about getting better (ambivalence).
4. **Massive global reversal**—when testing 'I want to be well' tests weak, and 'I want to be ill' tests strong (this is explored further in Chapter 9).

5. **Passive-aggressive unconscious emotions** such as envy, anger, and resentment where a person doesn't want to get well. For example, to spite the person whom they blame for their difficulty—'I don't want to give you the satisfaction of seeing me well, because this will let you off the hook …' etc.

6. **'Parts' reversals**: part of us might energy test strong to 'I want to be over this problem' but weak to 'All parts of me want to be over this problem'. Alternatively, our body may test as wanting to be ill, whereas consciously, our mind does want us to get well.

How to use the karate-chop (KC) for unblocking reversals

Fortunately, we *can* unblock reversals by using the karate-chop (KC) method to clear resistances. This changes the brain and neural pathways, so that clients become more 'available', open, and able to work in therapy. This simple technique involves tapping on the side of the hand with the fingertips on the KC 'self-acceptance point' whilst:

- **making a statement of conflict**
  o 'Even though I have this problem …'
  o 'Even though I don't deserve to get over this problem …'
- **followed by some form of healing intention such as a statement of self-love and acceptance**
  o 'I completely love and accept myself'
  o 'I'm OK' or some such variation.

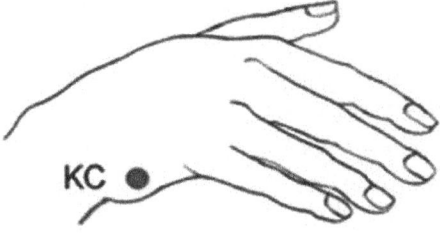

Figure 8 The KC tapping point

Reversals correction statement:

The simplest general reversals correction statement, which is said three times is:
'Even though I have this problem … I love and accept myself' × 3

People sometimes struggle to say they 'love and accept' themselves', though this statement is a powerful way of unblocking reversed energy. It may help to let the person know they can view this as an intention, even if they don't yet believe this to be true. It is also helpful to be aware that for some, the word love has been misused for purposes of abuse/control and so it might be triggering. Resistance to saying the positive part of the reversal phrase can in itself be a powerful moment of change in therapy. When a client can't stomach saying such a phrase and protests saying, 'but I *don't* love and accept myself', tears and distress sometimes emerge. At such times, saying 'I am working towards accepting myself'/'I aspire to love myself'/'I trust that my self-esteem is improving'/'I choose to accept myself', or just simply 'I am OK', are all nonetheless healing intentions.

List of commonly occurring reversals

There are several common reasons why someone may have a reversal, and not want to be free of a particular issue. Tapping the side of the hand to clear the negatively held self-beliefs such as 'I don't deserve to be well', 'It's not safe for me to be well', can clear dynamic inner conflicts where the client is torn between different views, or may have self-sabotaging inner voices guiding them. This profound but easy-to-use method can bring a client who has suffered massive trauma back into the flow of the 'life-giving' force of positive energy. The following are frequently occurring reversals:

- SAFETY   'even though it's not safe to get over x ... I love and accept myself'
- DESERVE   'even though I don't deserve to get over x, I accept myself and I'm OK'
- IDENTITY   'even though I'll stop being me if I get over this problem ... etc.'
- SHAME   'even though I feel too much shame to feel able to clear this'
- ANGER   'even though I'm too angry to get over this problem ...'
- WANT TO   'even though I don't want to get (over this problem) ...'
- POSSIBILITY   'even though it's not possible for me to ...'
- BENEFIT   'even though it won't benefit me to ...'

We generally tap through the whole list, saying each reversal out loud. We always end the reversals phrase with some version of self-acceptance such as: 'I completely love and accept myself', 'I'm OK', 'I choose to believe I am learning to love myself, etc.'

We energy test the phrase 'There is one or more reversal' and if this tests as strong, we can either energy test for specific reversals and clear them individually by tapping on the KC point, or simply run through the complete list above without any energy testing.

Different ways of working with reversals

The energetic equivalent of psychological 'resistance', reversals are an aspect of the defence system, protecting the person from deeper pain. Our defences are there for a good reason, so although the KC method for clearing reversals is relatively 'easy', working with these blocks forms a significant aspect of therapeutic work. They need to be addressed in the energy system before the whole of the client is fully available for healing, particularly when working with complex trauma. Asha Clinton's AIT contains a matrix of core sabotaging beliefs—including 'parts' who are fearful of change.

Reversals occur frequently, and there are several approaches for working with them:

We can *simply neutralise* them by speaking the reversal out loud and tapping on the side of hand.
We can *enquire further* about the nature, content, and origins of the reversal by asking 'what comes to mind?' This often takes us directly to childhood trauma and patterns of conflict which need to be cleared with energy methods.

We can *improvise and 'tell the story'* while tapping on the KC point. Speaking out loud and tapping frees the expression of blocked emotions and new associations arise.

'Mirrored' riffing in therapy: if a client is struggling to speak about their conflicts, both therapist and client can tap on their KC points, while the therapist names words and themes the client has been speaking about in the session for the client to repeat. This mirrors back and helps the client to fully register what they have been saying. It provides a powerful form of release and validation for the client. Once this is established the client can be asked: 'What other blockages might you have about this issue?', and it becomes easier for the client to voice their feelings while they tap. The wonderful benefit of KC tapping is that it untangles blockages and conflicts while at the same time removing them, which frees things up considerably. There is quite an energy about this practice which clients really feel, and it can foster a togetherness in the therapeutic relationship.

Self-help self-regulation: people easily take to KC tapping and can use it for self-regulation and 'clearing' issues as they arise. For example, a person can ad lib about their feelings while tapping:

> *'Even though* (e.g. I feel terrible shame/rage about my issue)
> I accept this is the way I feel
> and I choose to let it go now (or variations as necessary)
> and it's safe for me to let it go.
> *And I completely love and accept myself'*

Venting and owning hostile feelings. KC tapping is beneficial for venting hostile feelings especially when working with shameful feelings such jealousy, envy, resentment, or rage. This is an energising practice which helps people to accept their feelings whilst at the same time dissipating unhelpful aspects.

> e.g. *'Even though* I am in two minds about whether I want to get over this problem, because part of me benefits from leaving things the same and part of me is scared of change … and even though I am completely furious about xxxx so I want to sabotage myself to spite them … *I completely love and accept myself and forgive myself for my blockage about moving forward.'*

Using KC tapping to come out of dissociation and into the body:

> *Even though* I am so distressed I can't remain in my body, so I dissociate, I accept myself and my difficulty staying in my body, and *I am OK.*

The more you do KC tapping, the more easily and naturally you can improvise. It can be quite a playful way of integrating issues and conflicts. It is versatile, unblocks, gets the energy flowing, enhances self-acceptance, and is a non-shaming way of tackling painful conflicts. It can be used very simply and with more complex trauma. For example, KC tapping was the only energy method used throughout a two-year therapy working with a client suffering from DID, and she and her parts were enormously helped and harmonised by the process.

Meridian work (EFT/acupoint tapping)

Some will be familiar with tapping, which does many things. Tapping has calming effects on body brain and mind; it accesses a different realm of reality—the 'higher gauge' spoken of previously in Chapter 4 which is responsive to our intention; and it accesses places we need to get to in order to heal our issues. Tapping also calms and helps break up dysfunctional patterns. Any tapping on the body is a pattern disruptor which is particularly helpful in breaking down the repetition compulsions and stuck circuitry in the brain. It also engages the interpersonal neurobiology of the vagus nerve explored in Chapter 8. There are lots of videos on YouTube where you can see different ways that people tap—and you will see it is a simple, accessible approach.

There is a full diagram of the meridians (Figure 11) in Chapter 8

There are twelve main meridians and two additional vessels known as the governing and central vessels. The points we tap on are well known to acupuncturists and are mostly at the beginning or ends of meridians. We usually tap using a couple of fingers, about seven times on each point if we are going through a straight sequence, though sometimes tapping longer on a point feels beneficial.

The points connect with specific emotions and body organs. Gary Craig's EFT (Emotional Freedom Techniques) is the most widely known form of tapping—a tried-and-tested sequence which is extremely effective. There are also additional finger points which are very useful—it is good to tap on them all.

Tapping has a large evidence base demonstrating its effectiveness in clearing trauma of all varieties (ACEP[1]). In addition to EFT, TFT (Callaghan's Thought Field Therapy), and PEP (Mollon's Psychoanalytic Energy Psychotherapy) are also excellent. They work with more specific coding and are well worth learning.

> **BASIC ACUPOINT TAPPING USING 'REMINDER' PHRASE**
>
> 1. **IDENTIFY THE ISSUE:** There is an emphasis in acupoint tapping on focusing on *specific aspects*: e.g. 'what was it about the accident that most upset you?'
> 2. **ESTABLISH '*REMINDER PHRASE*':** This phrase names the problem or emotions and can be very simple such as 'this incident', or 'my shock', or 'the accident', or with more elaborate sensory details, such as 'the sound of the glass cracking' or 'seeing all the blood'.
> 3. **'GUESTIMATE' THE FEELING/level of triggering on a scale using SUDs** (subjective units of distress) where 10 is maximum intensity and 0 is none, using client's guestimate.

---

[1] The Association for Comprehensive Energy Psychology (ACEP) has a wealth of information on the latest research in energy methods. https://www.energypsych.org/

4. **CORRECT REVERSALS:** Repeat the following statement **1–3 times** (NB this is referred to as the **'Set-Up'** in EFT) while continuously tapping the karate-chop (KC) point on the side of the hand with finger tips:
   - **'Even though ...** I have this problem **I completely love and accept myself' or 'I'm OK'** or something similar.
5. **THE TAPPING 'SEQUENCE':** Tap a few times on each of the meridian points in Figure 9 starting at the top of the head (TOH) and down through all the torso points ending at the below nipple (BN) point while repeating the brief 'reminder phrase'.

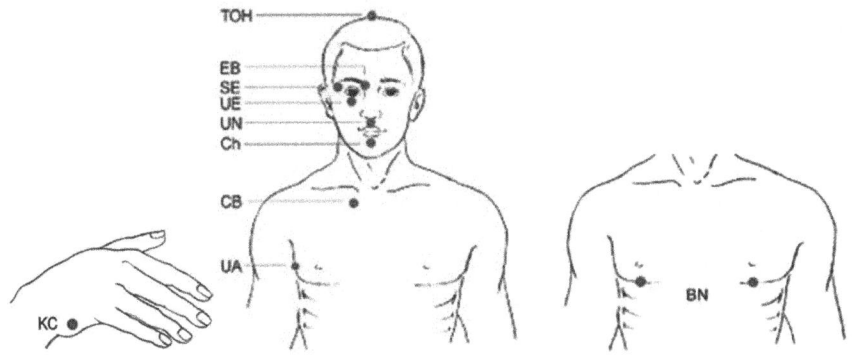

Figure 9 Tapping points

   KC: The karate-chop point is located at the centre of the fleshy part of the outside of your hand (either hand) between the top of the wrist and the base of the little finger, the part of your hand used to deliver a karate-chop. *NB Tapping is done with FINGERTIPS as there are chakras at the end of each finger.*
6. **'GUESTIMATE' SUDS:** On a scale of 0 to 10 again. **Do further rounds** tapping through the sequence with reminder phrase until SUDs go down to 2 or below.
7. **IF SUDs REMAIN HIGH:** Do more KC tapping while saying:

   'Even though I have some remaining ... (problem), I completely accept myself.'

Emotional correlates of meridian points for acupoint tapping

It is helpful to get to know the emotional correlates of the tapping points, since these act as 'codes' to release specific emotions. Figure 10 includes additional finger points which are very useful. To learn them all, look at the list of points with each emotional correlate to familiarise yourself, repeating out loud what each point releases while tapping on the point.

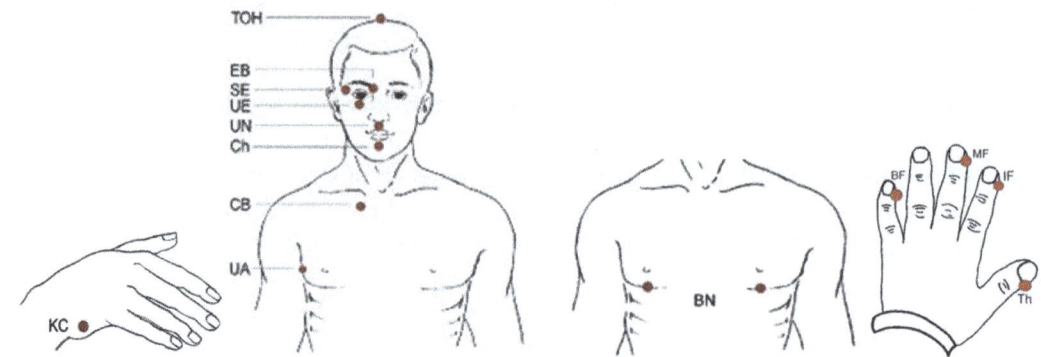

Figure 10 Tapping points and their corresponding emotional correlates (longer sequence with finger points)

Fingers and thumb: tap ON CORNER of nail (see Figure 10) on thumb, index, middle, and little fingers

These points are often linked with the following emotions so tapping on them helps to release the emotions associated with the points:

1. *Side of hand KC* ('karate-chop') point—*small intestine*—**conflict/self-acceptance point**: tapping here moves stuck energy and information, analogous to moving material through the gut, and facilitates reappraisal)
2. *Top of head TOH*, *governing vessel*—also known as 'a hundred meeting points' or the *thousand petal lotus*—**harmonisation**: links with the spiritual
3. *Inside the eyebrow EB*, next to the nose—*bladder meridian*—**shock and trauma**
4. *Outside the eye SE*—*gall bladder meridian*—**traumatic anger and rage**
5. *Under the eye UE*—*stomach meridian*—often linked to **anxiety and fear**
6. *Under nose UN*—*governing vessel*—often linked to self-consciousness, **embarrassment** and issues of autonomy and feelings of **powerlessness or helplessness**
7. *Chin Ch*, under lower lip—*central vessel*—often linked to **shame and humiliation**
8. *Ends of collar bones CB (K27)*—close together, either side of where a tie knot would be—*kidney meridian*—**tension, trauma, stress** and letting it all flow away
9. *Under arm UA side of body* where a woman's bra strap might be—*spleen meridian* often linked with **insecurity or feelings of being trapped**
10. *Under breasts, below nipple BN*—*liver meridian*—important in issues of **toxicity** and **toxic experiences**, where substances or experiences cannot be metabolised
11. *Side of thumb* by the nail—*lung meridian*—**grief, emotional distress** is often patterned in the breath
12. *Side of index finger IF* (thumb side) by the nail—*large intestine meridian*—feelings of **guilt**
13. *Side of middle finger MF* (thumb side) by the nail—*heart protector meridian*—often involved in our ways of **defending** and **protecting** ourselves emotionally and **blocked sexuality**
14. *Inside of little finger BF* by the nail—*heart meridian*—often involved in **anger, emotional wounds to the heart and terror**
15. *Gamut point, GAMUT* between knuckles of little finger and ring finger—*triple warmer/thyroid meridian*—involved in **physical pain, depression, cumulative stress, and the fight/flight system**

You can experiment when tapping by consciously associating relevant emotions with each point while going through either the EFT standard sequence or the longer sequence with finger points.

EXAMPLE

Clearing '*My fear of flying*' (reminder phrase) connecting the emotional correlates of specific acupoints where relevant, while tapping through the sequence.

Each tapping points relates to an organ or an emotion which can be helpful for releasing the specific emotional components of trauma.

Karate-chop (KC), side of hand (small intestine), self-acceptance point
Even though I am terrified of flying I love and accept myself × 3

Inside eyebrow (bladder)—shock and trauma
My shock and trauma around my fear of flying

Outside eye (gall bladder)—anger, rage, and frustration
My anger and frustration at being too frightened to fly

Under eye (stomach)—anxiety, feelings of sickness
All my anxiety and fear about flying

Under nose (governing vessel) powerless, helpless out of control
My fear of flying and the terror of being helpless and out of control

Chin (central vessel) shame or humiliation
All my shame about my incapacitating fear of flying

Collar bone point (kidney 27) accumulated tension, stress, and trauma
All my fear and trauma about flying

Under arm (spleen) I feel trapped, I am insecure
All my fear of flying and my anxiety about being trapped in the plane

Liver point (under breast/nipple) toxic experience
All the origins of these toxic fears and core beliefs that I have about flying

Thumb (lung) I cannot breathe—I am suffocating
My fear of flying

Index finger (large intestine) guilt
My fear of flying

Middle finger (heart protector/pericardium/circulation-sex) hurt, threatened, defensive, blocked sexuality
Defending myself against dealing with my fear of flying, by panicking about it

Little finger (heart) I am angry, my heart is wounded
My fear of flying

Finding the target—clearing difficulties energetically using tapping

The jargon of tapping talks about 'targeting' a problem. We follow the general therapeutic process outlined in Chapter 5.

Working with specific triggers (or perturbations) in the field

Powerful feelings of being triggered is often an indicator to start tapping straightaway. If the client is new to the work, the therapist will instruct the client to tap on the sequence of points while the therapist demonstrates by tapping on their own body, mirroring to the client.

> **EXAMPLE**
>
> Jenny was overwhelmed when she suddenly realised, *I don't have a family anymore.* We used this as a reminder phrase and tapped through the sequence (outlined in the guidance 'protocol'.) In the process of tapping, a flood of feelings, thoughts, memories, and associations were released relating to this issue. It connected her with a great deal of grief, and at the same time, although it was painful, facing the truth and reality of her situation brought considerable relief.

Another aspect of the relief is the shared experience where the therapist witnesses and mirrors back that they have understood the client's reality, which helps the client feel validated and recognised.

Reminder phrases: When tapping we generally use quite a short, charged phrase such as *I felt so ashamed*, which is called a 'reminder phrase'.

The tabletop metaphor: Someone may bring a 'global' issue to therapy, such as feeling depressed, social anxiety, difficulties speaking, or learning on a course. We explore this with the client, digging into all the details and nuances of their experience to establish the different aspects of the situation. Gary Craig uses the metaphor of the 'tabletop' to describe that we start with the surface of what is presented like examining the grains of wood on a table Once the details are established, we start to tap (if as therapists we are working on ourselves) or if we are working with a client, we invite them to tap, following basic acupoint tapping with a 'reminder' phrase.

Telling the story: We tap through all the details of the tabletop, 'telling the story' while tapping through the sequence of points in Figure 10 clearing with SUDs down to 2 or below

Table legs: Continuing Craig's metaphor, we then find the 'table legs'—the underlying traumas and issue which are holding the 'tabletop' in place. It is surprisingly easy to find the table legs—all we need to do is ask simple questions like:

> *When have you felt like this before?*
> *When was the last time you felt this?*
> *Do you remember feeling anything like this when you were a child/adolescent?*
> *What's the earliest time you remember feelings like this?*

Tapping on the side of the hand brings out free associations: If you ask the client to tap the side of the hand with those questions in mind, very rapidly the relevant experiences will come to the surface. If they are early adolescent or childhood experiences, they are likely to be particularly relevant. These are the 'table legs' experiences, and we work through them in the same way as the tabletop, tapping through the points while naming the details.

Tapping through the details of specific events: Clearing trauma involves working with specific events and tapping through detailed memories of what happened. Tiny details are important, including all the sensory details. If you take a road traffic accident (RTA), we clear all aspects of it thoroughly, by tapping through what is remembered, using new reminder phrases once the old ones have cleared and whichever elements of the experience stick in the mind such as:

- observations—what the person saw before the accident
- thoughts in their mind
- sensory qualities of the impact
- sounds such as crunching, smashing
- the aftermath
- what was heard, seen, felt—smells.

We follow the client's associations and their own healing process encouraging them to 'speak of whatever comes to mind'. It is amazing the wealth of unconscious memories which emerge.

Using global 'search phrases'

If we have a sense of a perturbation that we can't quite get at, tapping using a global search phrase like: *the priority issue*, or *when I was born*, or *when I was six* helps bring information to the surface.

To summarise, it's all a question of getting into the details of the experience or the problem, and most crucially, getting to the original experiences which contributed to it. Table legs are specific events which have been holding the problem in place. When you 'target' those specific events, the tabletop will collapse. In this way you reach deep into the heart of the problem and can clear it quite quickly. People who aren't naturally very verbal by nature often find this method very helpful in bringing out their feelings.

Waterfall-of-light chakra clearing

Working directly with 'source' energy and healing intention

I developed the waterfall-of-light chakra clearing from a tantric healing visualisation practice mentioned in Chapter 6. *Vajrasattva* (Sanskrit) is a 'light being' representing the pure energy and healing power of the universe—a direct connection with 'Source' energy, if you like: *Vajra* means the indestructible diamond-like essence of our enlightened nature and *Sattva* means being. In this healing method there is an inbuilt positive assumption and intention that our true essence/'higher' nature is essentially one of light and purity. With that connection we become one with Source, and the flow of that light purifies and heal us.[2]

Stressed energy is removed DOWN the body

Waterfall chakra clearing is easy to use, and very effective as a self-help resource for clearing distress and trauma via the energy centres (chakras) like a 'light' shower, releasing, cleansing, and clearing energetic blockages. It is not necessary to see the visualisation—you can just consider that the waterfall is flowing—the method also works by simply saying the phrases and moving down the chakras.

WATERFALL-OF-LIGHT CHAKRA CLEARING RELEASING TRAUMA AND STRESS DOWN THROUGH THE ENERGY CENTRES FROM CROWN TO ROOT

- Imagine a STRESSFUL EVENT/PATTERN that bothers you.
- Choose a SIMPLE PHRASE which sums up the experience. For instance
  - *Mum was often in hospital when I was young, so I feel lost when my partner goes away*
  - *Because of the stress at work, I am overloaded and easily triggered*
  - *All the times and ways I have been judged and shamed*
- SUDs: estimate on a SCALE 1 to 10 (where 10 indicates a strong level of distress) how strongly you feel the 'charge' of this now.
- CLEAR REVERSALS (KARATE-CHOP TAPPING) at the side of the hands: *Even though I have this problem I love and accept myself × 3*
- STATIONARY HAND: sense where you would like to place one of your hands on the central axis of your body, which will remain there during the clearing. This could be:
  - *On the chakra where you feel the most distress* such as the heart, the throat, the solar plexus and so on.
  - *OR you could place two fingers on the 'Blue Diamond' point* (Mollon, 2022) in the centre of the upper chest, just below the collar bone, the same location as the 'higher heart' and thymus gland. This activates the Blue Diamond healing field which connects us directly to high vibrational loving energy.
- MOVE DOWN THE ENERGY CENTRES (CHAKRAS) WHILE REPEATING THE PHRASE AT EACH CENTRE where the nerve ganglions also reside. This activity releases stress held in the body's nervous system at an energetic level. Start at the crown (top of the head) and go down the centres repeating the phrase at each centre:

  CROWN → FOREHEAD → THROAT → HEART → SOLAR PLEXUS → SACRAL CHAKRA (LOWER ABDOMEN) → BASE (of the spine—sit on your hand)

---

[2] When the Dalai Lama taught *Vajrasattva* practice in the UK several years ago, he invited people to share the essence of it, saying that whether done simply or more elaborately, the essential energy of this would benefit people. The waterfall chakra clearing is a development out of this practice.

- WATERFALL-OF-LIGHT VISUALISATION: imagine a waterfall of brilliant liquid light pouring down from above the crown chakra, while doing the above. The light flows down through the body, right into the cells, through all the chakras and into the ground, clearing out physical mental, emotion, and spiritual blockages and filling your body with fresh, pure, vibrant energy as it does so. The waterfall also flows all around your field, purifying and flushing away any dense energy in your energy bodies.
- TAKE A BREATH at each centre imagining that on the outbreath stressed energy is released. If you prefer to, you can also go down the chakras quite fast.
- SIGNS OF RELEASE: as energy clears people may yawn, sigh, or breathe more deeply and sometimes cry or feel tingling going down the legs. The method works even if people are not fully connected with their bodies and do not feel anything. The clearing is gentle, though there may be some abreaction.
- AT THE END OF A ROUND, 'GUESTIMATE' THE NUMBER you experience the level of trauma to be now. Do additional rounds as necessary to bring the stress down to a zero.
- REVERSALS (KARATE-CHOP TAPPING) at the side of the hands can be used to clear any blockages or aspects which arise if the SUDs reduce slowly.
  Even though I have this problem I love and accept myself × 3

Towards-the-end-of-the-waterfall clearing

OPTIONAL: The waterfall of light can be practised as a form of healing meditation. Simply rest in the waterfall of light and as things emerge from consciousness, consider that the light is healing them. Trust whatever arises and allow the flow of waterfall light to wash all past pain and hurt, cleansing and healing as it flows through.

Different ways of working with waterfall clearing

Issues/trauma can be addressed and cleared in a variety of ways:

- EMERGENCY work: If suddenly triggered, go quickly down the chakras visualising the waterfall of light, repeating an essential phrase such as *all my shock*, or *my overwhelm*.
- A single EVENT: e.g. *The sudden shocking news*—using a simple phrase to describe a distressing incident.
- AS A PATTERN of events or relational pattern: A useful phrase is *All the times and ways that ...* e.g. *All the times and ways I have been abandoned*.
- GETTING TO THE ROOTS: A previous trauma can make a current event more traumatic so it is helpful to identifying causal factors in earlier life where there has been a repetition (in some form) of the presenting trauma: e.g. *Mum had a road accident when I was in her womb, so my recent car accident has shaken me to the core*.
- ASSSOCIATIONS also need to be cleared. As with tapping, all the elements of the trauma are thoroughly addressed. If continuing to work with the RTA this might include:
  o **Components and sensory experiences of a traumatic event itself,** e.g. *the flashing lights of the ambulance; the crunching sound of bones breaking; unstoppable blood flowing from the wound.*

- ○ The **emotions,** e.g. *the panic of the nurses; all my terror that I was going to die; my distress that my husband was waiting at the theatre and didn't know what had happened to me.*
- ○ Subsequent **defences and coping strategies** connected to it or resulting from it, e.g. *my phobia of blood; all the ways I avoid being a passenger in a car now.*

The collaborative process of client and therapist developing 'clearing phrases' together can bring insight and clarity, and deepen the therapeutic alliance. After energy clearing, people usually experience noticeable relief and calm. Occasionally, if someone has been very dissociated from an experience, an energy clearing may connect someone with their experience, in which case, continue to clear through what arises.

EXAMPLE

Fleur was distressed over a family row where she had been grossly unfairly treated after her mother's death. Talking, exploration, and energy testing led back to unconscious roots of the issue. Fleur had played the role ascribed to her by her mother of being the 'good girl' who served others. She 'danced to her mother's tune' to try to gain attention, devoting her life helping others, whilst unconsciously sacrificing her own needs.

At a family meeting, her siblings, like her mother, had taken advantage of Fleur's 'good girl' qualities to do all the work around her mother's estate and probate. Fleur therefore felt utterly shocked and betrayed when they behaved viciously by ganging up on her and attacking her for the genuine help she had been giving.

Fleur was grief-stricken in that meeting to realise that everyone in the family had got on with their lives, had fun and been 'selfish', while she had devoted her entire life in service to 'mother' without receiving the love she craved. She had the devastating realisation that in always putting others first, thinking she was doing 'the right thing', she had missed out on many opportunities and 'wasted her life'. Making this link was very painful, but also brought clarity and insight. We summarised this experience, with the following formulation which Fleur cleared with the waterfall of light:

> *Mum pigeonholed me as 'the good girl' while also neglecting my basic needs, so I 'danced to her tune' to gain the attention she never gave; I am shocked and utterly devastated to realise I have similarly been taken advantage of by my whole family, and senselessly 'wasted my life' in self-sacrifice.*

Fleur felt considerable relief after clearing this. We then worked with the theme of the futility of trying to please her narcissistic mother, which had decimated her self-esteem. This involved facing the disappointment of co-dependence based on the need for approval; how she had been used by her mother and nearly all the family; and mourning her 'unlived life'. After a period of appropriate grief, during which time she became quite depressed as the reality of it all sank in, she separated from those members of her family who had been the most cruel. She went on to define herself in new ways, building on her natural talents and creativity, learning to love herself and generating a more pleasurable life.

Core beliefs

The core beliefs we hold play a crucial role in our mental health generally and working with them is key in CBT. Core beliefs in energy psychotherapy refer to more than cognitions; we include the whole interconnecting energy system—words, thoughts, feelings, emotions, and intentions—the whole 'thought-field' and *mindbodyenergy*.

People with safe, secure upbringings and 'good enough' parenting will generally develop a healthy sense of self through the positive messages they received. However, experiences of adverse incidents and neglect in early life negatively influence thought processes, schemas, and core beliefs, particularly when people have experienced preverbal trauma. When unmediated trauma is experienced in-utero/early life where there is no protection or boundary to that experience, deeply unconscious, negative, and distorted core beliefs develop as consequence.

> As Lipton has pointed out, the young child's brain state is such that he or she is, in effect, hypnotically receptive to the repeated messages, about self and the world, provided in the early environment. (Mollon, 2008, p. 355)

Such experiences create the unconscious beliefs that we clear in psycho-energetic reversals— *It's not safe to, I don't deserve to …*

Unconscious limiting beliefs 'run' our lives

EXAMPLE

Wendy came to therapy saying, *No one ever sees me*. During the process of our work in the first year, we cleared trauma after trauma relating to her life with an alcoholic mother who was so preoccupied with drinking that Wendy was barely seen.

Having a fundamentally limiting core belief running in the background is like being stuck with an old operating system in a computer. The experience of trauma results in both conscious and unconscious limiting core beliefs 'running our lives' and blocking and limiting our development. Such a vision of not being seen will tend to replicate itself until the underlying trauma is released.

Unconscious beliefs remain invisible to us

In Chapter 3 Lipton's experiments proved that beliefs are the primary factor shaping our biology. He also identified that we are controlled by subconscious 'programming' which is infinitely more powerful than the conscious mind, running our biology 95 per cent of the time. Since we are generally unaware of such subconscious beliefs, we rarely recognise that they are sabotaging our lives (Lipton, 2022).

Unconscious thoughts and beliefs determine our life's experiences. Entrenched limiting beliefs feel 'true' to the believer, so a client who holds fast to the idea that they are bad will struggle if you try to suggest otherwise and may well respond *But I AM bad*, not recognising that they are being 'run' by an old programme.

Specific experiences of trauma create an interweaving matrix of unconscious core beliefs (Clinton).[3] For instance, a neglected child may believe (often unconsciously):

- *I am bad*
- *I am unlovable*
- *I can't survive*
- *I have to be perfect (people-pleasing)*

Radomski, too, in her work with clearing in-utero trauma, holds that our earliest trauma creates a 'blueprint' for our expectations in life, which is explored in Chapter 9.

Core beliefs, identity, and the challenge of change

Our capacity to choose new beliefs plays a vital role in the possibility of change. However, when deeply set limiting beliefs become part of our identity, this can be challenging to work with therapeutically—first, in terms of bringing the beliefs into awareness, and second, in finding healthy alternatives. Functional alternative beliefs to the matrix above may seem quite radical to a client with a background of severe trauma, since the new options are so counter to the client's lived experience. For example:

- *My fundamental essence is good*
- *I am loveable*
- *I am able to sustain myself*
- *I am able to have relationships with people where I can be myself* ... and so on.

Resistance to change is largely due to the general human tendency to prefer the familiarity of what we already know, rather than facing the challenge of something new. Psycho-energetic reversals which block our movement forward reflect a commonly occurring range of limiting core beliefs such as:

- *I'll never recover*
- *I'm too bad to be helped*
- *It's not possible for me to get over this problem*
- *I don't want to be well*

Fortunately, KC tapping can help us move forward with healthily flowing energy.

---

[3] Asha Clinton has written numerous manuals on various aspects of energy psychotherapy, which are available to those who undertake her trainings. Unfortunately, I do not think she has as yet published her work more widely. The reference to core belief matrices comes in her 'Basics' manual, which I trained in, in 2006.

Aside from reversals, when working with core beliefs, is usually advisable to first clear the *traumas* which underlie the limiting beliefs using tapping or chakra clearing, and then clear the *core beliefs* afterwards before installing *functional core beliefs* to create new neural pathways.

Resourcing

Bringing in life-affirming beliefs after trauma clearing is a helpful way to end sessions, resourcing the client with new information about themselves which they can work with between sessions.

'Reprogramming' the mind and neural pathways from the negative consequences of trauma is greatly helped by working energetically. This embodied experience has a greater impact than cognitive affirmations:

> Energy Psychology (aka super learning) [is a] ... new belief modification program that engages the brain's super-learning processes, allowing programs to be changed very quickly. (Lipton, 2022)

Psycho-educational work with life-affirming core beliefs

The process of exploring core beliefs and finding functional alternatives is a valuable psycho-educational process in its own right—the insights revealed can be very beneficial. By uncovering unconscious attitudes to self, other, and the world, and developing greater awareness of the thoughts we unconsciously hold, choice and change becomes possible. For instance, if we simply take the phrase *I am bad*, this could be transformed into a variety of phrases which will have specific meanings for the client such as:

- *I love myself, all parts of me*
- *I am fundamentally a good person*
- *I welcome integrating shadow aspects as they arise*

The I AM 'Presence'

When creating positive neural pathways, the words *I AM* are very potent when followed by positive or negative words, with *I am bad* having a very different resonance to *I am loveable*. The '*I AM Presence*' is central to various contemporary spiritual teachings, bringing one to a state of being, embodiment, and connection with Source. Speaking out loud with full Presence from this space of '*I AM ...*' adds strength and gravitas to positive thoughts and beliefs, infusing our being with the relevant energy. When a client says *I AM courageous* with full Presence, and breathes this in at each energy centre, the message is transmitted to all the cells of the body. *I AM* is considerably more powerful than *I CAN be courageous* etc., which carries much less certainty.

> Assisting clients to formulate language patterns for their new beliefs is wonderfully empowering—both for them and for us. Blocks to creativity in the form of limiting belief patterns are usually self-imposed, but as their impediments are removed, vibrant energy for new endeavours can emerge. It is like a renewing breath of fresh air when clients permit themselves to see again the true jewel that resides within. (Hover-Kramer, 2002, p. 144)

Once we have identified the transformed phrases, we work with these energetically. We can repeat the phrase while moving up the chakras, taking a deep breath at each centre. Another powerful method is Sandi Radomski's *Ask and Receive* which works with the power of intention. This method differs from others in that it 're-writes' by bringing in new pathways whilst simultaneously dissolving old ones, similar to the Dzogchen metaphor 'like writing in water'.

Summary: thought processes, core beliefs and their traumatic roots

- *Limiting core beliefs develop out of trauma* and unconsciously 'run' people's lives.
- *Energy therapy enables us to 'reprogramme'* these conscious and unconscious default patterns.
- *When there is a heavy 'load' of trauma underpinning limiting core beliefs*, it is usually necessary to clear the traumas before the core beliefs can be fully transformed.
- *Core beliefs change physiology* as laid out in Lipton's 'biology of belief' and epigenetics.

Working with the creative power of positive intention

A developing phenomenon in energy psychotherapy is to work with words and intention alone without needing to use the meridians or chakras. While it remains a mystery as to how exactly all this works, there are various factors which play their part. Intention does not come from cognitions or the mind, but from the heart and soul, which resonate at higher frequencies than thoughts. The knowledge that flows through the subtle channels via our heart and soul enables us to access areas beyond the conditioning of our past, or our fears for the future.

Energy follows intention

The quantum paradigm is concerned with other, wider dimensions of reality which are not limited to distance/time phenomena. In Chapter 4, William Tiller's experiments demonstrated that consciousness/intention can and does alter outcomes. What we give meaning to—intention—is a choice. Our life unfolds according to that intention, and the more we condition a space with meaning and intention, the more it becomes so.[4]

Dr Joe Dispenza has brought excellent resources for understanding the creative power of intention into the mainstream, demystifying ancient wisdom and bridging the gap between

---

[4] You may be interested to watch a video on William Tiller's website: Background and Human Potential www.tillerinstitute.com/

science and spirituality (Dispenza, 2012a, 2012b, 2017, 2019). He teaches about the quantum field, rich with 'solution' energy, creating positive pathways and timelines towards realising specific wishes and goals. When we align ourselves with love and set intentions towards that which we desire—focusing on solutions rather than what we don't want—this creates a powerful healing trajectory in the 'unified field' of 'source' energy.

Since energy follows intention, we are constantly manifesting our intentions, whether consciously or not. Neil Donald Walshe (1995) said that Source energy says 'Yes' to everything—positive or negative—so it is helpful to develop habits where we affirm positive outcomes and seek solutions, rather than dwell on problems. If we wish to overcome the tendency to think negatively, a helpful habit to develop is to ' wonder what it will be like if …' and then imagine something good. When we aspire to feel the love, connection, and trust that the 'universe knows best' and focus on positive outcomes, difficulties often just dissolve.

When we trust in 'the universe' and our true nature, we reap the benefits of a solution-focused approach and the lower vibrations of fear and doubt gradually melt away. There are, however, paradoxical flip-flops between ego's ways, and fifth-dimensional 'effortless' manifestation. The egoic mind finds it difficult to address issues concerning consciousness and intention, because consciousness is a phenomenon beyond space and time. Our ego is largely preoccupied with our past or future experiences, and we struggle to be in the present, which means that we often re-create past problems in the present. When we take a short cut to higher dimensional fields by connecting with our Souls, plugging into the solution energy of positive intention is easy.

Naturally, for someone in the middle of a deep grieving process, positive intentions may be the last thing they want to hear about. Others may struggle to access high vibrational states, pulled down by cognitive worry and doubts of *can I?/can't I?/this can't be true/I'm kidding myself* often taking over—especially for those whose lives are filled with trauma. Working with positive intention therefore needs to be relevant and appropriate to someone's situation.

Some take issue with a positive approach, feeling it is potentially unbalanced—playing 'happy bunnies' is plainly ridiculous, ungrounded—dangerous even—and that people need to 'get real'. I have certainly been guilty of this myself on occasion. Years ago, someone shared a life vision with me which I felt might be a bit 'unrealistic' in terms of her earning her living. She came back to prove me wrong—I was delighted for her success in accomplishing her vision and it was a useful lesson for me. I have subsequently learned not to put my own limitations onto others' dreams.

What we focus on expands

When we give our attention to an intention, the energy expands and grows. This is a 'law' of the universe. Focusing on the desired outcome rather than the problem assists the positive flow of energy, helping us accomplish our aim. The Dalai Lama once said that instead of dwelling on all the suffering and war in the world, visualise world peace. Reflecting on peace brings the resonance to a lighter 'frequency'. When we reach a state of consciousness that vibrates beyond the level of problem, and are present in the moment, we contribute lighter energy to the world and help to raise the vibration.

We might try developing new habits of envisioning the reality that we wish for, rather than focusing on what we don't want. The discipline is to be aware of and apply mindfulness to change negative thoughts, so we learn to transform our thinking. As we dream into the unified field of all possibilities, we connect with all possible solutions. We put out the intention to the universe: 'This is my dream—make it happen', while holding our vision and vibration as high and steadily as we can. We also need to take action—taking a step in the direction we wish to go in—trusting that the relevant people and circumstances will fall into place from the Field.

> **SOLUTION-FOCUSED: SEEING THINGS IN TERMS OF THE DESIRED OUTCOME AND TRANSFORMING THE BELIEF**
>
> 1. **Start with the negative core belief**—e.g. *I sabotage everything I do*
> 2. **Transform the belief**—the intention becomes:
>   *I achieve what I set out to do and bring things to fruition*—then
> 3. **Explore and clear any blocks** using whichever energy method you like which is preventing the realisation of this intention.

Perception as a vehicle for transformation

All this underlines the importance of perception as a potent vehicle for healing in therapeutic work. Where we choose to place our attention makes a difference—working with positive intentions affirms wellness, which underpins the healing.

Perception is a choice: when our core outlook on life is imbued with positive intention things 'flow' more easily. So, it is useful to examine our fundamental perceptions as to how we perceive the world, including both our internal and external environment. It is not what happens to us but how *we perceive* our experience that makes the difference, and we always have a choice.

Creating new subconscious 'drivers': an underpinning belief such as 'all is well', when used as a mantra, can gradually become the 'driver' of our life, making a significant difference to the way our life unfolds. We do indeed create our reality with our intentions and thinking, so the more we believe in the power of transformation, the more we transform ourselves.

Ask and Receive—'using your higher being to heal'

Ask and Receive was created through experimentation by Sandi Radomski and Tom Altaffer. Radomski describes the method as being based on the discovery that we all have a higher part of ourselves that has the answer to all of our problems. *Ask and Receive* allows direct access to this 'higher state' information and then incorporates it into our body to use in our life. This method specifically focuses on intention and words alone as the medium for clearing, based on the premise that 'the universe gives us what we expect to see'.

Rewriting our 'narrative' whilst simultaneously transforming neural pathways

The focus on using words and phrases in *Ask and Receive* is a powerful demonstration of the creative power of mind/creator consciousness. As we create positive trajectories of healing intentions, the 'old narrative' is simultaneously dissolved whilst new neural pathways are created. Starting from a limiting belief such as *I am anxious*, we transform/overwrite this with a positive intention such as *I am calm and relaxed* and use the five sentences below to bring about transformation.

THE FIVE SENTENCES OF ASK AND RECEIVE

1. There is a part of my being which already knows that … (the solution is named e.g. *I am calm and relaxed*).
2. That part of my being is willing to inform the rest of me now.
3. It is doing so with Grace and Ease.
4. My mind, body, and spirit, my heart and soul are receiving this information.
5. Information transfer is now complete.

I encourage people to undertake Sandi Radomski's online training of this work—it is a tremendously valuable method to have in your energy psychotherapy tool kit. https://askandreceive.org

Miracles can happen

Ask and Receive harnesses the energy of love to nourish, heal, empower, and facilitate growth. When I did the *Ask and Receive* training, one of the trainees did a demo with Sandi concerning difficulties with her young daughter, who had suffered all her life with sleep difficulties, was deeply unhappy and troubled, and had struggled to fit into family life. Sandi worked with the mother as a 'surrogate' using *Ask and Receive*. The next day the mother reported that her daughter had slept very well for the first time ever in her life, had settled, and was in a much happier frame of mind. The whole family was happier as a result and follow-up showed that the change had lasted. The young child's life transformed, and it felt to everyone like a miracle.

Solution-focused energy

Ask and Receive emphasises the limitless aspects or our creativity. In third-dimensional egoic thinking, it is ego's view of limiting thoughts and beliefs which hold us back with the outlook *There is a problem, and I don't know the solution*. An open curiosity helps us shift from the mind to the heart, where there is more lightness, and the anxieties tend to dissolve. In the fifth dimension *There are infinite possibilities and there is a solution to everything.* Sandi holds that the unified field 'knows' there is always a solution out there, both in the physical and in the energetic space, even if our egoic mind doesn't know how we can achieve the outcome. If we can get beyond the limiting assumptions of the mind, as our awareness shifts and we trust solution energy, solutions manifest. Instead of replicating 'repetition compulsion' we reprogramme our neural pathways and transform our vision.

Our cognitive egoic mind is designed to protect our body and is concerned with survival (something which needs to be respected), rather than with awakening. However, fear is ego's tool which limits us and keep us under its control. A tendency to be fearful or to worry is often an indicator that we are coming from our egoic minds (unless we are experiencing 'signal anxiety' alerting us to danger).

Positive intention names things in terms of the solution and chooses words carefully so that the negative is not re-enforced in any way. So rather than saying 'I am able to get over these blockages' which contains the word 'blockage'—we could say instead: 'I am flowing through life with ease'.

CASE EXAMPLE

Marcel suffered from PTSD and had a habit of 'going hard' at his problems. He was about to attend an Ayahuasca retreat. His language—that he was going to 'blow the lid off'—made me wonder about his healing intention. Was it necessary to 'blow the lid off'?—could there be a gentler way? I wondered. Marcel replied that he was a fighter and felt he always had to fight. I asked him what he really wanted. What was his healing intention? He surprised himself at his response, which was: *To feel safe and inherently lovable and good.*

We then used the five *Ask and Receive* sentences to bring in those feelings:

> *There is a part of my being that already knows … **I feel safe, inherently lovable, and good**.*
> *That part of my being is willing to inform the rest of me now.*
> *It is doing so with Grace and Ease.*
> *My mind, body and spirit, my heart and soul are receiving this information.*
> *Information transfer is now complete.*

As we worked with this, taking in a deep relaxed breath after each sentence, Marcel could feel different parts of his brain releasing tension, and he felt tingling activity of the neural pathways as he felt them changing. At the same time, he felt a simultaneous release in his stomach. While doing this work, flashes of memory also flitted across his mind about his childhood trauma.

This brought him back again to his strong fighting will, and his fears of struggle and explosion. He defined this as:

> *My strong will—an imprint in me which wants to struggle and explode. I am so hyper-tense and alert to threat that I get tighter and tighter and can't relax.*

Together, we reformulated this to a positive alternative with the following phrase:

> *I'm relaxing and dissolving, trusting that my true divine blueprint is effortlessly unfolding, bringing me to safety, gentleness, connection, and love.*

This felt like a totally foreign idea to Marcel, and again, we worked with this using *Ask and Receive*:

> *There is a part of my being that already knows …*
> **I'm relaxing and dissolving, trusting that my true divine blueprint is effortlessly unfolding, bringing me to safety, gentleness, connection, and love.**
> *That part of my being is willing to inform the rest of me now and is doing so with Grace and Ease.*
> *My mind, body, and spirit, my heart and soul are receiving this information.*
> *Information transfer is now complete.*

On completing this, with long breaths between each sentence, Marcel recollected memories of being dropped off at his terrifying babysitter's while simultaneously feeling a soothing process occurring in the centre of his brain. In his free-association process, he also noticed *a hot iron rod through the centre of my brain going right into the brainstem*. We then cleared this association, using a 'Heal and Release' form of *Ask and Receive*:

> *There is a part of my being that already knows I am.*
> **Healing and releasing the feeling of a hot iron rod going through my brain and it is being dissolved and melted with soothing balm.**

As we cleared this, he tuned into a throbbing which had emerged in the centre of his head which he now recognised: 'It's rage'. We then tapped on the side of the eyebrow which is a useful point for releasing rage.

Marcel felt a huge sense of relief and a profound shift in his brain and whole being from this work. At the end of the session, he also reflected about compensatory reactions to trauma *which can make us do all the opposite things to those we actually need to do*. In his case, his mental and physiological knots were getting wound up more and more tightly, when what he actually needed to do was to relax, uncoil, and unwind in the opposite, releasing direction.

I shared with him the Dzogchen analogy of 'the snake effortlessly unwinding its knots'. He connected with this immediately and could see how he no longer wished to 'blow the lid off' on his retreat. Through the process of the session, Marcel reformulated his healing intention for the Ayahuasca Ceremony. Rather than tightening the coils tighter and tighter until the lid blew off and exploded in his brain, his new intention was to heal and release gently like the snake effortlessly unwinding its knots.

Reflections on Dzogchen and quantum methods

In comparing energy psychotherapy with the instantaneous natural quality in Dzogchen, experiential energy methods plug directly into the same high vibrational quantum field where miraculous healing can occur. We have taken a great leap forward so we can accomplish what previously took years of talking and analysis. Methods which relieve stress and suffering in an effortless flow of grace and ease are a real gift to humanity.

As Patrul Rinpoche comments, Dzogchen, 'The King of Medicines', is a state of self-liberation that:

> dissolves like writing on water—the writing and its disappearance are simultaneous. Likewise, as soon as thoughts arise, liberation is simultaneous … [so] One should abide by the flow of self-liberation without any trace, just as writing on water. (*The Three Words*)

I feel *Ask and Receive* is very much in tune with Dzogchen—'self-liberation without any trace'—where when working with the five sentences, trauma and limiting core beliefs dissolve effortlessly. The 'Apex Effect'—a term coined by Roger Callahan—describes how energy methods can dissolve the problem so completely, as if it never existed.

The universal wisdom in Dzogchen speaks of all accomplishing space, containing infinite possibilities and solutions—those we can imagine and those beyond imagination. To my mind, this is like the solution focused energy of *Ask and Receive* and other methods which work with intention. Characteristic of Dzogchen is the idea of instantaneous accomplishment—'instantaneous, as soon as you think of it'. What brings fruition is *intentionality*—our desire and aspiration. When we connect with this field of infinite potential and synchronous combinations of circumstances, new solutions to seemingly intransigent problems simply seem to manifest.

In *The Three Words*, the third word, which is 'Confidence directly in the liberation of rising thoughts' reminds me of the confidence in *Ask and Receive* that 'There is a part of my being which *already knows*' (that healing occurs).

Working with these energy modalities delivers healing directly into our cellular memory, dissolving—step by step—the 'stories' of fear, conflict, trauma, and loss and all that has kept us in limited states of consciousness. Several on the clinical training in energy psychotherapy, who were self-declared as 'not very spiritual', commented on the 'sacred' heart-opening quality of *Ask and Receive*. By reconnecting us with the creative power of our souls in the deepest and widest sense, the frequencies and techniques of such revolutionary healing bring us to states of balance, peacefulness, and as-it-isness. I am deeply grateful to Sandi and Tom for their gift to the world.

CHAPTER 8

Integrating *mindbodyenergy* and its many systems

T his chapter explores multidimensional aspects of the *mindbodyenergy* system. A particular feature of energy psychotherapy is that it elegantly combines attention to mind, body, and energy systems concurrently. All the components of *mind* are included—such as thoughts, beliefs, and emotions—as well as sensations in the *body*, and the patterning in the *subtle energy system.*

When therapeutic issues are explored in careful detail, this synergy of foci, not found in other approaches to psychotherapy, seems to allow an unusual depth and speed of change.

The subtle energy systems

Energy psychotherapy has made a significant contribution to the healing aspects of therapy by drawing on ancient traditions and integrating subtle energy. It is easier to comprehend this through personal experience, since energy work is essentially experiential and embodied, rather than something to be cognitively analysed. Once I had experienced the radical shifts in myself through energy psychotherapy, there was no looking back.

While those highly trained in acupuncture have a detailed understanding of subtle energies, we can use energy methods effectively with only a rudimentary knowledge of energy anatomy. As our experience develops, we become more finely attuned to working with the three main interconnecting subtle energy systems within *mindbodyenergy* which comprise:

- The meridian system
- The energy centres/chakra system
- The energy bodies (thought-fields, biofield, energy body, aura, light body)

The meridian system

In every culture and in every medical tradition before ours, healing was accomplished by moving energy.

Albert Szent-Gyorgyi, Biochemist and Nobel prize winner. (Reshel, 2016)

Meridians, which have been used in healing work for at least 5000 years, are low-resistance pathways carrying chi (Qi) to body and mind. They became better known in the West in 1972 when Nixon's press secretary had his appendix removed in China under acupuncture anaesthesia. Subsequent research, using light and radioactive isotopes, has shown the existence of these subtle meridian pathways, through which energy flows. Prune Harris,[1] described the meridian system in one workshop, as 'a network of channels in the body that carry information and energy from the energetic core through to the organs'.

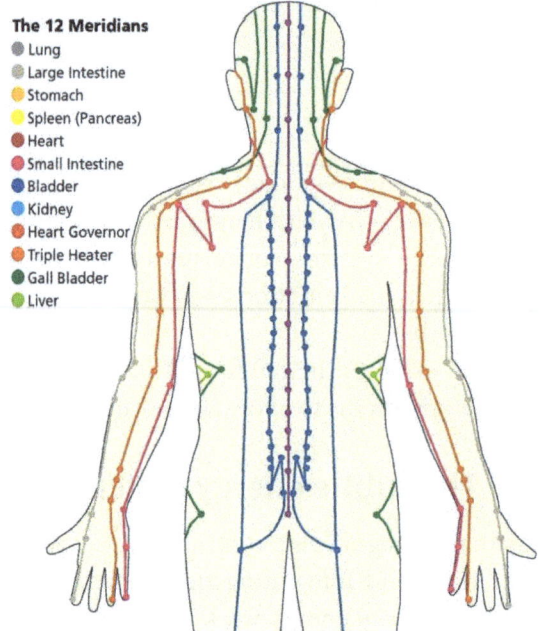

Figure 11 The twelve meridians

Twelve main meridians

The picture of the twelve meridians provides more detail than energy psychotherapists need to know, but it may be helpful to be aware that:

- There are fourteen channels (twelve organ-related meridians plus the central and governing vessels).

---

[1] Prune Harris of www.imaginalhealth.com

- Some flow from centre to periphery (yang), some from periphery to centre (yin).
- Some flow to/from upper limbs, some to/from lower limbs.
- Meridians are paired, e.g. kidney/bladder: the kidney meridian starts at the little toe, and the bladder meridian ends there.
- Where the meridians flow close to the skin, they can be accessed via acupoints.

Axiotonal lines

The axiotonal lines are meridians which extend outside the body and connect us with other subtle dimensions and the stars. Phil Mollon provides a fuller explanation of these in *Blue Diamond Healing* (2022, pp. 147–150 and other references) and axiotonal lines are also used extensively in the energy healing method in *The Reconnection* (Pearl, 2004).

Energy centres/chakras

A map of the energy centres has been described fully in Chapter 6. The word 'chakra' comes from a Sanskrit term meaning wheel, hence the idea of chakras as spinning vortices of energy. Energy psychotherapy accesses these in various ways—for example through touch, breath, visualisation, and intention. Some people are quite sensitive, so prefer to hold the palm of their hand a little bit away from the chakra. Others are happy to place their hands directly on their bodies.

Mini brains—neuron-rich energy centres

With our current understanding of the brain, we know that neurons are omnipresent throughout the body. The anatomical location of the energy centre/chakras often approximates to the site where there are major nerve clusters (or plexuses), hence Candace Pert referred to them as 'mini brains'. Neurologically, these are neurone-rich energy centres, such as the 'brain in the gut' which has the intuitive wisdom of 'gut feelings'.

The midline axis

The main energy centres or chakras are aligned vertically down the midline of the body along the spinal column—the *Line of the Light* (Levin[2])—and connect directly with the nervous system. We are often drawn to place our hands automatically on the midline of our bodies in times of stress, and our language speaks of these centres indirectly, for example, 'I felt gutted', 'I felt choked'. When asked, 'where do you feel this?' clients will often know and be able to point to or reference areas associated with the chakras, such as their heart, solar plexus, or throat. Others don't have such a sense and that is also fine.

---

[2] *Line of the Light* (Levin, 2001) see footnote 4, Chapter 2.

Contemporary reflections on the energy centres/chakras

- The chakras are 'sacred chambers of memory and consciousness' (Anodea Judith).
- Donna Eden regards chakras as energy stations, with memory encoded just as memory is chemically encoded in neurons. She understands each chakra as having seven layers.
- Hover-Kramer suggests that chakras can be thought of as energy transformation stations, rather like an electrical transformer, in comparison to meridians which carry electrical information to facilitate intercellular communication, and the biofield, which operates like an electromagnetic field. This threefold subtle energy system is continuously interacting within itself with physiological information systems (Hover-Kramer, 2002).
- Specific chakras link to different layers of the biofield, connecting:
  - Physically with the glands, organs, and other physical structures
  - Psychologically with emotions
  - Mentally with thoughts
  - Spiritually with different archetypal energies and spiritual development stages
  - At a subtle energy level with the meridians
- 'Stairgates' to higher dimensions: there are additional chakras above and below the body which connect us with higher dimensions including the stars (Phil Mollon).

Energy fields

In Chapter 2 I introduced you to subtle energy fields—known variously as aura, light body, energy body, biofield, and thoughtfields—to describe the field of energy and information that surrounds and interpenetrates the human body. In fact, there are many more terms. The essential feature is that this subtle energy field is composed of both measurable electromagnetic energy and hypothetical subtle energy, or Qi. Various 'versions' of energy fields seem to have many interconnections and overlap, although as Rupert Sheldrake points out, no one knows precisely how they all work. As this book is an introduction, I am not going into these in depth.

Thought fields

Callahan's Thought Field Therapy (TFT) forms a fundamental basis for meridian work and acupoint tapping. Thought fields are like a 'container' of all the information in the mind, body, energy system and environment. In TFT, thought is conceptualised as a form of energy, bound within an intangible system known as a 'thought field'. Different thought patterns are associated with different thought fields. Energy generally flows throughout each thought field, but the pathway can become blocked by conflicted thoughts or 'perturbations' which are information-encoded in the energy system. These 'perturbations' can be caused by negative life events such as trauma or a painful unresolved event, which results in psychological and sometimes physiological symptoms.

> The thought is encoded in the patterning of the energy field, which is expressed in the sequence of the meridians that require to be treated. This sequence is analogous to a code for a combination lock. (Mollon, 2008, p. 53)

The role of the therapist in TFT becomes that of 'decoding' the perturbation (disturbances in the body and troubling emotions), finding and tapping on the correct sequence of meridians to eliminate these perturbations, which shifts the signals which underly the perturbations. In this way, built-up energy can be released very rapidly, removing the cause of the symptoms.

Patterns in the morphic fields (Sheldrake) and the collective unconscious (Jung)

Sheldrake likened his concepts of morphic fields and morphic resonance with Jung's collective unconscious. He identified that an important aspect of the 'field' is the *repetition of patterns*. This is similar to Jung's concept of archetypal energies. He hypothesised that once a new morphic field—a new pattern of organisation—has come into being, through repetition the field becomes stronger. The same pattern becomes more likely to happen again the more often the patterns are repeated. The fields contain a kind of cumulative memory and become increasingly habitual (Sheldrake, 2020). Sheldrake also identified the principle of collective learning through the morphogenic field—that the learning acquired solely through a critical number of prior individuals now passes into the collective and enables subsequent generations to acquire these same skills and capacities much more easily. The collective aspect of consciousness is increasingly important these days

Mindosphere and interconnectivity (Siegel)

Dan Siegel emphasises the principle of interconnectivity—that we have many ways in which energy flows through our life experience. He calls this flow of energy and information the 'mindosphere' in which we live, which includes the body and our web of interconnectivity with the whole world (Siegel, 2012).

'The field'/the unified field/quantum field have been mentioned on many occasions.

Energy bodies

Biofields

Hover-Kramer describes biofields as 'a subtle form of electro-magnetic emanation that extends beyond the physical body' (2002). Our energy bodies intersect with the chakras and meridians providing routes through which energetic information is registered, transmitted, and communicated. In the insert United States and Canada, nurses have been trained to work with biofields and chakras through 'therapeutic touch'.[3] This is accepted as a valid clinical modality after well-designed research demonstrated how this work reduced anxiety and pain, increased haemoglobin levels, increased immune system responses, and accelerated wound healing.

Merkabah, astral, or light body

Another term is the astral body or Merkabah, our personal light body vehicle. We tend to associate this with other-worldly realms of multidimensional reality such as the astral world, the dream world, or the reality where spirits reside after death. The astral body—as all energy bodies—is not bound by space, time, or conditions such as heat, cold, or other physical conditions. During my early thirties, my partner Ulli and I were interested to learn how to astral travel. We 'put it out' to the universe that we would like to meet someone who could help, and synchronously found ourselves connecting with a man at Glastonbury who specialised in this. He taught us to how to astral travel in our Merkabahs, assisted by crystals. Knowing what I now know about energy, and the potential dangers of encountering not very pleasant energies in the astral field—especially if one is not balanced, aligned, or has 'holes' in the energy field (something I explore later)—I am somewhat horrified that we did this without more grounding and preparation. I am grateful that we were somehow protected and came to no harm. These days lots of people experiment with astral travel. I would tend to urge caution, since if a person is fragmented or traumatised in some way, it can be an unpleasant and destabilising experience.

The layers of our energy bodies

I shared a basic model of the four layers of energy bodies in the energy field surrounding us in Chapter 2. However, there is no definitive model of how many layers there are. The following ideas extend the discussion—and please also do your own research.

Barbara Brennan and Edgar Cayce speak of seven layers which connect with the seven-chakra model. Figure 12 illustrates this model. From the skin outwards these are (broadly):

1. Etheric body—acts as a bridge between physical and non-physical
2. Emotional body
3. Mental/cognitional body
4. Spiritual/intuitive body
5. Archetypal/human morphic field (Jung's 'collective unconscious')
6. Celestial/causal
7. Transcendental/soul

Donna Eden, who also 'sees' energy, understands there to be nine different layers which she describes in her book *Energy Medicine*, a generous and fascinating resource. Others speak of twelve chakras with twelve layers of subtle bodies and others, even more. Prune Harris, an energy medicine practitioner in UK, who like Donna Eden, also 'sees' energy, talks about the

---

[3] http://therapeutic-touch.org/

importance of the surrounding *membrane* of the energy body. This is like the concept of energy boundaries which is explored at the end of this chapter.

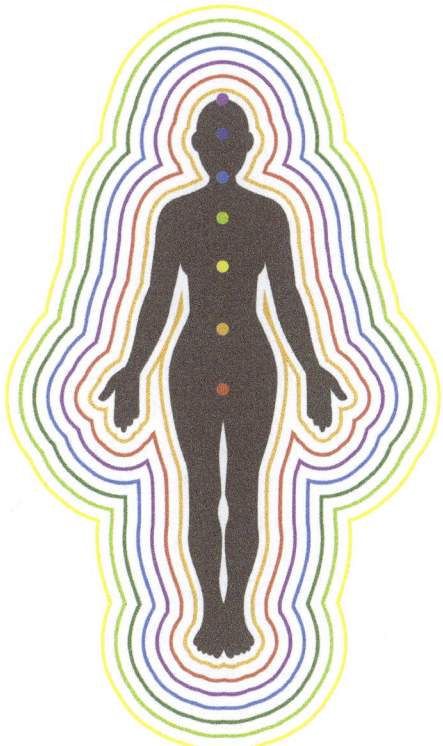

Figure 12 The subtle energy bodies/biofields around the body

I find that the widely accepted model I discussed in Chapter 2 is sufficient for energy psycho-therapy, so I will expand on it just a little here.

The 'band widths' of each principal layer—mental, emotional, and spiritual—vary from person to person, depending on their main mode of relating with the world. One client who was quite cut off from her emotions drew how she perceived her energy bodies. Her emotional body had a very narrow 'band', whereas her mental/cognitive body, the level from which she largely operated, was well developed and quite wide.

CAUSAL REALM—'Source' energy is furthest away from the physical body and resonates at the finest and quickest vibrations[4] flowing down through the bands of energy bodies around our physical body. Our 'Soul body' inhabits the causal realm.

---

[4] When speaking of the fine vibrations of the causal realm, at the time of writing this, one of the highest, finest, and fastest vibrations yet recorded are the gama rays identified in the Milky Way by NASA. This is the 'Fermi bubble'—a quantum energy field of gamma radiation in an infinite symbol of the figure of eight which spans sixty thousand miles.

SPIRITUAL BODY—the outer layer is the spiritual body or 'ideal' realm which has fine, fast vibrations. To be receptive to spiritual guidance, we need to clear any spiritual, mental, and emotional trauma so our subtle bodies are as clear and well balanced as possible. Many have experienced considerable spiritual/religious trauma and/or disconnection from our souls. When we die, hopefully we will have completed the work of clearing such blockages so that our spiritual body is at its peak, and we are in good 'energetic shape' (i.e. without distortions). Many years ago, I was privileged to sit with Dorothy De Chene, a mature Buddhist practitioner, while she was dying of cancer. Despite considerable physical suffering, Dorothy was deeply connected with her spiritual practice, and the doctors and nurses were astonished by the vibrancy of her energy, which had become very refined. It is a precious opportunity to be present when another passes, and I felt humbled by the extraordinary quality of her bright light.

MENTAL BODY—the thinking/intellectual body holds our mental cognitions, thought patterns, and beliefs. Western education is largely directed to developing the mental body, so those who focus on this at the expense of their emotional or spiritual development may have highly developed 'left-brain' functioning without necessarily having a balanced synergy between left and right brain. They may have intellectual but not emotional intelligence. For people who are 'in their head' it can be helpful to ask them to reflect on where their energy is predominantly located. A person will feel more balanced if they can centre their energy; this can be done by breathing through the navel, which brings the energy to a grounded location in the body.

EMOTIONAL BODY—emotion is 'energy in motion', and as our energies fluctuate, we experience mood swings. Energy work can clear the dense energy of trauma that influences mood, unhelpful thoughts, and reactive behaviours. Some connect the astral body with the emotional body.

ETHERIC BODY—closest to the physical body, the etheric body holds the slowest, densest frequencies. Unworked-through or repressed trauma at spiritual, mental, and emotional levels may eventually end up as blockages in the etheric body which sometimes manifest as physical illness.

PHYSICAL BODY—we experience fluctuating levels of energy and wellness in our physical body.

Working from a state of presence rather than empathy

Boundaries

Psychotherapists and counsellors are familiar with the idea that good boundaries are supportive of healthy relationships and bring clarity to the therapeutic frame as part of establishing a therapeutic contract. This contributes to the creation of a safe therapeutic space.

Since energy transmits, therapists need to regularly clear their 'field', otherwise psycho-therapy can sometimes be energetically quite draining, particularly when working with high levels of trauma. A study by Rössler (2012) found that therapists and mental health workers often become ill and burned out when they absorb traumatised energy into their bodies. If we resonate and overly empathise with a highly distressed person this can be problematic, whereas when our own energy field is coherent, and not muddled up with the 'other', we can be more helpful. (See Figure 6 in Chapter 5 to illustrate a healthy field between self and other.)

On a more ordinary level, however, if we get caught up in co-dependent relationships, it is easy for our boundaries to become merged.

Those who have suffered from complex or extreme and life-threatening trauma often have difficulties with self-soothing, so the phenomena of emotional dysregulation, fragmentation, and projection of unconscious material into 'the field' is a therapeutic 'given'. Supervision can help us avoid the dynamics of entanglements—certainly, if we do get caught up in such dynamics, we feel it intensely. Sensitive therapists and clients can easily become a 'clearing station' for others' unprocessed energy—it has certainly taken a while for me to learn how to manage energetically. Working from a higher-gauge state seems to help us from being adversely impacted by traumatised energy, but we do need to consider our energetic boundaries.

Energy boundaries

So, what exactly are energy boundaries? They operate in a similar way to ordinary boundaries but at the level of subtle energy. They pertain to the state of coherence of our energy fields in relation to ourselves, others, and the wider world and environment. These apply to all our relationships—with family, colleagues, intimate relationships, clients, and the community. Having a strong coherent sense of self can help to keep our 'field' more separated.

'Semi-permeable membrane'

Judith Swack (https://hblu.org/) first introduced the concept of the 'energy boundary' by drawing on her understanding of the role of the semi-permeable membrane in cell biology. The energy boundary is not a wall, but rather, a semi-permeable 'membrane' which allows healthy exchange of energies, information, and emotions, so it is no barrier to love.

Compromised energy boundaries

The energy boundaries between self and other can be impacted by a variety of factors:

- A rupture to the semi-permeable membrane causes tears, holes, and 'leaks' in the energy field. These are caused by traumatic experiences and, since like attracts like, can be an unconscious factor in drawing 'like' resonances into the field and creating what Freud termed 'repetition compulsions'.

- Intrusions from early attachment trauma, mergers, or co-dependence with others makes it difficult to operate as separate individuals in our own energy field.
- Invasive energies from people in our lives may result in carrying the energy of others or being taken over by energy which does not belong to us.
- 'Picking up' from the general thought fields of the mass collective—for instance when travelling on the tube or being bombarded by energy from the media and TV. When we get caught in 'the group soup' and absorb these (habitually) low vibrations full of all the latest fears and anxieties, it can be very draining.
- Intrusive thoughts, memories, nightmares, or flashbacks can 'flood' us.
- Empaths and sensitive people are adversely affected in quite debilitating ways and may have quite a 'porous' field so that, especially when working with complex trauma, there is a need to protect the field from taking in so much projection and fragmentation.
- Archetypal energies—severe and complex trauma often bring in archetypal levels of wounding of the spirit and soul. These impingements are outlined by Donald Kalsched in his work *The Inner World of Trauma* and *Trauma and the Soul*. Such energies are often powerfully visceral. Projective identifications can feel very disturbing, getting right inside us, leaving us ruminating about an event long after it happened.
- Inner 'attacking voices' are another biproduct of trauma which can affect *internal* boundaries between parts of the self.
- Re-enactments: the unconscious dynamics of the 'drama triangle' of *victim, rescuer, and abuser* roles may be enacted, with boundaries unwittingly becoming blurred in therapy. Frawley and Davies recognised that when working with survivors of abuse, transference and countertransference dynamics manifest where the client experiences their therapist as being like—for example—their sadistic abuser or betraying mother (Davies & Frawley, 1994). Naturally if the therapist is at fault, this requires acknowledgement and full-hearted apology. Energy psychotherapy can be helpful in repairing such traumatic ruptures directly using energy methods which bring relief, 'clear the field', and make the therapeutic space safe again: e.g. KC tapping *Even though I feel betrayed by* (name of therapist), *and I am feeling misunderstood and unsafe, and I am not sure if I can trust* (him/her) *again, I acknowledge and honour all these feelings and completely love and accept myself.* Then further tapping or chakra clearing can be undertaken to elicit and clear all the relevant feelings from this therapeutic rupture. Sadly however, such ruptures are not always repairable.

The process of strengthening energy boundaries

Freud spoke of our body ego as serving our first boundary with the world. It is interesting that when we strengthen energy boundaries—and there is an energy protocol following which facilitates this—this in itself is ego strengthening and contributes to a greater sense of self.

In the process of energy psychotherapy and trauma clearing we reduce the 'heavy' energies from ourselves and from the transgenerational trauma of others in our field. This work reduces triggering and helps us both to become 'lighter' while, at the same time, healthily strengthening our egos and our bodily ego. This reduces the porousness of our semi-permeable membrane, so we take in less dense energy into our field from others (the energy of others does not belong there).

As our energy boundaries become stronger, it becomes easier to deal with the natural flow and with the full palate and range of human emotions/vibrations as they arise—we become less impacted by triggering of past trauma or the heavy/denser vibrations of others. Through this process we become more sovereign in our own field—dealing with 'our own stuff'.

It may be that as we raise our vibration overall, the higher vibrations of 'love and above' flow freely to and fro whilst heavier or lower vibrations from other people, groups, collective unconscious are less able to pass through the 'semi-permeable membrane' into our field.

The importance of maintaining strong energy boundaries

When we develop this semi-permeable membrane around our own personal energy field this helps us maintain our own 'shape' and integrity when under challenge from a variety of intrusions. If people have weak or porous energy boundaries, they are very exposed, but when boundaries are 100 per cent intact, it strengthens a person's sense of identity and a knowing of 'this is where I begin and end'. Maintaining strong and healthy energy boundaries is an ongoing process which is as important in intimate relationships as in any other context.

Intentionality

Brockman (2006) refers to levels of awareness, intentionality, and choice which can help us to maintain our boundaries. He regards an energy boundary in terms of a limit that we intentionally establish to protect the integrity of ourselves and our life, which keeps us connected to ourselves so we can decide what energy, thoughts, emotions to let in or keep out. I find for myself that this work is constant and I regularly need to clear my field.

Changing our ways of working

In counselling and psychotherapy trainings, 'empathy' and 'resonance' are very much encouraged as ways of holding clients. However, empathy brings with it a potential for over-identification which can create a 'merged' porous energy field. This is energetically draining and unhelpful to both therapist and client. Alternatively, to keep our energy fields coherent and unentangled, mirroring back our understanding of our clients' issue from a heart-based state of presence and compassion provides a spacious but intimate way of helping the client to feel fully seen and recognised. Such a change, where the therapy relationship is subtly different, reflects one way that the energetic shift on our planet is impacting psychotherapy.

The outlook of the Piscean age involved taking on others' suffering, putting ourselves in their shoes, and feeling their pain. I regularly took in and metabolised others' experiences, feeding it back in digestible ways, which depleted me, and I was often ill. I eventually attended an energy training workshop. The trainer, a clairvoyant, 'saw' my energy and noticed that when people in the group were sharing, I literally left my body to be alongside the person who was talking; I was no longer fully centred and present in my body. The issue with empathy was that I needed to stop identifying with and 'taking on' the other's energy into my field. I am very grateful to him for teaching me another way, so that my energy boundaries are now more resilient.

In the Aquarian Age the trend is towards sovereignty and taking personal responsibility. The new way requires more autonomous relationships, where we maintain the integrity of our own energy systems, and relate with compassion in a state of Presence, centred in our own field. We offer support while clients do their own self-clearing, respecting the client's autonomy in taking care of and loving their child parts, an approach which, while acknowledging and honouring vulnerability, does not overly encourage dependency or co-dependence. Therapeutic work can also sometimes include an element of psycho-education where we can discuss and talk about healthy boundaries with our clients.

Presence rather than empathy

In a heart-felt state of Presence we remain centred in ourselves, while compassion naturally radiates. This spacious calm neutrality—perhaps similar to the state of not-knowing Bion described as 'without memory or desire'—facilitates healthy energy boundaries and takes care of the integrity of each person's energy field.

Our true essence is a non-conceptual experience of light and pure energy which can only be accessed when we are in the present moment. The more we shed our triggers and release the traumas and dramas of our stories, the easier it is to access this still point, the 'zero point' space where we are grounded, clear, and centred. Whether we see Presence as our connection with God, 'Source', our soul—or whatever—it is a universal principle that humanity has the capacity to access these expanded 'states' of consciousness.

Chapter 2 discusses some ways of accessing Presence.

Strengthening energy boundaries

The facility to strengthen energy boundaries is a valuable resource in energy psychotherapy. We can strengthen boundaries between:

- The traumatic event/memory and ourselves, which makes it easier to work on the details of the issue
- Relationships in the present where there are difficulties and enmeshments
- Relationships from the past which are still intruding
- Inner warring parts

STRENGTHENING ENERGY BOUNDARIES WITH SPECIFIC PERSONS OR EVENT(S)

Energy balancing methods and KC reversals in this protocol can be found in Chapter 7.

PROTOCOL: Use KC (karate-chop) tapping to clear each limiting core belief (reversal) which prevents you from having healthy boundaries. The simplest way to do this is without energy testing, assuming that you need to strengthen ALL of the core beliefs outlined and so you run through each one, adapting the template phrase below and tapping on the KC point as you do so.

> ***Even though I don't (or part of me doesn't) BELIEVE I DESERVE … to strengthen my energy boundary with X, I love and accept myself and ask for help in knowing that I DO DESERVE and am entitled to have strong healthy boundaries with X***

1. Start by doing some **energy balancing** exercises

2. **Guesstimate** OR use energy testing **the current strength of the boundary**, which ideally needs to be at 100 per cent (0–100 per cent) by asking the client to say:

   *e.g. **My energy boundary with the X is:** e.g. 5 per cent, 45 per cent, 63 per cent, etc.*

3. **Run through the list of reversals below**, saying each statement out loud. (If following the protocol using self-energy testing: test each statement for yourself, or, if working with another, self-energy test on their behalf.)

   o **I WANT to strengthen the boundary**
   If this energy tests WEAK, tap on the karate-chop point saying—for example—*'Even though some part of me does not want to strengthen my energy boundary with X, I deeply love and accept myself and ask for help with my ambivalence'*

   o **I DESERVE to strengthen the boundary**
   If WEAK, tap on the karate-chop point saying *'Even though I don't (or part of me doesn't) believe I deserve to strengthen my energy boundary with X, I love and accept myself and ask for help in knowing that I do deserve and am entitled to have strong healthy boundaries with X'*

   o **IT IS SAFE for me to strengthen the boundary**
   If WEAK, tap on the karate-chop point saying *'Even though it does not feel safe for me to strengthen my energy boundary with X, I deeply love and accept myself and ask for help in finding better ways of keeping myself safe'*

   o **IT IS POSSIBLE for me to strengthen the boundary**
   If WEAK, tap on the karate-chop point saying *'Even though it does not feel possible for me to strengthen my energy boundary with X, I deeply love and accept myself and ask for help in being open to the possibility that I can have a strong, healthy energy boundary with X'*

   o **I AM TOO ANGRY to strengthen the boundary**
   If STRONG (NB please note that depending on the statements, the correct healthy response will vary—in this situation STRONG indicates there is further reversal clearing to do) tap on the karate-chop point saying *'Even though I am far too angry to strengthen my energy boundary with X, I deeply love and accept myself, all parts of me,*

including my legitimate and healthy anger, and I ask for help in releasing myself from this bind of the anger'

- o **I HOLD TOO MUCH SHAME** to feel able to strengthen the boundary
  If STRONG (*NB please note that depending on the statements, the correct healthy response will vary—STRONG here indicates there is further reversal clearing to do*), tap on the karate-chop point saying '*Even though I (or parts of me) hold too much shame to feel able to strengthen my energy boundary with X, I deeply love and accept myself, all parts of me (especially the parts holding the most shame) and I ask for help in releasing myself from this shame'*

4. **Recheck strength of boundary** by guesstimating or energy testing. It should have gone up

5. **Use waterfall chakra clearing** with a phrase such as
   '***Everything that stops me having a strong energy boundary with xxx***'

6. **Recheck strength of boundary and continue to 100 per cent**

7. **Check if it would be helpful to maintain the boundary by a daily practice: This can be done by:**

   - Tapping on the heart chakra for about a minute each day with the **intention** of maintaining a strong, healthy, protective, and resilient energy boundary with xxx.
   - Set the intention to maintain a strong, healthy, protective, and resilient boundary.

Sometimes when we undertake energy work, we strengthen the boundary before going on to clear the trauma. Or we can do it the other way round. In the following example, we cleared the trauma first, which had created holes and tears in the client's field, and followed this with energy boundary strengthening.

EXAMPLE

Angelina was a kind, sensitive Polish woman who frequently visited her elderly parents at weekends. She would return to her flat drained and emotionally battered. Angelina's father had always been very abusive to her, taking out his anger on her since her childhood. Her boyfriend was similarly abusive. Angelina felt it was her duty to care for everyone, regardless of how they treated her. She had virtually no boundaries and her energy was constantly depleted. Caring and idealistic, she very much wanted to help her father who had never received love. After one visit to her parents, she arrived home in a state of total exhaustion, only to find that her partner, another emotionally 'starved waif' like her father, had also collapsed. Very jealous of Angelina for giving attention to her father, he often became extremely ill, competing for her attention while also being cruel to her.

During our work, we cleared various traumas around Angelina's abusive father. The following formulation was rather long, but Angelina was keen to have all the details in.

CLEARING PHRASE

Dad was verbally battered and shamed by his violent father, and starved of love from his withholding mother, so he was jealous of mum's love for me. He took it out on me by emotionally battering me, so I have holes and tears in my energy field. When I am with dad, I pick up his 'starving' energy which totally depletes me, and I carry the shattering weight of his unmet need.

We used a mixture of tapping and chakra work to clear this.

We also cleared similar types of traumas linking this pattern in relation to her boyfriend. During this work, Angelina recognised that in trying to 'rescue' her emotionally damaging father and partner, she was damaging herself.

We then went on to strengthen the energy boundaries between her father, and her boyfriend. Through this work Angelina became more aware of the ways she put herself at risk. She had previously been oblivious of her need for safety and self-care. Angelina noticed a significant difference in her energy and resilience. With some psycho-educational work around learning to set limits and boundaries, she reduced her predilection for going into and putting up with abusive situations and took better care of herself.

Self-care and protection from energy burnout

Working with energy requires developing self-care habits, so that we do not carry energy which does not belong to us. This is very important. I wish I had known these methods earlier on in my work so as to have better maintained energetic coherence and resilience. This selection of methods (there are many more) can be helpful for everyone.

Figure of 8 (mentioned previously): imagine/visualise that you are sitting within a figure of 8. You are inside one of the circles and the other person is in the other. In this way you are connected but separate which helps you to stop absorbing or taking in projections from the 'field' of the other.

Clearing your field at the end of the day (or after sessions) with a chakra waterfall using a phrase such as:

All that remains in my field that doesn't belong to me and doesn't resonate with love.

Clearing the field includes removing energetic relationship 'cording' which can link us unhealthily with others.

Resourcing with Presence and self-love: a significant step towards awakening is to find balance and love ourselves completely in all ways—not egotistical/narcissistic love but the love that aligns us and helps us to be open and balanced. Creating a space for regular meditation practice is also helpful.

Surround yourself in a light bubble

Imagine being enclosed in your own pulsating, translucent bubble that allows you to communicate effectively with anyone you choose and to be comfortable with intimacy, assists you in emotional and intellectual discernment, filters the cultural assault of noise, lights and toxins and enables, if you choose, a relaxed safe connection with the spiritual world. (Hammond & Crowley, 2008, p. 115)

Being mindful of the energy fields of others: as well as caring for our own fields, being sensitive to the fields of others is also important. My own energy can be quite 'big' at times. During the numerous energetic shifts occurring on the planet, I have been challenged in managing my own expanding energy and regret that sometimes I have been insensitive to others' energies. People can easily feel invaded, shamed, or vulnerable to being overpowered by others' energy, especially when working with trauma, which is why Presence is so helpful.

Trauma and the nervous system

The *mindbodyenergy* systems include subtle energy and nervous systems which both serve as a bridge between psyche and soma. Understanding how the nervous system is impacted by trauma helps identify what is required therapeutically.

Trauma, its impact on the body, and post-traumatic stress (PTSD)

Trauma is experienced at visceral, embodied levels, with stress, PTSD, and complex trauma affecting all bodily systems including the nervous system, immune, hormonal, respiratory, circulatory, digestive, and other systems as well as our subtle energy. When activated by trauma, our bodies are 'triggered' into 'heightened states', and our systems react in various ways. Energy psychotherapy addresses such states of psycho-biological 'arousal'—we look for and pay special attention to specific energetic charges or somatic states:

- Bodily signs of distress include physical symptoms—raised heart rate, shallow breathing, hyperventilation, panic attacks, heart pain, feeling sick, dizziness and others.
- The fight, flight, freeze, flop aspects of the neurological systems are widespread. For instance, when the frontal lobe becomes 'frozen' by trauma, people go 'blank' and are unable to think or find words. 'Stuck' trauma can manifest in various debilitating ways, causing difficulties in moving, making progress in life, or achieving adult 'developmental milestones' in relationships, work, finances etc.
- An inability to cope with affect (emotions)—the traumatised person may become emotionally dysregulated and unable to self-soothe, shutting down, disconnecting, or dissociating.
- 'Triggered' states of mind include debilitating shame and anxiety (another physiological condition); triggering of aggression/rage under stress; 'affect storms' such as states of uncontrollable 'ranting'; and extreme mood swings.
- Shattered states and fragmentation into parts. The ego may fragment, including into traumatised parts, such as young-child and dissociated parts.

- Archetypal energies: deep repetition compulsions bring out archetypal energies which can take over the ego's functioning such as 'victim', 'abuser', 'judge', 'wounded child', or the 'persecutor/protector' (Kalsched, 1996).
- Hypervigilance is common, with symptoms such as sleeplessness, nightmares, ultra-alertness, and a constantly scanning 'radar' looking out for potential dangers.
- Flashbacks—intrusive images of past trauma being experienced as though in the present, and 'unprocessed' memories which keep recirculating.
- *Overload and emotional flooding*—an incapacity to deal with people and situations on account of overwhelming anxiety and emotions.
- Somatisation—when events cannot be put into words, distress may manifest as physical pain, inflammatory response, auto-immune and other illness.[5] The nature of the illness or the part of the body affected may be a metaphor for what cannot be communicated in other ways, to themselves or others.
- Intrusive thoughts and flashbacks.
- OCD and other symptoms.

Unresolved trauma may result in people being stuck in 'survival mode', in one or other of the fight, flight, freeze, flop or fawn (people pleasing) trauma modalities of the nervous system. This can be life-shattering and life, limiting. It is with gratitude that energy psychotherapy and other bodily based methods help us resolve such states gently, harmonising mind and body so that significant numbers of clients find real relief and healing.

Polyvagal theory and the parasympathetic/sympathetic nervous systems

Our body and brain help us survive in the moment using the protective elements of the vagus nerve and the parasympathetic and sympathetic nervous systems.

Neuroception (Porges)—an intuitive sense of when we might be in danger

> Neuroception is the term used to describe the way our autonomic nervous system scans for cues of safety, danger and life threat without involving the thinking parts of our brain. (Dana, 2018)

Our bodies do things to protect us. The automatic reflexes of the vagus nerve responses are context-specific and protect us in times of danger. People sometimes reflect after an assault 'But why didn't I fight?' In some situations, immobilisation is the best defence, so this wasn't a choice—it was the neuro-implicit perception adapted for survival. Neuroception is that sense of intuition which warns us that someone or something around us is a threat to us. We are not

---

[5] A high incidence of severe depression, post-traumatic stress disorder, and medical retirement from South Yorkshire Police followed the Hillsborough Disaster (1989). An unpublished pilot study in an NHS psychotherapy service I worked in showed that 55 per cent of our patients suffered from PTSD and also had physiological illness and symptoms.

always aware of the external cues of danger, but our bodily cues 'know' and bring issues to our awareness via physiological responses, alerting us as to what needs attention.

However, as a result of trauma, neuroception may be faulty, misfiring, and detecting danger when there isn't any, setting our senses on high alert. Alternatively, when a person's neuroception and gut feelings have been traumatically overridden, neuroception may be 'switched off' so the person is unable to discern levels of safety and risk.

The vagus nerve, parasympathetic and sympathetic nervous systems: safety, danger, and life threat

Awareness of three broad states (or biological pathways of response (Dana, 2020)) of the *mindbodyenergy* system are relevant since we are regularly working with all these systems in energy psychotherapy when working with trauma.

1. ENGAGEMENT: the *ventral vagal* nervous system signals safety, enabling curiosity, play, and social connection.
2. MOBILISATION: the fight/flight survival mode, which cuts social connection, restricts, and narrows cognition and perception, and prepares the body for fighting or running away.
3. COLLAPSE: THE SHUT-DOWN, FREEZE, FLOP, DISSOCIATION state when the *dorsal vagal* nervous system is dominant.

ENGAGEMENT, SOCIAL CONNECTEDNESS, AND SAFETY—*via the downregulation of the ventral vagal system and parasympathetic nervous system*

Establishing safety is key. Polyvagal theory links the idea of social connectedness as a signification factor in facilitating recovery from trauma. It is concerned with:

- *safety*—how the vagus nerve reacts to safety
- *connectedness*—feeling attached to others helps us feel safe.

A neurological understanding about social interaction is particularly relevant when 'talking is not enough' and people are experiencing traumatic states 'beyond words'. The vagus nerve—which goes from brainstem to the heart—is concerned with our social engagement system and picks up signals from others via body language. The muscles of vocalisation, listening, and gesture are linked to the vagus nerve, regulating the heart, enabling our bodies to be in states of psycho-biological attunement which support growth and health. If those signals—such as positive facial cues and tone of voice—are friendly, they calm us via the down-regulating activity of the ventral vagal system which activates the parasympathetic (the 'rest–digest') nervous system and brings a sense of safety. 'Being' and 'Presence' aid social connectedness and attunement. A calm therapist with a calming voice helps to regulate stress hormones which gives rise to the implicit thought 'It is safe to be over the trauma now'. This brings about a slowing and increase of coherence in heart rate, the same social connection system that is active in the mother–baby nursing situation (Porges & Dana, 2018). In this way, the therapeutic relationship provides a safe 'other' which the senses react to through psycho-biological interconnectedness in the 'field'.

Energy techniques can speed up the process of establishing safety and relatively easily bring about emotional regulation. The client may feel empowered and able to take control through using self-care energy resources. This makes it safe enough to work through the trauma itself. Gradually the sense of safety extends into the lives of people as they recover from their traumatic experiences, finding other 'safe' people and developing a sense of calm, containment, and connectedness outside the therapeutic situation.

DANGER AND MOBILISATION—FIGHT, FLIGHT, FREEZE/DISSOCIATION
Sympathetic nervous system activates the fight or flight response, preparing for action:
Under danger and duress, the sympathetic system mobilises us into action through:

- increasing muscle blood flow and tension
- dilating pupils
- accelerating heart rate and respiration, and
- increasing perspiration and arterial blood pressure.

The freeze/dissociation response (a parasympathetic brake on the motor system)

- The freeze response is not a passive state but rather a parasympathetic brake on the motor system, relevant to perception and action preparation while deciding whether to fight or flee. It leaves us temporarily paralysed by fear and unable to move. In this response, rather than fighting off the danger or running away from it, we do nothing; the perceived threat causes a hypotonic or immobile reaction. Someone in a freeze response may experience numbness or the sense of dread or dissociation, thinking (the frontal lobe) goes 'off-line' and it is usually not possible to find words.

LIFE THREAT—*the 'flop' response: the dorsal vagal system and parasympathetic nervous system*

In life-threatening emergency, the *dorsal vagal system* engages the parasympathetic nervous system, a 'last-ditch' survival mechanism when the possibilities of both fight and flight are perceived as inadequate. In times of threat to life, the parasympathetic system goes beyond its 'rest and digest' function and closes down the body in order conserve energy, by

- slowing the heart rate
- decreasing intestinal and gland activity, and
- relaxing sphincter muscles in the gastrointestinal tract.

This reaction of physiological immobilisation—a life-saving protective shutting down for survival which might include passing out and total collapse of energy—is as a result of extreme fear beyond fight/flight stress. The functioning of the parasympathetic nervous system in this way is best illustrated by animals under attack: sometimes they 'play dead' so convincingly that the predator will walk away, leaving them to escape when the coast is clear. In working with trauma, if a person manifests total collapse and 'losing energy', it is an indicator of extreme fear.

EXAMPLE

Working with the 'flop' response

Ralph was sadistically tortured by his mother from babyhood. When he first came to therapy, he was highly dissociated. Ralph often 'collapses' into a total loss of energy and we have pieced together that this is because he is entering the territory of life-threatening early abuse. A simple method we use in energy therapy to bring him out of 'flop'—when he is ready to do so—is for him to rub all his chakras, which brings energy back into them. Ralph is very sensitive to energy work, so, little by little, we have been doing small pieces of trauma clearing using tapping and the chakras, facilitated also by his art-work, where he draws, paints, and communicates things for which there are no words. Ralph's dissociation is lessening and his ego strengthening through this process. He feels more of his feelings, can remain in his body, and is more in control about choosing how much he does—or doesn't—wish to explore and clear energetically. Creating safety and pacing the work slowly is key when working with complex trauma.

Hyper- and hypo-arousal and their relevance for muscle/energy testing

'The window of affective tolerance' (Siegel) is a valuable concept for understanding the hyper- and hypo-arousal of the nervous system experienced by people in times of distress.

- When in a state of '*optimum arousal*' people function normally, responses are manageable. and people can think.
- *Hyper-arousal*: when stress increases to the level of '*hyper-arousal*' people are mobilised for action. This state is associated with *fight and flight*, hypervigilance, anger, agitation, and freeze responses to trauma, or sometimes there is panic or impulsivity instead. Hyper-arousal, with its tendency to a *rigid* muscle state, can also impact energy testing.
- *Hypo-arousal*: when the person lose energy, collapses, and their muscles flop, they are numb and desensitised to external experience. This may result in poor self-care and boundaries, exhaustion, and on occasion, complete collapse, or shutdown.

Energy methods to balance and regulate the nervous system

Various methods can be used to bring the nervous system into a state of regulation and balance. When working with trauma, many therapists are familiar with employing the five senses to ground people, help them out of dissociated states and 'back into the room', so these methods are not explored here. If a person's alert system is set too high in constant *hypervigilance* or *hypo-arousal*, their nervous system needs to be re-set using bodily based rather than cognitive methods to calm down or re-energise the system.

Energy work and tapping—'combined cognitive and somatic' approaches

One way of doing so is through tapping on acupoints. When the mind is tuned to a relevant 'thought field', tapping has been shown to bring about benign changes in

- the *brain's neurobiology* and function
- the *body's physiology*
- the *subjective sense of well-being* (Feinstein, 2019, 2021a, 2021b)
- and *facilitating shifts of cognitive and emotional perspective.*

In the fight/flight or dissociation–freeze state associated with the dorsal ventral system, there is no safety. Acupoint tapping, targeting specific thought fields, has been shown to shift the *bodymindenergy* system towards the state of safety associated with activation of the ventral vagal nervous system. In this state, a person can review and reappraise current situations and their inner working models of the world. (Similar processes are involved in working with the chakra system confirmed by recent research (Brown et al., 2023).)

Thus, the NICE guidelines refer to acupoint tapping methods as 'combined cognitive and somatic' approaches.

> Preliminary evidence supports speculation, which is consistent with more than a hundred peer-reviewed clinical trials, that the procedure can send deactivating signals to areas of the limbic system that are in hyperarousal and can send activating signals to regions of the prefrontal cortex that support executive functions such as planning and managing stressful situations. (Feinstein, 2021b)[6]

Seven methods for working with dysregulation and triggering

All these de-stressing methods are helpful for both therapists and clients. Some have already been described in Chapter 7:

1. ENERGY BALANCING
2. KARATE-CHOP (KC) TAPPING
3. WATERFALL CHAKRA CLEARING
4. NAVEL TAPPING: This method quickly brings down triggering in the moment, helps to ground and bring the person back into their body. Simply ask your client to tap a little bit above the navel for about fifteen taps and you also can do so at the same time, modelling this. It is also possible simply to hold or rub the navel if tapping doesn't feel comfortable.

---

[6] Feinstein (2021b) summarises and illustrates how energy psychology modalities, such as acupoint tapping, can 'facilitate beneficial changes in the neurological underpinnings of:
  (1) mental states that impede immune function
  (2) emotional influences that contribute to illness
  (3) inner resources that promote healing'.

5. NAVEL BREATHING: The client is asked to bring their breath down lower into their body as though breathing in and out through the navel (the centre of the body).

6. VAGUS NERVE BREATHING: When people habitually live in hypervigilant states, they need to learn how to down regulate their system into the calming aspects produced by the vagus nerve. Otherwise, when the adrenal system becomes exhausted, the person will struggle to sleep. The vagus nerve breath practice is a useful resource for engaging the parasympathetic ('rest/digest') aspects of the autonomic nervous system, bringing a person out of 'triggered' states. This can prevent burn out.

7. BURN-OUT: In cases of burn-out, where people may end up not being able to sleep, vitamin supplementation is generally required, and sometimes adrenal glandular medicine will be needed to repair the adrenal glands.

VAGUS NERVE BREATH PRACTICE: 4–7–8 (or if these counts are too long, 3–5–7)
(The simplest form of practice is where the out-breath is two counts longer than the in-breath)

Vagus nerve breath practise 'down regulates' the body, bringing it into a state of calmness. It takes the nervous system out of hyper-arousal (where the sympathetic nervous system is activated) and into the calm 'rest/digest' state of the parasympathetic nervous system. When someone is 'triggered' it is a good starting place for introducing a simple energy intervention. Some people also find it helps them sleep better. If the seven or eight counts are too long, adjust according to breathing capacities, such as three–five–six, or somewhere in between. When you first start doing vagus nerve breathing, follow this pattern four times. Gradually you can build up to more. It is helpful to do these breaths in regular sessions during the day to entrain yourself, making this breathing a way of life. This is excellent for highly stressed people.

Calmness is the bridge which helps take us out of the lower mind of analytic thinking into the awareness of the higher mind. Breathwork brings us to this balanced calm state. The App https://appsto.re/gb/zZii8.i *Breathe–4-7-8 Method—Keep Calm & Get to Sleep In 1 Minute* by Slay is free. It provides two reminders per day, morning and evening.

- To start, do a deep breath in and out.
- Then breathe in through the nose, to the count of four (the counting is quite steady, less than a second).
- Hold the breath for seven counts.
- Breathe out for eight counts with open mouth and a gentle sigh—'HAAAAA'—with a slight restriction in the throat. This stimulates the vagus nerve which down-regulates the nervous system into a state of calmness.
- Then do another deep breath in and out to end.
- Repeat the whole process a number of times, as feels comfortable.

Other methods for settling the nervous system (see also Chapter 7)

- *Breathing*: navel breathing; lung meridian breathing; collar-bone breathing; heart-rhythm breathing, and two in-breaths followed by a long out-breath on a sigh—'Aah'.
- *Grounding* and physical exercise 'shaking off' the stress in whatever way is suited to the individual.

- *Energy calming methods* (such as 'triple warmer' or 'bird beak'), listening to music and other soothing activities such as being in nature.
- *Re-energising* by rubbing your chakras to bring more energy back into the system.

Somatisation

Energy psychotherapy provides new ways for working with somatisation. Ethically it's important that clients wishing to work on emotional aspects of symptoms have been to see their GPs and undertaken any relevant tests, so that physical issues are appropriately diagnosed. In my experience, people have frequently come to therapy in states of distress where medical tests have revealed physiological causes such as menopause, thyroid, iron deficiencies and so on.

People will be familiar with the idea of somatisation, where unexpressed emotions and conflicts in the mind can be transposed to a disturbance in the body. Most simply, stress impacts the body with the adverse effects of chronic flooding of the body and brain with stress hormones. In addition to the unhelpfully named 'hysterical' states, in deeper, more subtle forms of psychosomatic disturbance, the stress appears relatively absent from the mind and is expressed in the body through completely unconscious processes.

Energy psychotherapy facilitates the bringing into awareness of unconscious emotions. Somatic disturbance can often be worked with effectively and translated back into psychic disturbance, by identifying the relevant trauma so the physical symptom disappears. However, with deeply entrenched conditions, this is often not possible.

Free associations arising from work with the subtle energy systems of chakras and meridians can reveal how these processes occur. The twelve meridians all have links to bodily organs or to bodily systems and emotions. Energy testing helps us to find which meridians are particularly involved in a problem. So, for example:

- Gut problems can indicate difficulties digesting experience as well as literal digestion. These might involve the stomach meridian, small intestine meridian, or large intestine meridian.
- Experiences that are felt to be to be toxic—impossible to digest or metabolise—may be signalled through the liver meridian.
- Rage may show up in the gall bladder meridian—and so on.

When we tap on different points in relation to specific bodily, mental, and emotional states, this can shift proto-mental states (Bion, 1961; Sanders, 1984) moving then energetically through the meridians so they come out in the form of emotional expression, bringing relief and insight. For a chart showing the physical and emotional correlates with the meridian tapping points see Chapter 7. The chakras also have connections with physiological areas as identified in Chapter 6.

The following trauma was cleared before I had come across 'Tearless Trauma Techniques' though the methods we used worked perfectly well, following the client's free associations.

EXAMPLE

Vikki, a young Scottish woman who came from a rather dour Presbyterian background in the Highlands, came for therapy with sexual difficulties. She had happily enjoyed sex during her marriage, but one day totally froze when she saw a sex scene on TV and had been unable to have sex since. She had tried once, but it had been very painful because her body had not created any lubrication. Suddenly sex scared her, and she felt completely blank about it.

In terms of her history, Vikki could not remember much of her early life other than that she had a very strict religious father and an alcoholic mother. Both she and her younger sister had vaguely wondered if they might have been abused by their grandfather, though neither was sure. Aged around eight she had suddenly not liked wearing dresses anymore, and became a tomboy, calling herself Charlie.

A gynaecologist had diagnosed vaginismus and recommended a treatment plan to help her with this. However, Vikki felt so phobic that she could not contemplate any form of sex. Over six months she worked intensively with this issue in energy psychotherapy. Rather than approaching the abuse directly, the order of work was determined by following Vikki's free associations and incidents which had triggered between sessions. This work stabilised and strengthened Vicki's sense of self (ego strengthening).

I have come to totally trust the unconscious, finding that events which present in the moment are those which need attention (even though they may also be a form of avoidance). We energy tested to ensure safety: e.g. *It's in my highest interest to treat this trauma now* and started clearing issues such as

> *When I was young, I didn't want to be a girl, so I called myself Charlie and am still confused about my femininity now so I struggle with my femininity and can't allow myself to wear nice dresses, even though I long to do so.*

Once the therapeutic relationship was secure and Vikki was confident that energy work helped, we cleared a lot of early traumas using mainly tapping and some chakra work regarding her family. At a certain point, Vikki felt she would like to work specifically with the vaginismus. She shared details of her experiences, and we 'tapped while talking' as follows:

> Vikki's inability to have sex was putting a strain on her marriage
> Sex was agonising; her vagina couldn't accept her husband's penis and she was unable to lubricate or secrete any vaginal fluids
> She was upset by sex scenes on TV, feeling that if she watched something, it was actually being done to her.
> She had no sense of how to be around sexuality or femininity, feeling stuck at the age of a young girl rather than a woman
> She had an unpleasant feeling of dryness throughout her body where it felt that all her body fluids were drying up, including her face
> She felt inhibition and shame from childhood about sex

When undertaking trauma clearings, we worked with a healing/resource circle (explored in Chapter 9), which included all the parts of herself and aspects of her body and her partner's body which were relevant to vaginismus. This is to help integrate and harmonise parts.

CLEARING PHRASES

All my shame when I was very small and innocently took my clothes off at the beach and saw my grandfather leering at me.

My excruciating shame that everyone will know I was raped and have had sex.

HEALING CIRCLE

The Shamed One, The Rapist, Fire and Brimstone, Soul, Guardian Angel

Treating shame was an important turning point in the work.

CLEARING PHRASE

I felt so shamed and 'wrong' in my dour Scottish judgemental family for being natural and innocent, that I can't relax and feel the flow of my sensuality because I'm always trying to 'be a good girl'.

HEALING CIRCLE

The 'good girl', the 'bad girl', Dissociated Self, Innocent Child, Authoritarian Father, Absent alcoholic mother, Soul, Guardian Angel

She then associated to a sense of trauma in her female lineage.

CLEARING PHRASE

The transgenerational sexual trauma that women in my female lineage are uptight and repressed

The next association moved to treating her sexual trauma more directly.

CLEARING PHRASE

Because sex has to be repressed, my body freezes, my natural sexual instincts are frozen, and my body does not produce the natural lubricant I need

HEALING CIRCLE

Dissociated self, Soul, Guardian Angel vagina, penis, PTSD, vaginal fluid

This then moved to disgust.

CLEARING PHRASE

All my disgust at sex

HEALING CIRCLE

Vagina, vulva, penis, PTSD, vaginal fluid, Sperm, Disgust

And then shock.

CLEARING PHRASE

All my shock at suddenly realising how deeply sexually traumatised I am

It feels appropriate to conclude the vignette without going into further details of the early sexual traumas we cleared. During this work, Vikki had various abreactions and sensations, which passed through her body, such as tingling and dizziness, 'leaving' her body, or feeling sick. These experiences came and went in the moment without remaining problematic. After this energy work Vikki was pleased to report she was once again producing natural vaginal fluids and was able to have sex again with her husband. In a follow-up a year later, she was no longer plagued by memories of sexual trauma and was able to enjoy a normal sex life.

NB A caveat when working with severe sexual trauma.

If there are abreactions as the body memories release, it is helpful to respond to needs as they arise. I have a blanket and rescue remedy in my therapy room in case of shock, so if a client suddenly becomes cold/or their blood sugar drops after clearing large traumas, a cup of hot tea and a few raisins may be necessary for the shock and to raise blood sugar levels. This does change the therapeutic frame but is appropriate for this kind of work.

I am very thankful to my clients for allowing me to share vignettes such as this—naturally in disguised forms—and the wonderful ways in which energy therapy, quite straightforwardly, can make a huge difference, bringing healing into people's lives.

CHAPTER 9

The multidimensional clinical terrain: using energy psychotherapy to clear trauma at all levels

In the new paradigm, energy psychotherapy enables us to work quite easily at multidimensional levels. This chapter explores the extensive range of issues we can work with—though this is not exclusive to energy therapy and other therapies also address deep levels of work.

The roots of trauma

While attending a one-year introductory training in group analytic psychotherapy I experienced the powerful impact of unconscious birth trauma. It was just before the beginning of the second therapy group. The administrator was waiting outside the room to take me aside and inform me that I was to move groups because the one I was in was too large. I was so shocked. This triggered visceral anxiety and panic as though I were fighting for my life—my throat felt blocked, and I was gasping for breath. Fortunately, the group conductor came along and intervened, and told the administrator that I should stay in the group. I was grateful that I survived in the group.

This incident brought to mind the family anecdote that I nearly died at birth, half-strangled by the cord round my neck. Once conscious of this trauma, it made sense as to why I struggled starting ventures in life. Subsequently, after later clearing this trauma with energy psychotherapy, it's been so much easier to start things, and follow them through to completion.

Early traumatic experiences have a powerful impact on the body. Freud's idea of repetition compulsion is so true—we unconsciously re-enact experiences until they come to light so we can heal them. My strangled attempts to enter the therapy group demonstrate how helpful it is to get to the roots of trauma. If we only understand things at a surface level, the roots spread, and weeds grow.

Repetition compulsion and its multidimensional roots

How do we know when to focus on clearing deeper layers of trauma? Once we have established a good therapeutic relationship and engaged in regular energy clearings where the client is comfortable with the work, it becomes routine to look for the deeper roots of problems. For instance, if someone repeatedly experiences the same traumatic theme again and again of being homeless or repeatedly having to move, and several trauma clearings have failed to resolve the issue, this indicates the need to look deeper.

Energy testing proves invaluable in tracing the roots. We do a kind of detective work, where the therapeutic alliance can be quite playful, holding an open mind without any expectations regarding the results of the statements we test. The work is full of surprises and can on occasion be fun, such as when we feel we are getting lost and energy test phrases like 'We're barking up the wrong tree!' The resulting laughter deepens the intimacy of the therapeutic relationship.

We start by testing broad categories first. For example:

One cause for my (e.g. rootlessness) … has its origins in (e.g. trauma) from my current life.
Then we energy test one by one each element of the list:

1. trauma from current life
2. preverbal trauma including conception, in-utero, birth and infancy
3. attachment and developmental trauma during early life
4. transgenerational/ancestral trauma
5. cultural trauma
6. past life trauma
7. transpersonal trauma.

Often the client will energy test 'strong' to several categories in which case it is helpful to test:

The priority origin to clear now is …
We can work with one or more of these categories simultaneously (sometimes the past life trauma resonates with an ancestral or cultural trauma as well)

Another useful phrase to energy test is:

We now have all the information that we need to clear this trauma.

The clearing phrases we arrive at simply 'tell the story'. The classic psychoanalytic formulation of using statements which link past with present are particularly useful. For example:

> *I was traumatised by poverty, scarcity, and migration in my cultural background where I was constantly homeless, so I have a scarcity mentality, fear there will never be enough and keep finding myself lost and homeless.*

Later in this chapter I speak about Healing Circles, where, in clearing such a trauma, it would be useful to include the relevant archetypes such as 'The Homeless One' and 'The Refugee'.

Working with various categories of trauma

This section explores the multidimensional aspects of this work, illustrating how we can clear trauma on so many levels in so many ways—I hope this gives you some idea of the rich potential of this work.

1. Trauma from current life

People usually present for therapy with issues and trauma from their current life—birth to now. They may or may not have conscious recollection of specific trauma, but the bulk of energy clearing that we undertake is largely from these unresolved experiences.

2. Preverbal trauma—conception, in-utero, birth and infancy

'It is all in the first trauma—everything comes from the first trauma'—Sandi Radomski[1] holds that the earlier the trauma occurs, the more profound the impact on the trajectory of people's lives and how people unconsciously expect the world to be: 'The trauma we experience around conception, in-utero, birth and post birth creates "blueprints" for our life'.

As a matter of routine Radomski therefore energy tests whether an issue started at:

- conception
- in the first, second, and third trimester of pregnancy
- birth
- immediately after birth/bonding
- early life.

Three key themes relating to very early trauma: Helplessness, lack of safety and unconscious blueprints

1. HELPLESSNESS and HOPELESSNESS—if the infant has encountered very difficult struggles in the womb, during birth or in the first few months, they will be prone to feelings of helplessness and hopelessness.
2. LACK OF SAFETY is key, where life-threatening trauma and the infant's very survival may have been at stake.
3. FOETAL AND INFANT TRAUMA CREATE UNCONSCIOUS 'BLUEPRINTS' FOR LIFE—preverbal trauma creates unconscious associated core beliefs which relate to those traumas. When working with preverbal issues we also consider *what is/are the underlying limiting core beliefs which have developed as a result of the trauma?* The energies of these 'blueprints' become the unconscious 'drivers' for our life.

---

[1] Sandi Radomski taught about the importance of the first trauma in an online seminar I attended in 2017 on 'Allergy Antidotes'.

To overcome these deeply engrained traumatic patterns we need to clear both the preverbal trauma and the related 'blueprint' core beliefs associated with that trauma.

Conception

Conception trauma may result from difficult circumstances around conception, or the soul's trauma of not wishing to incarnate in the world, such as:

- *I was conceived to repair a failing relationship*
- *I was conceived when my mum was forced to have sex*
- *I was conceived to replace a sibling who died*
- *I was happy where I was and didn't want to enter the earth plane.*

These traumas all impact the developing foetus.

In-utero stress

If the mother is herself unsafe/in danger, and her stress levels are unmediated by the support of others, the baby resides in the stress hormones and conflicting feelings of the mother, with no barrier to protect it. This can result in 'blueprints' such as:

- *I am bad*
- *Life is stressful and overwhelming*
- *I soak up other peoples' stress.*

Birth trauma

A range of mishaps and difficulties can arise during birth, including life-threatening experiences.

Stuck in birth canal

- *I am helpless*
- *I can't do it on my own*
- *I feel stuck in life*
- *I will never get through this.*

Cord caught round the baby's neck

Feeling terrified, stuck, unable to go forward or back, resulting in limiting beliefs such as:

- *Life is scary*
- *I can't move safely*
- *My efforts to start/complete things are strangled etc.*

Bonding, early attachment trauma, and relational patterns

Clinical emergencies, premature birth requiring incubation, postnatal depression of the mother and so on, can threaten the fundamental survival need for attachment. These will also have their attendant blueprints such as

Because … mum suffered postnatal depression (or whatever the trauma …)

- *I am isolated and alone*
- *I blame myself for everything*
- *I am unlovable*
- *I put others' needs before mine and grew up feeling responsible for others.*

Resetting the body to feel safe

Our bodies are programmed for survival, with safety and protection taking precedence over other considerations. Preverbal and early trauma creates the body's 'set up'—the predisposition to be fearful, stressed, or flooded with PTSD. This impact on the baby's body results in the tendency to feel fundamentally unsafe, or stuck in one of the *fight, flight, freeze, and flop* survival responses which continue to operate until the trauma is cleared.

We honour the body, which to some extent operates independently from the conscious mind. It has its own history, wisdom, and communication system, and so in energy testing, we might test it separately with such phrases as: *Body, I feel safe now.*

We can connect with, communicate with, and/or 'reset' the body so it learns that it no longer needs to be stuck in PTSD or stress-surviving strategies. I experienced this after surgery. Although the procedure went well, my body had 'picked up' on the surgeon's anxiety during one tricky moment and was still holding onto this fear, which made it difficult for my body to fully relax and recover until I had cleared the trauma to reset it.

Communicating lovingly with our bodies

Many have negative attitudes towards their bodies. Our bodies hear what we say to them. Consider the impact of words transforming water crystals in Emoto's images (Chapter 2). We have a similar impact on our bodies when we speak to them. Developing habits of loving self-talk, sending positive messages, and viewing our bodies compassionately is therefore very important.

We can 're-set' our bodies in various ways:

- Neural pathways are changed by clearing trauma and transforming our unconscious blueprints.
- We can resource ourselves through self-care, using energy balancing and other energy self- help methods for self-soothing and calming the body.
- It can be helpful to address the body in its own right, including the body—or body parts— as separate components in the healing process.

EXAMPLE

Preverbal trauma—fear of flying

Monica came to therapy saying she was 'constantly in a state of panic and easily shaken up by things'. She was about to go on holiday the following week and had experienced a panic attack on the last flight she had been on, when there had been bad turbulence, and she had been 'beyond terrified'. She had heard that energy methods might be able to help.

In talking through the details about her experiences, Monica reflected 'I realise this panic has happened a couple of times before although less severely'. She also recognised that while she found flying very stressful, 'actually, I was worrying about all sorts of other factors in life as well, which are causing me stress and which I can't seem to manage'.

It didn't take long to find the earliest trauma. Her mother had told Monica that she had been at her wits end when Monica was a baby, and had shaken her.

The connection was very clear, so we formulated the following phrase and did chakra clearing

> *Because I was shaken by mum as a baby, I find turbulence on planes beyond terrifying, so I panic at the thought of flying.*

We then used *Ask and Receive* to install:

> *I and my body are safe and remain calm and centred in the eye of the storm.*

Monica came back after her holiday reporting that the flight had been easy, and apart from a little bit of deep breathing to calm herself, she had managed the flights successfully without any fear or panic. This illustration shows how when we find the exact pattern and clear it energetically, it removes the disturbance and we ca 're-set' the body.

3. Attachment and developmental trauma

Relational patterns and difficulties with attachment and developmental trauma in early life are often key. Energy psychotherapy is especially well placed to work with these traumas, which otherwise can be difficult to shift in conventional therapies.

'Repetition compulsion' is painfully evident in people with unhappy attachment histories who unconsciously re-enact childhood traumas of insecure, anxious, avoidant, or disorganised and chaotic attachments which continue into adult relational patterns (Ainsworth, Main & Solomon, 1978). Although these patterns can be intransigent, it is possible to heal early relational attachment wounds using long-tern energy psychotherapy.

When people have experienced specific developmental trauma, clearing these can be surprisingly fast. One such example concerned a man whose trauma carried a transgenerational component. His situation demonstrates the importance of knowing the history in relation to the presenting issues so that it is possible to formulate connections for the energy clearings.

EXAMPLE

Antonio was an Italian waiter who wanted help with his panic attacks. He was off work, couldn't function, and was too scared to leave the house. He described his mother, who lived in Italy, as rather over-involved and overindulgent. His father had died when Antonio was a child.

Antonio lived with his girlfriend in London, who 'called him out' on his laziness. After a row at the cinema where he thought she might leave him, he had a big panic attack. He couldn't breathe at all, felt pains in his chest and was scared he was dying or having a heart attack. The situation escalated with daily panic attacks and difficulties breathing. His mother came over to visit and took him to the doctor for an ECG which was normal. However, despite various attempts to get help from doctors in the UK and Italy, his panic attacks continued.

In telling his story, Antonio wasn't happy with his girlfriend. Although she was sincere, he felt she was too direct and didn't let him get away with things, and that sometimes the truth is too harsh and critical. His father had been like this as well. Although his father had certainly loved him, was fun and had played basketball with him, he had been strict and punished Antonio which had felt too severe.

The energy of the conversation became 'charged' at this moment as an association arose and Antonio suddenly said *I am afraid to die*. His anxiety was intense and palpable in the room. It felt it was time do some energy clearing.

I asked—'How old was your father when he died? And how old were you?'
Antonio replied that his father had been twenty-seven and he had been four. He then had the dawning recognition that he was now twenty-seven, the same age his father had been when he had died, something of which he had not previously been conscious.

It energy-tested strong that it would be best for Antonio to clear this trauma in the language of his childhood, so he went straight into tapping, first using the phrase:

> *I have panic attacks* in Italian.

> A healing circle included:
> His four-year-old self, Antonio, his Father, and the archetype of Death

A formulation/phrase came very quickly which we cleared through the chakras:

> *All my anxiety and unconscious fear that I'm not allowed to live longer than my father, so I am having panic attacks.*

Antonio's panic attacks ended after this session. He went back to work and came back for a second session the following week to treat some more trauma about his father. He reported feeling so well with his panic attacks gone, his breathing normal, being back at work, and able to go out of the house that he felt he didn't need any more sessions.

Attachment trauma: developing a sovereign self

Since our primary need is to be healthily connected with other human beings (Fairbairn, 1944[2]), depriving, abandoning, and terrifying attachments are nothing short of catastrophic. Attachment trauma presents in the consulting room with an extensive array of symptoms.

---

[2] Fairbairn's structural model (1944) proposes 'that the libido is not primarily aimed at pleasure, but at making relationships with others'.

Chronic relational insecurities manifest as emotional dysregulation, lack of a healthy sense of self, low self-esteem, dissociation, self-sabotage ('self-abandonments'), avoidance, and disconnection.

Terror, where nothing is safe, is a powerful driver, manifesting as avoidance of intimacy and attachment, and fear of separations and abandonments. Disorganised attachment brings further difficulties, where 'fear without solution' (Main & Solomon, 1986) results in disorientation with simultaneous and contradictory behaviours to approach and flee at the same time. A survival-mode type of existence is common when it doesn't feel safe to express true feelings for fear of rejection. When a compliant 'False Self' (Winnicott, 1960) is presented to the world, it compromises the capacity for healthy power and autonomy. Insecure attachments result in a life driven by need, with difficulties maintaining stable relationships, co-dependency, and an impoverished capacity for love.

Clients with a history of traumatic separations often cling to unhealthy relationships and put up with demeaning treatment from the 'other', lacking the self-respect to feel they deserve better, persecuted by internalised self-attacking voices of shame and self-judgement ('I must be bad because I was abandoned'). Attachment patterns often stretch back over generations and whilst some clients show remarkable resilience, many fall into hopelessness, feelings of emptiness or isolation, and the despair of ever being loved. The following describes a section of work with a long-term client.

EXAMPLE

George was a caring gay Jamaican who worked as a manager in retail. His parents had to work long shifts when they emigrated to this country, so had been unable to offer him consistent care as a child and George constantly felt abandoned by both. When he came out in adolescence, his parents were ashamed of him and strongly rejected his sexuality.

Initially we focused on ego strengthening work by clearing early traumas concerning the homophobia of his parents. On account of the racism they experienced in the UK, they felt insecure and wanted to fit in and be 'normal', so they felt threatened by George's homosexuality. Clearing this trauma helped George develop confidence and resilience.

However, he had a major setback after falling 'madly in love' with a man who treated him very badly. George felt he had made a rare, meaningful, and truly intimate connection with 'Tom'. After a passionate fling, he was desperate to hear from Tom, who hardly responded to any of his messages and kept George 'dangling on a thread'. Terrified of being abandoned, George was triggered into states of frantic catastrophising. He knew his obsession was unhealthy, but he couldn't stop looking at his phone for messages. George became so anxious and distracted, and in danger of unravelling his life. Struggling to focus at work and lost in daydreams about Tom, he started making mistakes. The more George felt rejected and abandoned, the more obsessed he became. George's sister recognised that his mental health was deteriorating, and persuaded him to take some sick-leave as she was afraid he might lose his job. This woke George up to the seriousness of his situation.

Although he didn't want to give up on Tom, George knew his addiction to this rejecting man was destructive. He also recognised that his wounded child had been traumatised by this encounter. We first cleared the reversals:

CLEARING PHRASES

Even though my wounded child isn't safe enough to let go of Tom and I have become destructively obsessed with him, I completely honour the feelings of my child self and love and accept him. Even though part of me wants to let go and part of me doesn't, I love and accept all my parts.

George's free associations led him to the roots of the problem, where he remained with his GramMa in Jamaica when his parents came to the UK. He was very close to her during the first three years of his life, and felt desperate when he had to leave her to join his parents. He had suddenly been cut him off from all contact with the person closest to him. She died in Jamaica without George ever seeing her again. His free association led him to the roots of the problem.

We then co-created the following phrases to clear.

CLEARING PHRASE

Because my little self was so traumatised when I was torn away from GramMa, my terrified heartbroken child self is preoccupied with longing for Tom.

HEALING CIRCLE

Abandoned Child, dissociated self, Soul, GramMa, The Gay Man, The Homophobic parents, The Universe, Soul

Because I was constantly rejected, abandoned and don't feel I really bonded with my homophobic parents, it feels unbearable to be rejected by Tom with whom I felt close, so my child self is preoccupied with longing.

We used a mixture of tapping and chakra work and suddenly George felt a surge of terror at the prospect of losing Tom forever. The intense longing was so familiar, it provided a perverse sense of security. George suddenly understood how this relational pattern was exactly the same as his never-to-come-true phantasies that 'one day I will see my GramMa again', and 'One day my parents will turn round and love me'. In this key moment, he realised that his habitual pattern of clinging would only stop if he put an end to it.

A psycho-educational component involved making the distinction between pain and grief. George was so used to being in a state of longing that he mistook this pain for love when it was largely unresolved attachment trauma. We discussed how there is no end to pain which goes round in circles, whereas grief lets go and flows like a river. George reflected about this and came back at the next session saying he wanted to 'cut the cord' of his connection with Tom.

Overcoming this trauma, which had gone right to George's very core, was a considerable milestone in his healing, an emergence out of co-dependence into his sovereign self.

4. *Transgenerational/ancestral trauma*

The concept of transgenerational transmission of trauma is widely accepted these days. Studies in genetics and epigenetics show that the environment of parents and grandparents have an effect on the as yet unborn generations, through the expression of the genes. When people suffer unresolved life-threatening experience, such as through slavery (Gump, 2016) and the Holocaust (Grand & Salberg, 2016), the unconscious residue of such trauma manifests in the observable problems of subsequent generations. Social research demonstrated that depression is passed down across the generations in the 'cycle of deprivation' (Brown, Hilderbrand, & Harris, 1978) and in adverse childhood experiences (ACEs) (Felliti et al., 1998).

Patterns of trauma often go back over many generations and lifetimes, creating traumatic patterns in our 'fields' where we are carrying more than the weight of our own personal (this lifetime) trauma. For some, to be fully free of trauma, it is necessary to clear these deep 'karmic miasms' and complexes at a transpersonal level, including ancestral trauma and traumatic patterns going back through the paternal and maternal lineages.

To clear the patterns of generational, ancestral, or past life roots we can use straightforward clearing phrases, such as the following, which are usually sufficient:

> *Because of all the generations of postnatal depression in my mother's lineage, women in my family are subject to low mood and depression and have difficulties attaching to their babies*
>
> *The debilitating shame of unmarried mothers throughout generations in my mother's family meant that I was bathed in her shame in-utero, and so struggle to feel worthy of love and nurture*

HEALING CIRCLE

Saboteur, dissociated self, baby self, inner child parts, Shame, The Terrified Child, The Unloved one, The Unmarried Mother, The Scapegoat

PATTERNS: We can clear generalised patterns using phrases such as 'All the times and ways that … 'which creates a broad funnel to catch and release considerable amounts of traumatised energy.:

> *All the times and ways in all my lifetimes and in my ancestral history that (e.g. there has been a pattern of bullying and violence)*

EXAMPLE

The following transgenerational trauma illustrates hypo-arousal (the flop response) which is an aspect of the ventral vagal system. In this work, we cleared trauma related to the themes below, and then did a final piece which changed his 'flop' trauma response and re-set his body.

James was a mixed-race client, presenting with sleep problems, anxiety, loss of energy, and difficulty motivating himself at work. He was a senior director in a large corporation and wanted to be more active and connected but found he was easily overwhelmed and would 'close down'. His issues were gradually resolved by working through layers of transgenerational trauma on both sides of his family. The trauma that we cleared included:

- *Transgenerational abandonment* in his family through migration.
  - ◦ James' mother had abandoned her mother when she moved countries
  - ◦ his father had similarly abandoned his father.
  - ◦ James had been abandoned by his mother when he was three
  - ◦ he also felt he had abandoned both his parents when he moved continents as a young man.

When his abandonment issues were triggered, James went into 'hypo' responses where he felt passive, collapsed, and unable to mobilise himself. Both he and his mother felt guilty about abandoning parents on other continents. James felt he was carrying an additional heavy load of his mother's and his own guilt.

- *Transgenerational race issues*: Like his mother James also experienced transgenerational trauma regarding migration and his dual nationality. Both he and his mother had 'passed easily for white'. James had largely ignored and denied his Black self, and became grief stricken about his identity confusion, when he recognised his internalised racism where it had been easier to 'pass for white' than protest and put up a fight. We also went on to clear his guilt about this

- *PTSD collapsed states*: When James cleared deep guilt, anxiety, and fear about having abandoned his own parents he gradually reconnected with his own abandoned disconnected child. His collapsed internal child-self became extremely distressed. After weeks of in-depth trauma work, clearing of the following trauma finally helped him be free of his 'hypo' response:

  My mother left me when I was three, and without anyone to hold me, I fell into myself and became passive and cut off. Consequently, I am terrified of not having structure in my life. At such times, I fall into myself and become passive, disconnected, and unable to mobilise myself.

HEALING CIRCLE

Three-year-old, His loving grandmother, Unavailable mother, abandoned child, Collapsed self, Terrified Child, Disconnected Self, Parasympathetic and Sympathetic nervous system, Vagus Nerve, Soul

In his final session, James commented that the healing circle had helped integrate his wounded child parts so 'I can be whole and fully adult'. His previously disconnected anxious child parts used to wake him up during sleepless nights, but he now experienced them as settled and integrated, so he no longer had sleep problems. James's outer world reflected these inner changes. He was much better able to handle stress at work and as he became stronger he recovered his energy and resilience. People at work noticed this, and he was offered promotion with significant success in launching a large innovative project.

5. *Cultural trauma*

Historical and cultural patterns of trauma include the traumatic themes of slavery, displacement, migration, genocide, and starvation. The depth and breadth of cultural trauma has not been sufficiently addressed over the years. 'Black Lives Matter' is one area where society has awoken to debilitating levels of racism and prejudice, shamefully endemic for generations in our society. Such trauma can be addressed in energy clearings by naming and clearing specific traumas. For example the following are some clearings clients have worked with:

- *Because of all the times and ways people are unconscious of their own racism, I suffer repeated trauma when people make remarks without even realising that they are being racist.*
- *I was very conflicted being brought up in a traditional Pakistani family while being educated in a Western school so I am confused about my identity, who I am and what my values are.*
- *There is much homophobia in my culture and homosexuality is viewed as dangerous, so I am traumatised, living in fear of expressing my sexuality.*

6. *Past-life trauma*

Many people are understandably sceptical about 'past lives'. Patricia Cory gives some helpful insight into the illusory nature of time and quantum reality where there is only one moment—the present moment. This means that 'past lives' are occurring simultaneously, with everything existing on parallel timelines. In this space of multidimensionality, all is being expressed in the same moment of existence:

> When we speak of 'past lives' or 'ancient civilisations' we are, from our perspective, actually describing an entire panorama of simultaneous experience. It is no different when we speak of the future … what you perceive as a string of chronological lifetimes and fixed events, we recognise as consciousness simply manifesting at different co-ordinates in the time-space continuum. (Cori, 2000, p. 77)

Reincarnation is a challenging idea for many unless one has viscerally remembered or had access to one's past lives. We respect the belief system of the client we are working with, so for those who are unsure, past lives can also be represented as a metaphor without making categorical claims that they are real. However we understand them, energy work can resolve these complex issues relatively simply.

We often access such trauma through our body memories. When I needed to confront the Buddhist teacher about his abusive behaviour, I felt sick with terror, feeling I would be betraying him by speaking out against him. This triggered an old murky memory in the pit of my stomach and my gut told me I needed to understand something about a past life. I had never previously thought about past lives, though as a Buddhist, I did accept the idea of reincarnation. I had also read—and recommend—a book by an American psychiatrist, Dr Brian Weiss, called *Many Lives, Many Masters* (1990) which outlines how traumatic patterns 'bleed through' from previous timelines. Dr Weiss provides a fascinating account of how intransigently 'ill' mental health in-patients made apparently miraculous recoveries when the deep origins of trauma from previous incarnations were recognised and released.

I phoned a psychic friend to ask if she could help me with a past-life regression—most of my other friends would have thought I was completely mad. I would never have believed, had I not experienced it, the visceral memory of my body as she guided me through a very unpleasant 'cloak-and-dagger' experience. Some people when they talk about past lives seem to remember being Joan of Arc or someone glamourous. I am afraid my own experience was shadowy and very unflattering. I was in medieval clothing in a dank cold stone building—I could smell the moss—and there was a heavy velvet curtain. I was about to go through the doorway when I felt a piercing pain from behind as a dagger was thrust through my neck. I was gasping, re-experiencing my violent death throes, and I can still hear the guttural sounds now as I write this. It was utterly real. After this traumatic 'death', I left my body, and my friend guided me to a light peaceful place with violet light where I received healing. The cells of my body were shaking and trembling, so we used some Aura- Soma orange 'etheric rescue' which my friend gently massaged onto my jangled, traumatised body, which calmed it down. She explained that out of this Machiavellian intrigue, I had been tasked with the responsibility of being a Trustee in this life, to address the teacher in the Buddhist community. Apparently I had been involved in dilemmas of 'church and state' many times, but in a different form this time—by retaining pure motivation and integrity I would expiate my karma. Without re-experiencing that past life, I would never have had the strength or courage to stand up to that overpowering narcissistic teacher.

There were also other significant lives to heal. At my next session, my friend passed on the message from her 'guides'—'don't doubt your experience'. (I had in fact been convincing myself that I had made all the previous session up.) We cleared some extremely unpleasant lives where I had been both Master and slave in the galley ships where I was either whipped or wielded the whip. Part of me just wanted to gloss over the past life thing as ridiculous. The following week I went wild swimming with a dolphin with my friend Hilary, when suddenly a police barge went by, and the dolphin was caught in the boat's propeller, revealing bloody gashes on the side of its body. It was horrifying. In case I doubted my slave experience, this synchronous message underlined the truth of it. Hilary came home with me and looked after me as I wept ceaselessly. I no longer doubted the veracity of 'past lives'.

Compared with the drama of the above story, working with past-life trauma using energy clearing tends to be quite straightforward, undramatic, and matter-of-fact, and makes a remarkable difference to our state of well-being.

7. *Transpersonal trauma*

People experience various forms of transpersonal trauma, a phenomenon which increasingly presents in the consulting room. Being stuck in between incarnations, not wishing to incarnate onto this earth, experiences of trauma 'off planet' or working with 'soul fragments' where the soul continues to hold a traumatic imprint of other incarnations are fairly common examples.

I asked William Linville his view on transpersonal trauma and multidimensionality in a personal session in 2017. He said that this work concerned gathering up reclaiming and integrating all our soul fragments and facets of ourselves through a process of recollection, clearing and purifying our psyche. We bring together all aspects of our consciousness—our conscious, unconscious, and soul levels—into the present, and into our body. Our body is the physical vehicle which embodies our soul and carries the experiences of all our lifetimes, different timelines and parallel 'life streams'. (A parallel life stream is another term for past incarnations, since the past present and future are all going on simultaneously within the current moment.) This is a process of working with the 'particles and facets', bringing soul fragments back from all 'bases and places of our existences' into this life, healing the traumatic fragmentation of all that has been split off. When we tune in, bring back and integrate these multidimensional levels of ourselves, we become stronger, more resilient, and whole This reclamation also includes releasing ourselves from limiting vows, contracts, and agreements—decisions made previously when in despair about difficult life circumstances.

Linville emphasised that 'past life' work isn't concerned with 'bringing back gunk' but about reclaiming beautiful facets of ourselves which were adversely affected by traumatic blockages from other lifetimes, which continue to affect us now. By clearing all the roots and origins of our trauma and integrating these experiences, we develop 'a clear pristine fully embodied integrated life stream within and throughout You, your higher levels and your creator levels'. No longer dragged down by old density, we have more light in our being, and manifest effortlessly and spontaneously 'in the flow'. Linville went on to say that this process involves

> radiating and purifying all the way into the quantum world, a space and a place where everything is open and amplified—without the old baggage, sequences of events align easily to receive beautiful gifts in the quantum world—and also, in the physical world.

I think William Linville's exposition pretty much describes the work we can do in the multidimensional terrain of energy psychotherapy.

Working with PTSD

In Chapter 8 we looked at the impact of trauma on the body, nervous system, and resulting therapeutic issues. Please read the section here in conjunction with Chapter 8 which lays out physiological states of stress responses when working with PTSD.

Energy—a 'language beyond words'

Phil Mollon's reflection that talking can make trauma worse highlights just how helpful energy psychotherapy can be when there are no easily accessible words, and our bodies are exhausted by overworked nervous systems. When clients become overwhelmed, their nervous system is flooded, cognition is knocked offline, and they may not be able to process much in words. In such situations, cognitive behavioural approaches, psycho-education, and analytic interpretations are likely to be ineffective, or even counterproductive.

Energy is like a language beyond words. It is particularly helpful when treating PTSD or preverbal areas of experience, where deep layers of trauma are held unconsciously in the body, and states of frozen terror make it impossible to speak. Free association and dreamwork can facilitate access to these experiences which cannot be spoken of. Working with imagery contains the energetic information symbolically, so creating artwork which puts experience into pictures and working with dreams are powerful vehicles for healing. It can be very effective to look at an image and tap or clear through the chakras—the process still works. Energy testing also supports nonverbal work—you can ask a client to simply think of something without speaking and the energy testing will reveal the required information to work safely and clear the trauma.

Working with PTSD—particularly preverbal trauma—is visceral. Paradoxically when clearing preverbal trauma—for instance for foetal or baby trauma—we can nonetheless construct the 'story' of what happened in words which names the trauma when doing energy clearing. The therapist can speak these words on behalf of the foetus while the client taps of does chakra work: for instance, *Mum was terrified of dad while I was in her womb, so I live in a permanent state of PTSD.* The actual experience of energy clearing of such deeply embedded layers of PTSD is similar to the 'trance state' referred to by Tom Kenyon in Chapter 4.

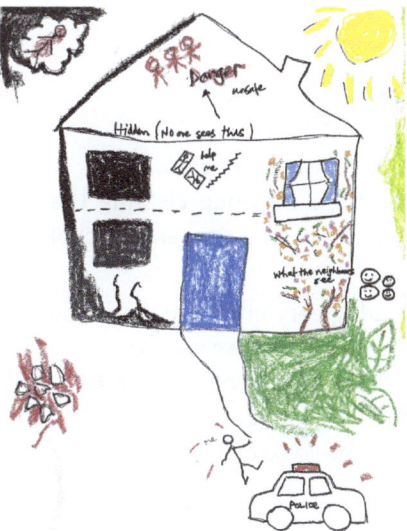

Figure 13 Energy work using imagery when there are no words

Therapeutic dissociation

When people are particularly fragile and vulnerable, The EFT 'Tearless Trauma Techniques' works in a therapeutically dissociated manner with those who may be potentially de-stabilised by addressing their trauma directly. The techniques use a modified form of EFT for clearing trauma and experiences which are too disturbing to feel or name. We emphasise to the client that there is no need to think about the trauma or go into it in any way at all.

TEARLESS TRAUMA TECHNIQUES

- The client is asked to identify a *specific traumatic experience*
- The client is asked to *'imagine a container "over there"'*. They may like to describe this container (e.g. a trunk at the bottom of the sea; an impenetrable bubble in outer space; a steel safe with a padlock on it; a bejewelled carved wooden box etc.)
- They are invited to put *the trauma(s) in the container*
  'Any part of you, can put anything you like in that "box over there" without specifically speaking of its contents'
- *A lid is put on* the *container*
  - ask the client to *'give it an innocuous label'* relating to the contents. (e.g. the box; the 'stuff'; at the lake; the barbeque; the school bus etc.)
- Without connecting with the memory
  - Ask the client to *guess at the SUDs* rating of how intense the memory would feel if s/he were to imagine it
  - *Don't actually feel the SUDs*
- Meridian tapping through the basic sequence is restricted to the three points of information:
  1. There is a *container over there*
  2. It has a *label*
  3. There is an estimated SUD rating

- Tap until the estimated SUDs are at 3 or below
- If desired, the client can then continue clearing the remained of the trauma through whichever energy method—for instance a waterfall chakra clearing with the phrase: *'All that remains of this trauma'*

Another useful 'tip' when clearing very intense trauma: the client can use karate-chop tapping using very general words in the set-up phrase such as:
- *Even though I can't even think about what happened …*
- *Even though it feels too terrible to imagine …*
- *Even though thinking of this would be overwhelming* (I love myself, I'm OK and etc.)

Clearing PTSD with words and energy

PTSD can of course also be worked with while fully naming the trauma.

EXAMPLE

A fellow of the Royal College of Surgeons, Mike was recommended energy therapy after being severely bullied by another senior surgeon in his team. He was astonished to find that energy psychotherapy was so gentle and non-traumatising. Mike had lost all belief in himself and was suffering from debilitating stress and migraines. He was on sick-leave, and was considering throwing in the towel—another colleague who had also been bullied had left the profession altogether. External consultancy had been called in to address the aggressive culture in the team, which was wrecking people's careers.

As a surgeon, dealing with life-and-death situations was the norm. Mike was used to relying on his skill and intuition to make emergency split-second decisions about the right thing to do during surgery. However, since the bullying, he had totally lost all faith and confidence in himself and was paralysed at the thought of making wrong decisions. He also felt terrible shame at being reduced to such a state by a woman and was paranoid that people were whispering about him. Barely functioning, fragmented, and unable to cope with constant flashbacks of bullying, a psychiatric assessment had deemed Mike to be suffering from PTSD. Mike's condition was debilitating. He lived in constant anxiety that 'when the flashbacks come back you are broken, nothing works, and you feel a total loss of confidence'.

Mike had been off sick for several months when he came to see me and was facing a 'back-to-work' scheme on reduced hours. This filled him with horror, not least because he feared having to work again with 'Christine', the bullying consultant who remained in post. The work culture was not supportive. People were not given time off duty to recover after serious incidents and 'with the amount of bad things we see at work, there is no mental health support for the stress and trauma, or proper debriefing after adverse incidents and it isn't safe to share such feelings anyway—we just have to tough it out'.

In our work together, it became clear that bullying at work had re-triggered various traumas in Mike's life: bullying by his mother when he was a child; and also, by his volatile former wife 'Jenny', which had led to the breakdown of his marriage. Like Christine, Jenny and his mother had frequently undermined and attacked him, whilst also gaslighting him, which led him to doubt his sanity.

We started with some energy boundary work between himself and his work situation to strengthen his fragmented ego. Initially these boundaries were around 5 per cent but after getting them up to 85 percent he noticed a significant difference, feeling a bit more his old self again.

We worked with a series of traumas around bullying, bringing in supportive energies at the each of session with *Ask and Receive,* such as 'Confidence, balance, and pride in my work'. Key traumas that we cleared were:

Jenny [wife] constantly abused and gaslighted me and I doubted my sanity, so the similar experience with Christine [surgeon] triggered me and brought it all back, and I now have PTSD.

Jenny gaslighted and projected onto me so much that I still doubt my memories and whether I am inventing things.

Because Christine's bullying was cruel and sadistic, it has dragged up memories of being curled up in the dark, terrified of mum who came in and hit me when I was little, even though I begged her not to, and then she denied it had ever happened.

Because of all the times and ways in childhood I was traumatised by being let down in relationships and it wasn't OK to ask for help, it feels safer to rely on myself, and be independent and in control, so I struggle to ask for help now as it feels shameful to be in need or appear weak.

Because of trauma and PTSD, my instincts and intuition took a hit, and I no longer trust myself.

Mike realised during this last clearing that he had lost connection with his 'inner voice', his instinctual guidance. Previously he had always 'been able to trust my own instincts and have the inner peace in myself to "know" those things—this was what used to keep me safe in my work'. Mike felt that connecting back up again with his 'inner voice' was a key piece of the work. To my mind, this was his reconnection with his soul.

After eleven sessions in all, clearing early traumas and the bullying at work, Mike reported that his stress levels were hugely reduced. He was successfully back at work, had regained his former confidence and his 'anxiety symptoms have just gone', including his flashbacks. Being someone who was generally 'rather sceptical about things like energy psychotherapy', Mike decided to look into it and discovered that in the research literature 'the evidence is really good for energy therapy'. He was impressed at how gentle it was and how well it worked, and he felt it should be a standard form of care in the NHS.

Complex trauma

Complex trauma and fragmentation

Wamser and Vanderburgh (2013) defined complex trauma events as 'chronic, interpersonal traumas that begin early in life'. Complex trauma exposure:

- involves chronic/multiple traumas during developmentally vulnerable time periods
- is a common occurrence for children and adolescents
- causes disruption of early attachment relationships
- adversely affects brain development
- results in significant difficulties with dysregulation—emotional, behavioural, somatic, and cognitive
- gives rise to disconnections of the body and mind, including dissociation, not being embodied or grounded
- fragmentation can occur on all levels.

People who have experienced complex trauma vary a great deal. While some may be ready to go straight into clearing trauma, others need a slow, gradual structured approach. Supervision, energy testing, and your therapeutic experience will help you to think about how to safely introduce energy therapy with your client, so that survival defences are not unravelled.

As well as the fight/flight/freeze/flop models, we are now alert to a greater range of defensive 'cues' and strategies which people use to survive complex trauma. However, the ways we've been trained to establish safety and build rapport may fail us when working, particularly when the client feels relationships are unsafe and eye contact is frightening. Perhaps most challenging is the level of triggering, fragmentation, dissociation, disintegration, and 'shadow' energy that can arise.

Staged treatment plan

There is a lot of literature about complex trauma.[3] The classic phases of Herman's treatment plan for working with complex trauma provides a safe frame. The first stage concerns safety, grounding, and stabilisation (with undertaking risk assessments being another possible prerequisite). The second stage is concerned with remembrance and mourning. In energy psychotherapy we do this through clearing traumatic memories and the roots of trauma while simultaneously integrating and stabilising the sense of self in the process. The final stage concerns reconnection with life and self. As the PTSD is gradually and radically reduced, the client is free to focus on building and developing their life.

The stages in complex trauma are not linear but 'inherently turbulent and complex' (Herman, 1992). Her cautions are pertinent and succinct: 'safety always begins with the body' and 'Exploring trauma memories … by moving directly into the work of Stage Two … without any previous attention to the work of Stage One … can be downright harmful'. Herman concludes that 'In the course of a successful recovery it should be possible to recognise a gradual shift from unpredictable danger to reliable safety, from dissociated trauma to acknowledged memory, and from stigmatised isolation to restored social connection'. (Herman, 1992, p. 155)

Energy psychotherapy brings new ways for helping clients feel safe, grounded, and regulated, and the client's nervous system benefits greatly. When people set the intention to heal themselves, this work facilitates the repair of the profoundly debilitating impacts of complex trauma including developing a healthy sense of self (ego-strengthening), being more embodied, and experiencing greater states of calm and well-being. As with other forms of therapy, the motivation to be well is key.

The therapeutic relationship remains crucial as a safe container, as is the delicacy of timing and pacing of the energy work. Sadly, particularly with complex trauma, we sometimes get this

---

[3] I found that *Skills Training for Patients and Therapists* (Boon, Steele, & Van Der Hart, 2011) includes helpful resources for developing inner safe places (pp. 82–89). Walker (2013) in *Complex PTSD: From Surviving to Thriving: A Guide and Map for Recovering from Childhood Trauma* also offers very practical skills.

wrong—attachment theory speaks of the phenomena of 'rupture/repair', which is sometimes unconsciously enacted when working with complex trauma. It is very distressing if the rupture cannot be repaired.

Useful energy methods for working with trauma fragmentation

Trauma creates fractures, wounds and disconnections. Fragmentation of the ego results in an unstable sense of self; there may be severe fragmentation into parts and 'alters'; and there may also be spiritual disconnection/separation from the soul. Internal divisions in our psyche cause added suffering and misery, where the 'Judge' or 'superego' becomes a critical inner voice, harshly undermining and punishing our child parts and sense of self. The 'persecutor/ protector' perversely attacks the vulnerable inner self in an attempt to be safe. In *Trauma and the Soul* (2013) Kalsched provides a vivid account of the archetypal world of this fragmentation and splitting, and the truly heroic journey involved in recovering from complex trauma.

The universality of archetypal experience helps us connect with the wider picture of our human condition, where we all play out our roles in life. Archetypal energies represent our collective shared experiences—we can potentially identify with a vast array of characters on the human stage: we have been everything—saints and sinners, villains and healers. To evolve from unresolved trauma, we need to recognise and accept these archetypal energies as parts of ourselves—not only the obviously wounded fragmented parts, but also benign and shadow parts—rather than disowning or projecting them out.

Archetypes 'taking over' the ego (e.g. Judge, Victim, 'Righteous one')

Countless traumatic repetitions of a particular pattern, including those from previous lives and our ancestral history, cause the energetic pattern of an archetype to become deeply embedded in our 'field'. This imprint can be so engrained that it becomes the dominant energy, so, for example, our 'Judge' might take over our ego, permeating how we appear to the world. This phenomenon— of coming across as a 'lost child', a 'martyr', or a bit of a 'princess'—is easily recognisable by others. Such characteristics generally indicate unresolved trauma from past life or transgenerational pattering. Releasing the dense frequencies—for instance of judge, persecutor, or zealot— through energy clearings makes space to access more joyful vibrations.

On a personal level it is easier to integrate potentially challenging energies through the lens of an archetype. Working with healing circles (explained shortly) enables us to bring in shadow elements such as 'The Bully', 'The Victim', 'The Princess', 'The Narcissist' and so on. Archetypes help us tread more lightly so we can 'play' undefensively at a little bit of distance, as compared with a direct confrontation with these energies. We can learn to accept ourselves with good humour—for example—'there I go again, being a bit of a victim!'—without crushing the sense of self/ego. Many who work with energy psychotherapy very much appreciate feeling more whole and balanced through this non-shaming way of accepting and integrating our energies.

1. *The integrating power of healing/resource circles*
Mandalas—the ancient origins of 'healing circles'

I developed the energetic method of working with 'healing circles' from my experience of Buddhist spiritual practices which employ central *mandalas*. The non-dual inclusive principle of the mandala is to invite into the circle all beings without discrimination for purification and healing—both friends and 'frenemies' alike. The 'sacred space' of the mandala[4] represents the absolute purity of the unified field in which all is contained.

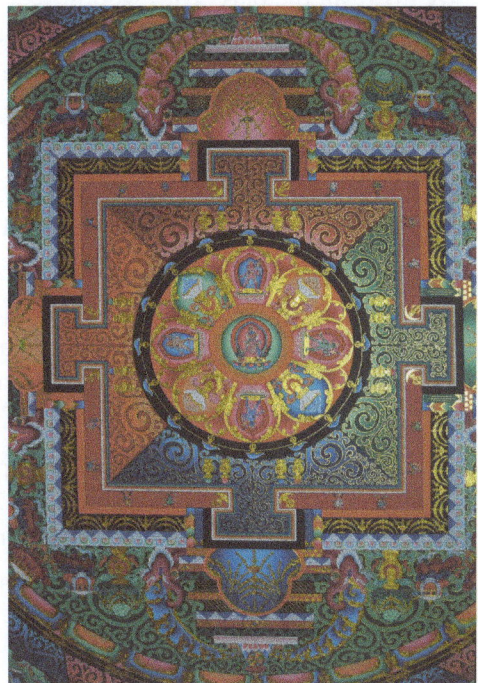

Figure 14 Traditional Buddhist mandala

The energetic signature of archetypes within the healing circle each carry their own unique vibration. Like the frequencies of the spectrum of colours, we don't label green as 'good' and red as 'bad'. Each colour—or each 'part' or archetype—is simply pure energy. Our energy system recognises and 'reads' the words/vibrational resonances, thereby including them in the healing process, without judgement. Naming the elements in the healing circle brings the vibrations of each energy into the 'field' of the trauma being cleared, which harmonises and integrates them. Being inclusive of all parts facilitates the integration of 'shadow' into the whole.

---

[4] This is the same as 'the fifth dimension' of the unified field.

From a higher-dimensional perspective, all energy is *as-it-is* and all beings—both peaceful and wrathful energies—are held in a space of peaceful expansiveness, neutrality, acceptance, and allowance. There are no 'splits' in the unified field because the fifth dimension is not polarised by judgements of 'good' or 'bad'. Like the *yin/yang* sign which represents pure energy and balance, the circle creates a harmonising space of wholeness and purity. As it says in the Dzogchen teachings, at this (vibrational) 'level' 'even the name of negativity does not exist'.

Healing circles provide a safe inclusive way of containing and integrating parts by creating our own personal mandala. We invite all the parts with whom we feel a resonance—both from our personal life experience and at the wider level, from the collective unconscious. We then do energy clearings while we sit in Presence to all these energies. This process is effortless—we simply consider the parts are there in the circle, and the work is already done.

CO-CREATING A HEALING CIRCLE

SUMMARY—WHY, WHEN AND HOW—explaining healing circles to the client:

Healing circles are 'mandalas'—or safe spaces—which represent the client's world and provide a way of containing and integrating traumatised child parts, dissociative aspects, archetypes, 'alters', and supportive energies. Healing circles may be used with any clients at any time while clearing trauma. Once we set up the circle, the energies remain present in the field while we use energy methods to clear the relevant trauma.

- *Some of the parts of the circle require healing, others provide* support to the process
- *Naming the elements is enough*—simply by putting the intention into the energy field
- *The healing circle safely contains positive and negative parts* in a neutral space

WHY: in order to have a more complete energy clearing, to make the clearing easier, integrate energies, and help the client to feel more stable.

WHEN: after identifying the trauma to work on,

- either when working with current triggers or explicitly working with deep traumatic roots. Once the focus of the work is established, we then set up a healing circle.
- Healing circles can also be used in a 'stand-alone' way as part of talking therapy to identify different aspects of the client which are involved in a particular 'complex'.

HOW: A collaborative process, co-creating with therapist and client

- *Client reflection*: invite the client to sit comfortably and spend a little time seeing which parts and elements come up naturally
- *The therapist may suggest particular parts* or archetypal energies which the client has not thought of which may be helpful to include
- *Bringing in higher vibrational energies to support the work*: each client has a unique perspective on positive and comforting resources. These might include: Source/Soul/Higher self; Guardian Angel; 'nature' or 'mother earth'; 'the universe'; or specific 'spiritual beings' who carry personal meaning for the client: teddy bears, animals and etc.

POSSIBLE ELEMENTS TO INCLUDE IN A HEALING CIRCLE

(Capitalised words represent archetypal energies, and lower-case words designate personal parts)

- CHILD PARTS such as: The Wounded Child, The Traumatised Child, The Silent Child, my little self, infant, baby self, The Abandoned Baby, The Lost Child etc.
- DISSOCIATED PARTS such as: The Dissociated Self, my cut-off self, my disconnected self, my dissociated body etc.
- ARCHETYPES come from myths and legends in the collective unconscious, and include key 'characters' which everyone recognises such as The Judge, The Witch, The Martyr, The Saboteur, The Trickster, The Victim, The Abuser, The Bully, The Orphan, The Scapegoat, The Parentified Child, The Guardian Angel, The Loving Parents, The Archetypal Mother, The Absent Father, Friends, The Rebel, Cinderella—and so on, the list is infinite
- CONTEMPORARY AND PERSONAL ARCHETYPES (e.g. TV, Book, Film etc.)
- UNIVERSAL AND ENVIRONMENTAL FACTORS: nature, the universe, Gaia, the environment, Trees, the Sea etc.
- SUPPORTIVE PARTS e.g. Guardian Angel, Soul, Grandma, Source, my teddy, my dog
- BODY PARTS AND BODILY SYSTEMS—we often include the body and its wounded aspects as separate elements within the healing circle, especially when working with psychosomatic conditions and physical symptoms such as 'The Sympathetic Nervous System'; The adrenal glands etc.
- ENERGY 'TOXINS': this might include allergens or archetypal triggering energies. Naturally perpetrator and 'shadow' energies need to be worked with carefully and sensitively as they may feel toxic and terrifying to have in the field. Nonetheless, as the work progresses, it is helpful to include these shadow archetypal energies as part of the work.
- 'ALTERS' and dissociative parts

Once the circle is created energy test statements such as

- *There is one or more to add to the healing circle*
- *There is one or more to take away*
- *We have all that we need to clear the trauma now*

A NOTE: including body parts in the energy field (relevant to specific trauma) alongside energy clearing helps strengthen, harmonise, and integrate the named parts. Physical symptoms also often carry metaphorical meaning such as:

- sore throat—difficulty having a voice and speaking out
- digestive system—difficulties 'digesting' experience or emotions

METHOD:

First, identify the trauma to work on. Then invite the client to set up a healing circle by shutting their eyes (if they feel comfortable doing so), and spending a little time seeing what comes up naturally for the purposes of inviting parts into the circle. We have different sensory modalities so not all have visual senses—some people may come up with feelings, others have thoughts, or hear messages. Some free-associate and memories float past, whilst others have clear images.

Initially there may not be many elements in the circle, which is completely fine—there will be small circles and big circles, and one is not better than the other.

This is a collaborative creative process—both client and therapist may consider which parts might be helpful to have in the circle, honouring the client's unique way and 'cast of characters'. Naming the elements is enough since this puts the intention into the energy field.

Use of healing circles:

- Alongside whatever energy methods you are using with your clients—chakra clearing, tapping, working with Intention or *Ask and Receive*.
- Can be used with any clients in clearing trauma at any level.
- They are best introduced as simply as possible.
- It is the experience that is important
- The idea of containing parts is a useful starting point for introducing healing circles to clients.
- People have favourites who nearly always turn up in their circles, whereas others may have completely different circles for different clearings.
- Some do not connect with the idea of healing circles and prefer not to work with them which is fine.
- As a caveat for working with complex trauma it may take a while before the more challenging archetypal energies can be included in the circle since these can feel 'toxic' and frightening to the person. This especially needs to be born in mind for child parts in the circle who need to feel safe and protected.

EXAMPLE

Clearing a 'witch' complex to integrate shadow energy

Sometimes archetypal energies form complexes so we need to work with the group of archetypes and their dynamics to heal the complex. One client was struggling with envious 'witch attacks', so after exploring in some depth, the envious undermining situations which had caused considerable triggering, distress, and paranoia in the client's life, we co-created the following phrase, and a healing circle to convey the energies of the complex. The bulk of the time in this session was spent talking and discussing, considering all elements and formulating the core of the problem. Then we cleared this quite quickly through the chakras with an extensive healing circle.

CLEARING PHRASE

All my guilt, shame, and sadness that because of the cultural trauma of intergenerational fall-outs and witchy in-fighting, it is normal to weaponise the gift of insight to attack others, peppering relationships with malevolent disowned swipes, and this comes out in me as hormonal surges of bitchiness.

HEALING CIRCLE

Witch, Bitch, the Celtic goddesses, the Warrior woman, the Martyr, the Sacrificial Lamb, the Bully, the Victim, the illusion of the 'Ideal Family', the Judge, the Inquisitor, the Shamed one, Soul, the Dishonest one, the Disillusioned one.

2. Working with dissociation

In *The Girls Within: A True Story of Triumph over Trauma and Abuse*, Gill Frost (2020) offers a moving account of working with severe dissociation using energy psychotherapy, which demonstrates how effective these methods can be.

Integration

I find energy methods astonishingly helpful in facilitating integration using 'group therapy' with severely dissociated parts and alters.

EXAMPLE

Charlotte's 'group therapy' with her alters: 'It's the wisdom of all of us when everything is channelled in to I'.

In the following example, the client desired integration. During therapy the different dissociative parts and alters were energy tested separately and each part agreed to undertake therapy as a group—'group therapy'. This resulted in the integrative work with 'Charlotte', a DID client. However, one baby part did not feel comfortable with this, so she was taken to a 'safe space' while the rest undertook energy work together.

While treating all her alters simultaneously, Charlotte, who was the 'caretaking' alter, was very pleased during one big clearing, that a new part emerged which she called 'I'. In free-associating, Charlotte had the following experience of this integration, when 'I' started talking with a new-found clarity as follows:

> **'I'** is the healthy me, integrating myself on earth—**'I'** wants to be the face of being whole—**'I'** wants to stop being an addict and wants to be whole and out there with all the parts of her speaking in unity and being allowed a voice and a name whenever she needs it—'through I'—it can be any part of her—rather than having to hide behind 'Charlotte', and not being allowed to say things.
>
> **'I'** wants to walk out of the door now instead of having to put on the mask to face the world.
>
> All of us know that all of our conditioning has just been a lie and that we can and should and need to talk with freedom and clarity, and there are appropriate places to talk.
>
> **'I'** needs more places to talk which are safe and healthy. There is fear in finding those places, which means leaving certain work securities, and trusting **'I'** will find other places.

> *'I' wants to be balanced and take her time to research and be relaxed and feel and know her choices to be right from her centre—when she follows her centre it always tells her the right thing, and then we are safe and healed and fine and we do well and prosper in the way we want to—it's the wisdom of all of us when everything is channelled in to 'I'.*
>
> *It's difficult to do this at the moment because 'I' as a whole knows she is an addict and is still in difficult places and hasn't got the use of as many spaces as she would like and may fall back into an addiction space. So, the work is helping 'I' to abstain and have awareness, and find balance, and 'I' needs to bide her time and learn what she needs to learn.*

In reflecting afterwards, it seemed that Charlotte and the family of her alters actually tapped into her centre, her inner wisdom and her soul. Her wisdom 'flowed' and found a voice through 'I'.

Integration is not the only way

The degree to which integration occurs is to some extent a matter of choice. Some who have lived with inner voices all their life, may prefer to keep the companionship of their parts. With extreme trauma and DID the idea of integration is sometimes unhelpful. Some clients prefer to accept and live with their 'alters' in better ways. Those who have had many years living with a variety of identities of both outer and inner parts and alters may fear the potential loneliness of being a 'singleton'. It may feel preferable to accept and keep their parts as they are, so that 'you are never on your own', as one client said.

3. Releasing 'massive reversals' to affirm life energy
Massive/deep/global reversals

Another important phenomenon when working with complex trauma is when the energy of a person is massively reversed. This is when the energy of the whole energy system is flowing in the opposite direction to being well.

With care, and within a relational approach where we might be exploring the client's stuckness and their difficulty moving forward, we can energy test using the phrases:

- *'I want to be well'*
- *'I want to be ill'*

If the person tests WEAK to *'I want to be well'* their system is severely compromised at the energetic level and will not be able to benefit from energy psychology methods until this reversal is corrected.

An even more severe indicator would be to energy test:

STRONG to → *'I want to be dead'*
WEAK to → *'I want to be alive'*

Obviously care needs to be taken when energy testing such statements, since the results can be very shocking if the client is completely unconscious of such wishes.

Reasons for a global reversal can include that the person is:

- severely depressed
- in thrall to 'the death instinct'
- affected by an energy toxin, such as alcoholism, chemotherapy, or various allergies, including allergy to a person
- the person's energy system has flipped into reverse in response to a trauma or series of traumas.

Energy testing for reversals can also be related to more specific reversals around a particular goal.

Mini reversals

Mini reversals refer to a reluctance to let go of *all* the emotional distress—and can be tested with sentences such as:

- '*I want to be **completely** over this problem*', vs
- '*I want to keep some of this problem*'
- '*All parts of me want to be over this ...*'

EXAMPLE

Susan and the massive reversals of her body

Susan, in her late forties, worked in a department store in London. She presented with a phobia about driving, having had several car accidents. This example focuses on her car traumas and their link to underlying issues.

Her mother became pregnant accidentally, so Susan felt, *I was unplanned and unwanted and I was an accident*. We treated both these traumas during her first session.

Aged seven, Susan's parents divorced, and she believed it was all her fault. When she went to stay with her father in his new home, she was desolate to find he hadn't prepared for her visit—there wasn't even a bed for her. She went out briefly for a walk in the park feeling unloved and unwelcomed, and walked straight out into the road without looking and a car ran her over. It was a very bad accident in which she nearly died, necessitating many painful surgeries during childhood and adolescence to repair all the damage.

Susan reflected: *Being run over confirms my belief that I deserve bad things to happen to me.*

After clearing this as a reversal and other general reversals using KC tapping, such as, *It's not safe for me to be well*' and others, we went on to clear the following traumas.

CLEARING PHRASES

The accident when I was seven and all the terrible consequences.
All my terror and trauma at all the times and ways I have been in car accidents.

During the clearing, the terrible shock of the first car accident came out—and her detailed memories of the accident, seeing everything in slow motion, being out of her body watching what was happening in limbo and not knowing if she would survive. I felt there might be massive reversals so asked her if she would mind if we energy tested her body separately and we tested

- Body I am alive—NO.
- Body I am dead—YES.

Susan was surprisingly relieved about this because it felt so true—she felt she had been living a half-life. We used *Ask and Receive* to help her heal and release from the terrible shock of all these experiences, using such phrases as: *I heal and release from the trauma of my body feeling it is dead, and I no longer need to feel the way I did when I was seven.*

Her body had various abreactions around the shock and so we then used *Ask and Receive* to install safety. After this body 're-set', her body now tested as being alive.

However, she now felt that her emotions were numb. We then energy tested *Emotions I am dead* which tested strong. Susan had various associations. She felt that her anger was close to the surface all the time but as a child there was nowhere for it to go. She energy tested strong to: *I have been living in a state of PTSD since the accident* which helped her understand how her anger and anxiety were closely linked in her PTSD fight/flight responses. It was at this point that a free association came through about the underlying cause of shock about the accident. She reflected that *I didn't want dad to be angry with me.* She suddenly connected with the shock of emotional abandonment when she first arrived at her father's house which had caused her to dissociate and had led to the first accident. After clearing this underlying trauma—that the cause of the RTA had been the shock of abandonment—there was a big shift in the work, and she made rapid progress in her healing.

CHAPTER 10

Evolving consciousness—awakening clients and transpersonal experiences

New Earth relationships

Egalitarian, co-operative, inclusive and diverse

New Earth favours egalitarian rather than hierarchical structures, and as collective consciousness evolves, so too has the nature of the therapeutic relationship. In the old 'doctor knows best' model, disagreeing with the therapist's interpretation was often discounted as 'resistance', but these days we work together more collaboratively. Contemporary heart and soul-based psychotherapies actively share power, honouring each person's sovereignty, combined with attachment-based understanding which invites playfulness and curiosity, building greater trust, intimacy and authenticity.

As power relations in New Earth evolve and transform, the therapy world is also working to develop better intercultural awareness in the therapeutic relationship. However much more progress is needed in examining our prejudices Therapy is still not as inclusive as it needs to be regarding diversity—age, gender, class, disability, sexual preference, race and so on. For instance, most therapy training environments are still disproportionately white. In a field of learning dominated by white Western theorists/practitioners which replicates 'old' power relations, the impact on black, Asian and minority ethnic learners is enormous. Several of my black therapy colleagues continue to have very painful experiences not least because, (for those of us who are white), our racism is often largely unconscious.

The spiritual and transpersonal is another area of diversity requiring further exploration. With wide-ranging cultural and spiritual/religious beliefs and differences, it would seem wise to inform ourselves about today's awakening clients, so we are not thrown by unfamiliar phenomena such as 'speaking in tongues' or 'light language'—which may be quite outside our own experience.

An expanded therapeutic remit

The range of clients coming for psychotherapy has changed considerably since the time I first started in clinical practice. People increasingly present with complex spiritual and transpersonal issues which break through conventional norms and paradigms. Therapeutic work in this field is often mixed with trauma so there is a significant tension between being open to the unknown and holding a base of grounded reality. We may not have the answers to various spiritual conundrums, but if therapy is to remain a safe container, we need to be open to those seeking solace and support so that we offer a space where clients will not feel pathologised or deemed unstable if they bring out-of-the-ordinary transpersonal or multi-dimensional experiences. This, then, is a call for a broader framework for therapy and counselling trainings, so therapists are better equipped to understand today's clients.

Complex spiritual and transpersonal issues

When someone awakens we celebrate this as an expansion of consciousness. However, we also need to understand the potential pitfalls. People with backgrounds of complex childhood trauma who experience a spiritual opening, may fall into states of borderline fragmentation and splitting (Kalsched, 2013; Schwartz-Salant, 1989) and fluctuate between different states of mind. Glimpses of 'higher' states of consciousness might intermingle with early trauma, dissociated parts, ego and soul aspects, and the wounds of traumatised 'child' selves. Each stage of the therapeutic process needs to be attended to in order to help the client back into a balanced state. Energy psychotherapy's approach is well placed to facilitate integration and containment; it can effectively address the client's overwhelm by taking things a bit at a time, clearing traumas piece by piece. However, this is delicate work, and we may not always get it right, given that clients in such states are often very sensitive and exposed.

Since transpersonal presentations frequently have roots in trauma we need to discern if an issue is purely spiritual or has psychological/developmental underpinnings. Splits in the psyche stemming from early developmental trauma and internalisation of the 'bad object' may form a good 'fit' with the 'punishing God' of fundamentalism, which may be accompanied by emotional dysregulation and 'borderline' features. If stuck in the 'paranoid–schizoid' position, a person will be polarised by extremes of good or bad with little room for integration (Klein, 1946). Furthermore, childhood neglect sometimes results in undeveloped brain function and the incapacity to mentalise (Bateman & Fonagy, 2004). The person will not have developed a sense of 'psychic equivalence', so that beliefs such as *I am* bad' (an 'evil sinner') might border on the psychotic. Consequently, if therapeutic work encroaches on 'faith' or spiritual beliefs, a person with such a mindset may easily become paranoid about 'instant karma' or feel debilitating shame as their sense of self is hijacked by their harsh superego, or 'persecutor/protector' (Kalsched, 1996, 2013). Daemonic internalisations of shadow archetypes alongside complex trauma may increase risk of self-harm and/or suicide.

People who experience 'kundalini awakening' alongside untreated early trauma are also especially vulnerable to fragmentation. 'Spiritual emergencies' can arise if a person lacks egoic integration and development to ground the 'altered states'. Awakenings can also trigger states of egoic inflation (what Chogyam Trungpa termed 'spiritual materialism'). Sadly, people who become narcissistically grandiose are unlikely to recognise their deluded state.

Another phenomenon is an obsessive search for spiritual 'signs' and synchronicities, (exacerbated if there are autistic/ADHD traits). Manic activity may ensue if 'divinations' are sought by excessively throwing tarot cards or the 'I Ching' until the desired-for 'reading' is obtained. While not inherently dangerous, such behaviours can tip over into—for example—an obsessional search for 'twin flames'—if unchecked, this could lead to stalking and potentially psychotic states of mind.

A very specific form of spiritual trauma occurs in cults. Those with backgrounds of attachment and abandonment traumas may be drawn to the certainty offered by charismatic spiritual teachers and cultic gurus. Someone with an insecure or disorganised attachment may easily project their desire for a loving God/Universe onto an abusive guru, who replicates patterns similar to their original abusive caregivers. The 'devotee' then becomes enslaved in 'people pleasing' which compromises their capacity for free and individuated thinking. In cults (of any kind) people develop an increased dependence on the abusive other, trapped in idealisation and defensive denial of what is actually going on (Newland, 2019; Shaw, 2013; Stein, 2017). Co-dependent relationships are prone to infantilisation and coercive control; if gaslit by a supposedly trustworthy leader, the resulting spiritual trauma is immense. Narcissistic cult leaders also tend to promise spiritual 'solutions' which bypass emotional process. For example, it is highly damaging when spiritual teachings—such as *all experience is empty*'—are misused. Repressing their emotions, the confused spiritual student may dissociate and bypass necessary psychological growth in favour of 'magical thinking' to keep their ideal alive.

Starseeds

'Starseeds' are a little-addressed transpersonal dimension in therapy. Sherri Divband (2020), a therapist who works with young star children, describes them as the 'anchors of New Earth' who have incarnated with a prior mission to help the planet.

> Star children are these masters that come in to teach and guide us. They have astronomical intelligence and are here in all aspects of life to help humanity—how we operate in medicine, education and innovative technology. They are much more advanced than us and come in with this innate knowledge to show us a better way. (Divband, 24 June, 2021)

Mary Rodwell names Starseeds 'The New Human' (Rodwell, 2016). Dolores Cannon (2011) speaks of three different 'waves' of Starseeds, including Indigos, Crystals, and Rainbow children. Today, large numbers are incarnating, bringing in extraordinarily advanced technologies or energetically 'activating' and awakening people with their enhanced intuition, high frequencies, and healing gifts. They are helping to raise the vibration and transmute negative energies to prepare Earth for 5-D reality.

The Starseeds I have worked with faced turmoil and challenges growing up, feeling they just don't belong here. Their struggle to fit into life and their families can make their sojourn on Earth highly stressful. One—in Corporate IT—vividly remembered her multidimensional experiences in other incarnations. Like many Starseeds, she was consciously connected with her intergalactic origins, feeling affinities to stellar systems such as The Pleiades, Arcturus, and Sirius. Her difficulties on Earth were debilitating because other people could not understand her well-intentioned but radically different approach to relationships.

5-D visionary states

Despite differences in spiritual and transpersonal states of mind, there is a remarkable convergence, reported across centuries and cultures, about fifth-dimensional (awakened) heart-based consciousness. People awaken through many routes. As well as via meditation, shamanic journeying takes us into different dimensions with nature spirits, power animals, and other worldly beings; Jung's 'active imagination' can lead people into an archetypal mythopoetic world of visions and expanded views of reality; American psychiatrist, Brian Weiss (1994) explored the multidimensional states of past lives/parallel realities; Stanislav Grof (1998) worked with expanded states of consciousness using hallucinogens; and recently increasing numbers are entering visionary states by attending ayahuasca ceremonies. Research in the clinical use of psychedelics also indicates very positive mental health benefits.

Unfortunately, however, some people's psyches shatter and fall into terror and fragmentation when they experience 'altered states'. Working therapeutically with transpersonal consciousness therefore requires a great deal more consideration.

Relevant clinical training and spiritual development

With 'the shift' occurring on our planet, what are the most helpful approaches to adopt in the quantum world of the twenty-first century? Relatively few therapy trainings have a transpersonal component—most do not. To be relevant for today's clients, as a baseline, psychotherapy and counselling trainings need to consider humanity's evolving consciousness to the fifth dimension.

Trainings in both arcane schools of wisdom and in-depth psychology are thorough, requiring that trainees undergo a solid grounding in their disciplines. This involves a long apprenticeship through a process of graduated learning and development which helps embed a stable foundation—comparable with a secure root chakra, or Bowlby's 'secure base'.

Ethics and shadow in the new paradigm

When we integrate shadow, we arrive at wholeness. However, unconscious, unworked-through shadow results in distortion and lack of integrity. We live in an age of narcissism—of service to self—which is why it is so important that we thoroughly address our developmental issues and trauma—otherwise, there is a danger that the transpersonal becomes glamourised.

Nowadays, there is a tendency for people to look for instant gratification and this also features in ways people seek to access higher states of consciousness. It is not uncommon for people to attend a weekend workshop and be introduced to powerful shamanic rituals or drug ceremonies including the use of LSD or ayahuasca, with little to anchor their experience. Learning esoteric skills without proper grounding or adequate follow-up might bring about transpersonal openings with unintended and potentially drastic consequences, bringing out early, destabilising childhood trauma.

This becomes ethically more complex if the workshop participant happens to be an inexperienced therapist or therapist-in-training, who is excited to try out their new skills with clients. Training organisations therefore need to offer clear guidelines for their therapy students; for instance, prioritising skills in holding, containment, and developmental work before mixing with different disciplines such as shamanism. To avoid such muddles and potential damage to both therapists and clients, is why we only accept experienced qualified therapists on our energy psychotherapy clinical trainings.

Intuition is another tricky area. Naturally, following the client is vital in any therapeutic endeavour. However, if the therapist becomes too fixed on 'following their own guidance' they may, unwittingly, in the service to their own ego, override their client's wisdom. If shadow inflates the therapists sense of self-importance, there are even greater risks. Even if, as therapists, we have a sense of inner 'knowing', we might be and often can be wrong (especially if one is out of alignment). 'Intuition' can be ethically problematic unless, as a therapist, one keeps this to oneself. There is a delicate balance to find between healthy scepticism, 'knowing', and trusting one's intuition/guidance. Phil Mollon, former Chair of the international organisation ACEP (Association for Comprehensive Energy Psychology), and Chair of its ethics committee, speaks of the 'Dangers of idealisation and illusions of knowing' (Mollon, 2008). In Chapter 19 of his book (pp. 467–474) he explores how certainty can be dangerous, and a degree of doubt is healthy. Phil suggests to therapists: 'Allow yourself to be guided by a combination of your own deepest wisdom and the client's deepest wisdom—but giving priority to the indicators from your client's system'.

Getting carried away with the powerful effects of energy work is another risk if this inflates the inexperienced therapist's perception of themselves as a 'healer'. It is always important to emphasise that any healing which occurs is as a result of the *energy*—it is *not* the therapist 'healing the client'. The powerful results of energy work can also lead to unrealistic expectations of 'quick-fix' solutions. Certainly, new energy approaches do make healing swifter and easier. Nonetheless, many of us have needed to be in therapy for several years to work through our difficulties and traumas—developmental integration takes time.

Finally, in working with the transpersonal, for the safety of both client and therapist, the ethical standards promoted by regulatory bodies may not be sufficiently informed. What is perceived by some as completely normal, might be deemed inappropriate by others. Each therapist's Code of Practice is governed by the ethical guidelines of their regulatory bodies, so these codes need to be reviewed, clarified, and updated to reflect changes in contemporary therapeutic practice, to include an understanding of energy and transpersonal work. Similarly, complaints procedures also need updating.

The therapist's own psychological and spiritual development

Neville Symington argued that instead of considering spirituality as outside the realm of therapy, the therapy profession needs to adapt and be supportive of the journey of spiritual evolution as a core aspect of life's experience. Whether a person—therapist or client—feels comfortable with this area may depend on their own level of spiritual engagement and awareness. It therefore seems essential that therapy trainings which do not already do so, review their training 'brief' to include a psycho-spiritual/transpersonal component. Continuing professional development could then invite reflective practice, so that therapists keep abreast of new developments in this field and are better placed to serve today's awakening clients.

The concept that spiritually open therapists and supervisors need to experience their own journey of evolution and expanded states of consciousness is like the expectation that counsellors and psychotherapists need to have therapy themselves as part of their training before being considered a 'safe pair of hands'. Long trainings mature therapists, so that they can listen openly to their clients without unconsciously projecting their own issues. Similarly, in terms of spiritual awareness, attending to our own disbeliefs about spirituality or transpersonal experiences—our scepticism, fears, prejudice, or ignorance—is a useful starting place. If we are not able to understand our client's world, there is no shame in recognising our limitations or needing help to learn how psycho/spiritual work can be meaningfully addressed and integrated.

Since transpersonal experiences are 'beyond analysis', the journey of awakening is not cognitive, but *embodied*. The developmental work of 'psychotherapy in a new paradigm' extends to include the evolution of our consciousness, by releasing density and raising our vibration, so that we can hold more light in our cells. In this way, awakening is well served by energy psychotherapy.

Love—the interconnecting frequency

We can only fully perceive another when we resonate at the same or a higher frequency/level of chakric development. So if (for example) a high vibrational Starseed is in therapy with a less spiritually evolved therapist, they will look for a suitable 'wavelength' which they can both tune in to. The client will want to know that the therapist can understand and perceive them accurately without judging and can help them with whatever they are going through. This is why it is so important that the therapist has an open heart. Since the universal inter-connecting point is the frequency of love, even if the therapist has not done much spiritual work on themselves, if their heart is open, they can provide a safe space for meaningful therapeutic exchange.

Spiritual practices within psychotherapy

'The therapist's presence ... generates, or evokes, a field of spiritual energy which envelops client and therapist and activates the client's connection to their own soul' (Yeomans, 1994). When working with energy, it is helpful if the therapist has developed presence through having some kind of meditation or spiritual practice/connection.

The therapist can bring presence into therapy sessions in various ways:

- *Meditation*: meditating with the client for a few minutes cultivates presence. In energy psychotherapy, we can do this during energy balancing exercises or after a clearing. Such moments of stillness help us be open to our wise self—our true authentic nature. 'Being' takes us out of the fight/flight axis of survival mode while 'simply remaining' (a meditation term) and cultivating awareness, establishes harmonious interconnect-edness in the field.
- *Breathwork* is excellent for grounding and balancing energetically. If clients tend to dissociate, conscious breathwork done together by therapist and client can bring us home to ourselves so we become more regulated and embodied.
- *Visualisation, chakra meditations, and light practices* are expansive, and clients can find such visualisations transformative.
- *Resourcing using healing circles*: creating an alliance with our inner parts and energies facilitates containment, acceptance, and integration. Bringing in both positive resources and challenging archetypes enables us to harmonise our energy field and heal our wounds.
- *Reframing and retrospective gratitude*: finding meaning in painful experiences, in the service of greater understanding, brings about post-traumatic growth and deeper spiritual connectedness.
- *Mindfulness, awareness, and 'witness consciousness'*—when we view from the soul's rather than ego's perspective, the soul's 'witness consciousness' brings a higher-dimensional compassionate and accepting attitude.
- *Cultivating self-love and self-compassion*: learning to accept and experience love and self-compassion creates a natural healing space.
- *Embodiment and connectedness*: trauma clearing using energy methods helps us become more present and connected with our bodies, and facilitates the integration of feelings and experiences.

Incorporating energy work in therapy trainings

Since vibration and frequency are at the heart of the new paradigm, the therapeutic discourse expands from one of 'understanding' and analysing our problems to include clearing trauma and dense energies from our bodies and energy fields. To bring this understanding into therapy trainings, in addition to core training in therapeutic skills and psychological development, a transpersonal/energy component of therapy trainings (many of which are outlined in this book) might include:

- rudiments about energy and resonance
- essential balancing exercises for self-regulation
- simple energy methods for clearing trauma
- intercultural, spiritual, and transpersonal perspectives about consciousness
- mindfulness and awareness—simple practices using breath
- the use of healing circles to integrate all parts of the client in therapy
- skills training at graduate and postgraduate skills levels, working with *bodymindenergy* to address trauma held in the body and facilitate integrative work
- Specific topics:
  - gathering together the souls' disconnected fragments
  - active imagination (Jung); working with imagery and archetypal energies
  - out-of-body experiences—working with disconnection and dissociation
  - transgenerational and past life trauma
  - working with Starseeds

- Understanding energy boundaries
  - porous boundaries/lack of energy boundaries/boundarylessness (which is increasingly prevalent with ADHD and autistic traits)
  - trauma violations and the creation of leaky tears/holes in the energy bodies resulting in depletion and energetic draining
  - self-care methods for retaining healthy energy boundaries

Depth assessment skills

Transpersonal states of consciousness may arise in any form of therapy. First, we seek to understand a person's history—the mental, emotional, spiritual, and cultural issues within their personal matrix. The road maps outlined in Chapter 6 provide developmental frameworks for recognising what might be happening, and assessing the therapeutic priorities which need attending to.

When spiritual awakening is part of the picture, 'assessment' can be quite complex. Clarke (2010) and Miller (2024) cite how spiritual emergencies may be classified in many ways—as peak experiences, past-life experiences, channelling with spirit guides, kundalini awakenings, dark and night possessions, near-death experiences, UFO encounters, or drug and alcohol addictions. A cultural bias might determine whether such experiences are labelled psychotic or spiritual. Shamans, prophets, spiritual teachers, saints, or luminaries may be perceived as having enlightened qualities, whereas others having similar experiences might be labelled psychotic, even though both groups might benefit from, and become transformed by, the experience. In such instances, having a healthily functioning ego may be the determining factor which indicates if the experience can be stabilised and integrated.

This somewhat overwhelming list of classifying factors shows how important it is to respect the client's world view when trying to make sense of their spiritual dilemmas, transpersonal experiences, or 'altered' states of consciousness. With such a wide range of possibilities we need to be able to hold simultaneously contradictory perspectives, such as being open, 'not knowing,' and having the capacity to discern.

Suspending disbelief and not being too hasty to 'diagnose'

Any of us can temporarily go off the rails at any time. A healing crisis and new integrations may be occurring and sometimes things just right themselves, so it is helpful to stay open and avoid jumping to conclusions too quickly. If someone presents in a disintegrated state with a fragmented ego, they may simply be trauma-triggered. It is usually possible to stabilise them quite quickly with energy therapy by treating the relevant trauma(s).

However, when traumatised people dissociate or leave their bodies, they may present with a variety of transpersonal and/or 'spiritual' phenomena. How do we differentiate between spiritual/transpersonal experiences and intensely dissociated, troubled states? Listening to our countertransference—especially that of our body—and using energy testing, can provide useful information:

- Does this person's experience feel to be out of balance? In which case, undertaking simple energy balancing exercises (see Chapter 7) can be profoundly helpful and calming.
- Might an early trauma have been activated, borne out of extreme pain and distress breaking open early splits in the psyche?
- Is this a borderline/or inflated state?
- Is this a transpersonal experience or a potential psychosis?

These points raise important questions. For instance, when a client is 'seeing things', we need to be able to differentiate between a psychotic disturbance, the visions of someone with a genuinely intuitive or psychic state of mind, and spiritual emergence/spiritual emergency (Grof, 1998; Jung, 1973a; Levin, 1998).

As an example, an intuitive client from a family gifted with 'the sight' was very distressed to see moths and creatures flying out of her skin. A psychiatrist diagnosed her as psychotic and prescribed anti-psychotic medication. The client felt she hadn't been fully 'seen' so she had a consultation with a past-life regression therapist. This process revealed that she had been buried alive in a tomb in a previous life and her current visions were of traumatic memories of grubs hatching out and flying out from her body in the coffin. In her psychic state of intuitive fifth-dimensional consciousness (where the past, present, and future are contained in the present moment), she was experiencing this past life in the present.

There may be many ways of understanding such experiences. To my mind, though the client was very distressed, I did not feel her sanity was in question. In this instance, she felt relieved to be seen—by accepting her experience, she felt recognised and validated. A psychoanalytical perspective might interpret that her psyche had been 'buried alive' by intergenerational trauma—a key question might be: does the client find this interpretation helpful?

Common sense and balance

When people seek therapy to address difficult spiritual experiences, they are sometimes very ungrounded (as described in an early case vignette), with nowhere to live, no money, and no job—they have no 'secure base'. In determining how best to help, common sense is important. While energy work generally helps to integrate both ego and soul, if someone is on the borders, we need to consider carefully what might be needed to stabilise, what intervention would be containing, and whether there is any risk which necessitates seeking additional support.

Even though we do not want to be too hasty to 'diagnose', sometimes common sense requires that we intervene, so that a situation isn't allowed to deteriorate. However, this isn't always possible. In one instance, a woman developed a powerful spiritual mystique. Seduced by her beauty, people colluded with her grandiose portrayal of herself as a 'crazy wisdom *dakini*' ('crazy wisdom' is a phenomenon in Dzogchen and *dakini* is an aspect of the 'divine feminine'). She went on to bankrupt her husband and seduce many others, obtaining several thousands of pounds from various people, although 'common sense' indicated that she was severely mentally ill—she was eventually sectioned as psychotic and hospitalised.

* * *

I trust that in considering the challenges of transpersonal experience, this does not detract from the truly positive aspects of awakening—the wonderful unfolding expansion of consciousness which ultimately brings us to states of light, peace, and love.

Supervision for transpersonal work

A creative supportive space

An exciting development within the world of energy psychotherapy is that as more and more therapists train in this innovative field, a creative community is learning together, sharing our discoveries about energy psychotherapy and transpersonal issues. In terms of being a supervisee myself, I very much appreciate a kind, open-hearted, and collaborative supervisory space where I explore the work with a supervisor who has skill, insight, and wisdom. Let us set the intention for the development of well-informed supervisors, experienced in energy work and transpersonal issues where supervisees can feel confident to share the complexities of their work, and explore their uncertainties and 'not knowing' without fear of being judged or viewed as an unsafe practitioner. Moreover, it is particularly helpful when supervisor and therapist tune in together to 'higher guidance', seeking assistance directly from Source. This greatly facilitates the collaborative flow.

Traditional diagnostic frameworks and analytic thinking in supervision

So, what other supervisory elements might be helpful? Whatever their clinical orientation, the supervisor is there to support the therapist in providing a secure base for their clients and to think about 'levels' of therapeutic intervention. Both humanistic/person-centred approaches which work in the here and now, and neurobiological understandings, contribute to safety, which is a key factor when working with complex trauma. Analytic perspectives provide a useful frame for understanding the roots and 'repetition compulsions' of trauma, developmental stages, unconscious defences, ego strength, and how to establish groundedness. The development perspective of the chakras is also very helpful (see Chapter 6).

Underlying theories/approaches contribute to recognising vulnerabilities and discerning how to work safely and assess risk. Sometimes it may be neither advisable nor ethical to work with a severely traumatised person. As one example, a psychic whom I worked with briefly, was paranoid about the black and white floor tiles in her kitchen, doing everything possible to avoid stepping on the black tiles. From a psychoanalytic perspective this phobia might suggest the 'paranoid–schizoid position' (Klein, 1946) as a factor. However, this client had endured extreme group abuse which often causes DID, out-of-body experiences, and greater sensitivities to energies and psychic phenomena. Black and white tiles feature strongly in satanic ritual abuse, so her phobia may well have been linked to this. Living as she was with a terrifyingly abusive partner in circumstances of coercive control, this woman was particularly unsafe. All these indicators suggested that she was not sufficiently stable and lacked the support necessary to undertake therapy at this point in her life. Neither was she ready, nor wishing to work at a deep level—a delicate situation where there is no 'right answer'.

Examples of 'transpersonal' work

The following examples illustrate multidimensionality, where past, present, and future coalesce in the quantum field of zero point, in the moment of now. Working in this field sometimes feels a little dreamlike and 'light'—or alternatively, energetically very 'heavy' and trance-like—but whatever the experience, transpersonal work feels very real, and is deeply embodied, visceral work. When in 'presence' with the client, the work flows quite easily, normally, and naturally and it is surprising how quickly and effortlessly the trauma clears.

EXAMPLES

'Krys' and her devastating past (parallel) lives as a warrior in battles over many centuries:
Krys was a psychic Starseed who remembered her recurring roles as warrior and army general throughout many lifetimes, both on earth and off-planet. We used energy testing during all our work together to verify the traumas which she needed to clear. Krys reported feeling responsible for great devastation and mass killing, felt irredeemable for all the harm she had caused, and was struggling to rid herself of intense guilt. She lived her current life on a continuing battle ground—various wounds and injuries kept manifesting, which, she felt, were repetitions of wounds from the battlefields. She gained considerable relief from energy clearings of these and other past-life traumas. Following this, she experienced a radical improvement in her health, her sense of integration and well-being. While, to an outsider, Krys may have seemed a little grandiose (the commanding quality of having been a general was quite in evidence), the visceral quality of the work and very evident changes demonstrated to me the importance of clearing these deepest multidimensional roots of trauma.

'Jane's neck injury—'bleeding through' from a past life
Jane was a retired nurse in her mid-seventies, a proud courageous woman with considerable presence. She had survived complex trauma and abuse as a child and presented in therapy with PTSD, terrified and anxious all the time and in permanent states of hypervigilance. She hated feeling vulnerable, and largely hid this from those around her. Following a car crash, Jane lived with a debilitating injury which caused permanent neck damage and pain. One day she commented on her morbid fascination with beheading which led directly into an energy clearing where she viscerally re-experienced being beheaded (though she felt no physical pain). She 'relived' the details as the executioner failed to cut her head off at the first strike of the axe. She commented on the exact replication of the pattern of severed nerves, a symptom in her current neck damage where many nerves were disconnected, causing agonising nerve pain. After this energy clearing, the intensity of Jane's PTSD and fear considerably reduced. Her husband sent a message via Jane that he was happy to see her so much more relaxed, and that 'whatever we were doing, keep on doing it'. However we understand Jane's presentation— that she was re-experiencing unresolved traumatic energy bleeding through from a previous timeline, or as a metaphor for her pain and distress—the energy clearings helped relieve her distress, and brought her to a state of calm.

'Ahmed'—disturbed by energies of the 'shadow world'
Ahmed was an intelligent gifted young Arab who had taken too many drugs and was confused about his perceptions. He frequently saw terrifying visions of 'end-of-the-world' scenarios with much death and suffering. He and his girlfriend regularly took drugs together and discussed their 'mental health issues'—he could never be sure if he was psychic or suffering from drug-induced psychosis. He was eventually referred to me for energy work to help him deal with his depression, anxiety, and a general feeling of lack of grounding, where he was 'floating' much of the time. In telling me his history, it transpired that throughout his life, his father thought Ahmed was a 'loser' and had been highly critical and undermining of him, giving intense 'verbal beatings'.

When Ahmed was a baby, he was taken to clinics in Europe to help with life-threatening asthma. Almost by chance, he told me that the first remedy his parents sought was with a local healer. Ahmed had been taken to a blind man who burned his skin to 'take the devil out of him'. At this point in the session, the 'charge' in the room was very high so we cleared the trauma in the moment, using the words:

> All my trauma and terror at being burned and tortured by the blind man when I was a baby, 'taking the devil' out of me to treat my asthma.

During the clearing Ahmed realised he had completely left his body when he was a baby to cope with this torture and had felt disconnected most of his life. However, during the energy work, he strongly experienced his soul coming back into his body. The following week, he reported feeling 'whole and good'—his 'true self'—for the first time in his life. His mind had cleared dramatically after the session; he no longer felt confused, he had clarity, and was grounded. As therapy continued, Ahmed began to unpack more of his visions and realised that some of them had actually been prescient—including knowledge of the Covid-19 pandemic well in advance of it actually happening.

'Geraldine'—was bullied for her intuitive abilities and so shut them down
Geraldine was bullied and ridiculed for being different by those from the rational culture in which she grew up. After this trauma she shut down and disconnected from her considerable psychic and intuitive abilities. Outwardly she appeared to grow up, but secretly she suffered a great deal from her loss of spiritual connection. Treating this soul-wound—which was at a transpersonal level quite distinct from the personal—was as important as clearing the more obvious traumatic wounds—such as bullying—from childhood. We also cleared patterns of repetition compulsions from previous lifetimes where Geraldine had similarly shut down after being persecuted for her psychic and healing gifts. As Geraldine reclaimed these lost soul fragments into herself and reconnected with her soul, so her healing and intuitive gifts began to open up again.

Wholeness, trust, healing, and love

We know that everything is energy, and science reveals that the essence of this energy—the divine matrix—is love. The God code is written into every cell of life (Braden, 2004). Source energy is present throughout the fabric of the entire universe flowing throughout our being, just as we are part of this whole. Our soul—our original unique blueprint—is a holographic fractal of the divine. When we learn how to open our hearts, fully connect with our souls, and experience the divine love that we truly are, we realise that ultimately, we are all one. Even though our life circumstances may vary quite radically, we are all interconnected in this vast field of energy.

Awakening—if we choose this path—is a possibility for us all. We might have an epiphany when, through blessing and grace, we realise that our true nature is of light. We feel very grateful to overcome our ceaseless mind-chatter and experience instead our innate goodness—it is blissful. In the quantum field, just one glimpse of enlightenment instantaneously cuts through aeons of suffering in the eternal moment of now—though for most of us, we lose this state of unity consciousness fairly quickly and discover that learning to stabilise the experience takes years of practise.

The ordinary 3-D world is completely different. Although mystics talk about the 'illusory' nature of reality, suffering feels only too real when we are in pain or disconnected from love. We might turn to therapy for help and discover that energy psychotherapy provides wonderful opportunities for healing. I am so grateful for the 'ease and grace' of these methods, which, after releasing dense energy, help us to feel so much lighter.

***

As I look back on the quest to find myself—as a musician, a psychotherapist, and an energy worker—there have been many turning points. We all learn from our experiences, so in sharing these reflections, it is in recognition that you too will have learned much from your journey.

My beautiful sensitive sister's illness and subsequent suicide had the most profound influence on my life. Many readers will have had to deal with devastating grief where we do not know how we will be able to get over the loss. During that period of mourning, I was so touched by simple acts of human kindness—such as being invited to eat with friends who were gentle and loving when I could do little but weep.

A pilgrimage to Nepal and visiting the sacred sites of India provided space to mourn. I wanted my sister's suffering to serve a greater purpose. Her death put things in perspective and galvanised me to change. I wanted finally to overcome the engrained habits of my early upbringing and instead value the preciousness of life and the fundamental purity, goodness, and light that is common to us all.

Since then, it has been a continual roller coaster of awakening. Ego fought back and I kept losing my way. Transcending dualistic perception and viewing life with love and compassion rather than judgement is constant 'work in progress'. St Francis of Assisi's prayer, 'Lord, make me an instrument of Your peace' has offered balm and healing. Although as 'creator consciousness' there are many opportunities to choose high vibrations and envision what I would like rather than falling back into negative habits, it takes self-discipline to practise mindfulness and awareness, and to remember to choose love.

Individuating—no longer following others and being a sovereign self—was a big challenge. After leaving the spiritual community there was much emotional clearing out to do—of grief, regret, anger, and disappointment … rather than externalising my guides as the source of wisdom outside me, I also needed to trust in myself and in my inner guidance (though, paradoxically, I still pray and invoke the blessing of God/Source, Jesus and Buddha—honouring that ultimately, we are one).

Another catalyst for change occurred after developing a minor heart condition, which pushed me to leave the security of my NHS job—I think it would have killed me if I had stayed.

I struggled to find the courage to overcome fears and doubts, where I had no control of the outcome, and simply allow the universe to guide me. Stepping through doors into the unknown was terrifying. However, I discovered that when you take a leap of faith, the universe *is* there to catch you—it has been a revelation just how much guidance there is to support us, providing for us each step of the way. For instance, during the period of financial instability which followed, large bills of thousands of pounds accumulated, and I did not know how I would pay. I set my intention to trust (without being sure that I believed) and then out of the blue one day, my conveyancing solicitor (long after completing on my property), phoned up and said, 'I've been thinking you should be due back several thousand pounds VAT on your purchase—would you like me to try and reclaim it?' A tax expert had previously told me this was impossible. However, my wonderful solicitor managed to do so, and after paying him, I had *exactly* the right money to get me back into solvency. This proved beyond doubt that trust does overcome fear and there *are* solutions to problems even if we do not know how they will manifest. Learning to trust has helped me unwind and 'relax in the arms of the universe', knowing fundamentally that all is well.

Finding integration and balance between light and shadow has been another major theme. In facing unpleasant archetypal roles that I have 'played' in this and other lifetimes, I really struggled to arrive at neutrality—or zero point. The biggest revelation about past lives is not so much that terrible things happened to me, but that I, too, could be the one who did terrible things. I found it so challenging to accept and integrate frightening shadow energies as part of me—but also, as I go deeper into clearing layers of trauma and negativity, the brighter is the light. Recognising the universality of our archetypal human experience (whilst also honouring our specific personal and cultural roots) makes it easier to embrace these facets and bring them home to unconditional love—though again, this continues to be 'work in progress'.

Triggers used to totally dysregulate me. However, I have learned to value them as opportunities for growth, bringing to our attention wounds that need healing. I like to dedicate this personal work (something I learned from Buddhism) as a contribution towards healing the collective field. Although I no longer formally follow Buddhism, I really honour its wisdom. I have found many Buddhist teachings—such as the teaching on impermanence—immensely helpful. I used to try to hold onto everything. However, understanding that impermanence is the natural order of things—the cycle of life and death, where winter dies so spring can be reborn—helped me let go. Another inspiring teaching, The Five Perfections, invites us to trust in life itself as the path (see Chapter 6). However hard and painful the situations and circumstances which manifested on my soul's journey have been, as I reflect, they really have helped me evolve. The under-standing that life's circumstances—including its 'obstacles'—ultimately benefit us, has been transformative.

Forgiveness, compassion, kindness, and gratitude all play their part on the path of joy. I find acceptance, however, particularly astonishing. It has taken years to learn that 'what you resist persists'—avoidance just brings more pain. Acceptance more than anything has helped me find peace of mind. By simply accepting present reality, problems just fall away, and life becomes so much easier.

We are all at different ages and stages on our journeys. I feel very humbled by dear friends who have died of serious and painful illnesses yet still managed to transform their suffering. One, Tracy, a spiritual practitioner, cleared her energy so completely that when a Dzogchen Master visited her after her death from a brain tumour, he recognised her in her passing as one of the first Western students to arrive at enlightenment—the ultimate healing and transcendence.

**

I have always been a seeker of the new energy. Globally, during the early 2020s, we have been experiencing the greatest shift in cosmic history as several major galactic cycles concurrently came to an end and we simultaneously birth and create the new world … how extraordinary to witness and be part of such history-in-the-making. As the influx of plasma light increases and light is cast on the shadows of the old world, we are appalled at the revelations of so much darkness and corruption, leaving many disheartened and overwhelmed. And, at the same time, if we can stay in the flow of this high vibrational energy our fears and doubts melt away. In all this, how we choose to perceive the world is key. As we are one with creator, by steadily holding a positive vision of how we would like things to be, we can create a better future 'with ease and grace'.

I feel blessed to be alive on earth at this exciting time in our planet's evolution. I am very grateful for all that I have been given, and the dear friends and soulmates I have met along the way. Meditation, energy work, and connecting with my soul have brought love, sacredness, beauty, fulfilment, and creative expression into my life. And as the path unfolds, it becomes simpler and clearer.

Many people find that the experience of energy work brings them to a peaceful feeling of completeness—we come home to ourselves and embody our souls. I do hope that you too will come home to experience the light of your soul, find joy and inspiration to guide your lives—and know that all is love.

Epilogue

Synchronously, at the exact moment of completing this manuscript, an email winged its way across the world from the Khyentse foundation in India (the lineage of Dilgo Khyentse Rinpoche) sending a photograph of the Heart Sutra ceremony. So I end as I started this book, invoking *Prajnaparamita*—the divine feminine—who emanates love and blessings, and opens us to the vast spaciousness of awakening.

May we all realise the Awakened heart!

Epilogue.

Glossary

Acupoint tapping: A generic term for those energy psychology approaches that involve tapping on meridian acupoints (TFT, EFT, and various other methods).

Additional vessels: In addition to the twelve meridians, there are two important additional vessels—the governing (tapping point under the nose) and the central (tapping point under lip, on chin). These vessels do not have alarm points.

Advanced Integrative Therapy (AIT): The approach developed by Asha Clinton, involving work with chakras, integrating themes and insights from a range of traditions and approaches, and including protocols for many different applications. https://www.ait-uk-europe.com/

Akashic records: A record of all the experiences we have been through in all our lifetimes during the soul's journey, sometimes referred to as a library of information.

Alarm points: Each of the twelve meridians has an 'alarm point', mostly not on the meridian itself. These can feel tender when the meridian is out of balance. They are used diagnostically to locate relevant meridians to treat but can also be used therapeutically (for example, in lung meridian breathing).

Allergy antidotes: A range of methods developed by Sandi Radomski to alleviate allergies and sensitivities.

Ascension: The purpose of ascension is to bring all multidimensional aspects of ourselves into one embodiment, in oneness, in our human body. We do so by raising our frequency and gathering the multi-faceted aspects of our being into our body—integrating the divine aspects of us within the physical. There is a 'collective' ascension occurring for all humanity, where those who hold the values of 'service to others' are said to be evolving to fifth-dimensional consciousness known as 'Heaven on Earth'. 'Ascension' may be somewhat of a misnomer, since it is not so much a process of 'going up', as *embodying* the higher frequencies, embodying spirit in matter. As we connect with and integrate different parts of ourselves—our soul, our higher self and so on—i.e. the multidimensional aspects of us—our consciousness expands. As we return to source-light and embody these higher frequencies in the cells of our body, our whole reality changes.

Ask and Receive: An approach developed by Sandi Radomski, Pam and Tom Altaffer, relying on a series of carefully formed statements, to 'Ask' and 'Receive' the desired change.

Association for Comprehensive Energy Psychology (ACEP): The professional body for energy psychologists of all kinds.

Awakening: Awakening has two principal meanings. One concerns the dawning realisation as people wake up to the truth of what has been happening on our planet—the 'Great Awakening'. The second meaning concerns the opening of our hearts, lifting the veils of egoic reality (our state of separation) into the 'awakened state' of oneness, in the quantum field of the fifth dimension.

Axiatonal lines: These are hypothesised vertical energy flow lines which extend above and outside the body into the wider field. These have a kind of parallel equivalence to the meridians; Phil Mollon teaches tapping fingertips and thumb tips, which uses these lines. They are also used in Eric Pearl's *The Reconnection*.

Biofield: This is the word chosen by a team of scientists in 1994 to describe the field of energy and information that surrounds and interpenetrates the human body. It is composed of both measurable electromagnetic energy and hypothetical subtle energy, or Qi. This structure is also called the human energy field, aura, and energy body.

Chakra clearing: Procedures for clearing emotional information via the chakras. Many different methods have been developed, including holding, tapping, spinning, singing, holding tuning forks, coloured light, Tibetan bowls, use of intention, and Blue Diamond work.

Chakras: Energy centres down the midline of the body. These were originally described in traditional Indian yoga but have been explored in various ways within Western traditions (Leland, 2016). They are described by those who can see them, as vortexes/whirlpools of force that swirl rapidly and give the effect of a fiery wheel. Although not physical or anatomical, the chakras do have neuro-physiological correlates in the form of high concentrations of neuropeptides.

'Chasing the pain': A technique in EFT, whereby the focus is upon following the shifting somatic sensations (not necessarily actual pain).

Church, Dawson: A researcher, trainer, publisher, author, and speaker who has greatly facilitated the field of energy psychology. He owns the *Energy Psychology* journal, the Energy Psychology Press, and the www.eftuniverse.com website.

Clinton, Asha: A Jungian Psychotherapist in the USA, who developed Seemorg Matrix, subsequently renamed Advanced Integrative Therapy (AIT).

Collar-bone breathing: A breathing procedure developed by Roger Callahan that is often helpful in states of systemic energetic disorganisation. It is calming and helps to bring the energy system and brain into coherence. A simpler version was developed by John Diepold and colleagues, and also modified by Phil Mollon.

Cook's hook-ups: Various postures and procedures developed by chiropractor Wayne Cook, to correct energetic disturbances.

Craig, Gary: The developer of EFT.

Cross crawl: An old Applied Kinesiology technique to correct homolateral energy flow. There are various forms of this, all involving some kind of alternating arm and leg movement (rather like normal walking).

Dzogchen: Known as the 'Great Perfection' or 'Great Completion', Dzogchen is a tradition of teachings in Tibetan Buddhism aimed at realising the ultimate nature of reality or enlightenment. It is also termed *Atiyoga*—or utmost yoga—since it operates beyond the cognitive mind of ego in the realm of 'pure awareness' or *Rigpa*. It is also somewhat confusingly referred to as 'The Nature of Mind'. This level of consciousness, called 'The king of all Medicines, is similar to 'zero point' in the creative quantum unified field, wherein lies the vast expanse of all possibilities.

Eden energy medicine: The brand name of the approach developed by Donna Eden and David Feinstein.

Emotional Freedom Techniques (EFT): A derivative of Thought Field Therapy, developed by Gary Craig. At the energetic level, it is a simplification of TFT, but in its application there can be considerable psychological sophistication.

Energy: Quantum physics identifies that physical atoms are made up of vortices of energy that are constantly spinning and vibrating. The universe is one indivisible dynamic whole in which energy and matter are so deeply entangled it is impossible to consider them as independent elements. There are two distinct forms of energy that are involved in energy psychology. Electrical and Electromagnetic energy is well understood. Subtle energy, while outside the Western paradigm has long been recognised in other cultures e.g. in China as Qi—the basis for acupuncture.

Energy balancing: is sometimes referred to as neurological regulation in other energy psychology systems. Systemic energy disturbances can occur if there is:
- 'Neurological disorganisation' (also known as 'polarity reversal') and
- 'Homolateral disorganisation' (when the energy flow across the body and between right and left brain becomes confused)

The body's energy system needs to be in correct balance and alignment, otherwise this prevents the body's energy system from flowing naturally, either in terms of electromagnetic polarity, or in terms of left- and right-brain functioning. (See also neurological disorganisation.)

Energy psychology is a collection of mind–body approaches which focus on the relationship between thoughts, emotions, sensations and behaviours, and the known bioenergy systems (meridians, chakras and the biofield). These bioenergy systems and processes interact within individuals and between people and are also influenced by cultural and environmental factors.

Energy psychotherapy is an integration of energy psychology methods into psychotherapy. It is a particular feature of depth psychotherapy integrating trauma clearing that has been developed in the UK.

Feinstein, David: A clinical psychologist, well known for his summaries of research and his lucid talks and papers on possible modes of action of energy psychology. He is married to Donna Eden and together they have developed Eden Energy Medicine.

Fibonacci sequence: Sometimes termed the Golden Ratio, in the Fibonacci sequence each number is the sum of the two preceding ones. This creates a spiral, the fundamental growth pattern which is pervasive throughout the universe, in nature, music, biology, and other disciplines. A fern leaf, the internal structure of spiral seashells, or the swirling spirals of galaxies offer good visual examples.

The fifth dimension: This refers to the quantum (unified field) which operates at a high vibrational state. It is also a state of consciousness which can only be accessed through an open heart, a peaceful balanced state of equanimity sometimes referred to as 'zero point'. It is the state of 'pure awareness' beyond egoic mind which opens out into a new reality, which some term 'Heaven on Earth' where time ceases to exist and post present, and future all exist within the present moment. This is contrasted with ego's state which operates in the 3rd dimension of Newtonian physics, the world of duality, cause and effect, and egoic mind.

Gallo, Fred: The clinical psychologist who proposed the term 'energy psychology'. Gallo has been a major figure in the EP world.

Goodheart, George: The founder of Applied Kinesiology, which gave rise to many offshoots, including energy psychology.

Great Awakening (The): This refers to the awakening of consciousness, which is currently occurring on planet earth, and is also linked with the idea of Ascension.

Grid lines: There are various energy grids, like ley lines, which conduct subtle energy around the earth. One is known as the Crystalline Grid, which links the crystals in the earth. There is also a third dimensional grid, and a new fifth-dimensional grid, like a 'super-information highway' which is anchoring in higher dimensional energy and plasmic light, assisting planet earth and its inhabits in the ascension process. When we link together as lightworkers in mediation, our intentions travel via this subtle energy grid.

Healing from the body-level up (HBLU): The approach developed by Judith Swack, previously a cell biologist.

Higher self: The higher self is a term associated with multiple belief systems, but its basic premise describes an eternal, conscious, intelligent being, who is part of the multidimensional self. According to Micheila Sheldan, in essence, human beings are present on many levels in fractals of 'reality' simultaneously, as an aspect of Source/Creator expressing itself.
- Our Soul is individual, embodied in our physical body
- Our Higher self is an energetic, collective being
- The Oversoul is our cosmic self

Homolateral energy flow: Homolateral energy flows *across* the body. A test to check whether the homolateral flow is balanced, is to have the subject look at a large X and also at two parallel lines. The X should energy test strong and the parallel lines weak. If these are out of alignment, one correction is to do any variant of 'cross crawl'.

Hydration: Many energetic disturbances are caused by a lack of sufficient water or de-hydration. Our bodies require a lot of water to conduct the electrical current through the body when undertaking energy psychotherapy. If we are dehydrated, it is not possible to conduct efficient energy therapy, but this can easily be remedied by drinking water.

Individual energy toxins: A term used by Roger Callahan to denote substances that disturb (scramble or reverse) a person's energy system. They are specific to the individual—commonly including perfumes and grooming products, laundry products, air 'fresheners', and other pollutants.

Introduction to the nature of mind: In the Dzogchen tradition, this is the 'pointing-out' instruction which helps people experienced the awakened state. As the lama gives the instruction, the ordinary nature of egoic mind dissolves and consciousness opens out into the nature of true reality or *Rigpa*—pure awareness. This is an embodied experience of light consciousness, beyond categorisation or concept—*No words can describe it.*

K27 points: Important points on the kidney meridian, ends of the collar bones under the throat—known as the 'house of associated points'.

Kinesiology: (see also muscle testing or energy testing). Kinesiology is the monitoring of subtle variations in muscle tone, as indicators of states within the body, mind, or energy system. Relatively simple forms of this are used in energy psychotherapy and are referred to as muscle testing or energy testing. It is an easily learnable skill.

Kundalini energy: In Hinduism, kundalini means 'coiled snake', a form of energy or *shakti*, located at the base of the spine. When awakened through tantric practice, kundalini yoga or through spontaneous awakening, this energy rises up the spine which is termed 'kundalini rising'. The power of kundalini energy is associated with the divine feminine and leads to spiritual liberation.

Lung meridian breathing: A breathing procedure developed by Phil Mollon involving fingertips resting on the Lung Meridian alarm points.

Massive reversal: A term used by Roger Callahan to denote the state in which a client muscle tests weak to the most global statement of intention towards well-being—e.g. testing weak to 'I want to be well' or 'I want to be happy'—perhaps strong to 'I want to be sick' or 'I want to die'.

Meridians: Hypothesised channels that carry the flow of subtle energy, as described in acupuncture and traditional Chinese Medicine, and as used in energy psychotherapy. We can make use of these without knowing quite what they are. According to acupuncture, they connect the internal organs with the body extremities and are thought to play an important role in regulating the body's functions.

Mini reversals: A term used by Roger Callahan to denote the way in which a person's system may have allowed most of the perturbations to clear but is resisting letting go of the final residues—for example if the SUDs have dropped to 2 or 3 but are not dropping further.

Morphic fields/morphic resonance: Information-holding energy fields. Sheldrake defines them as 'self-organising regions of influence, analogous to magnetic fields and other recognised fields of nature' and considers that morphic-fields are equivalent to Jung's 'collective unconscious'. Callahan considered the 'thought field' was of this nature.

Multidimensionality: As humanity awakens, we start to encounter quantum reality and multidimensionality, where past present and future co-exist in the present moment. Eckhart Tolle calls this *'The power of now'*. Different timelines—the different possibilities and trajectories of our lives—are occurring simultaneously. There are infinite possibilities for both personal and collective timelines. Each time we make new choices and decisions we create new potentials/timelines. As souls, we have the potential to live within (at least) twelve dimensions, reflected by the twelve strands of our DNA. Our soul carries us through this journey as we expand through consciousness and energy throughout all our lifetimes. As people wake up into 5-D consciousness they start to recall past and parallel lives. According to Perez (2022) we are here on earth to integrate spirit and matter and bring our higher levels of consciousness into our physical reality. We also heal our soul by bringing all parts of our experience together—past life traumas and soul fragments, as well as higher dimensional aspects of us. Being here on earth gives us the opportunity to integrate all these multidimensional aspects into one body, one consciousness until we become one with Source/the Creator/God.

Muscle testing, or energy testing: Simple forms of kinesiology are employed in energy psychotherapy and energy psychology to make enquiries of the energy system and gain information about processes in both mind and body. It is a kind of bioenergetic feedback. Muscle testing/energy testing is based on the finding (subsequently verified by computerised muscle-strength testing devices) that muscles are stronger when responding to a true statement, and weak when responding to a false statement. Muscle testing is more of an art than a science. It provides information but not 'the truth' and can be distorted, like any form of communication, by error, misunderstanding or lack of skill in the tester. However, used sensitively and respectfully it can help to guide the work by providing working hypotheses on how to proceed and to track progress.

Neurological disorganisation: An old and rather unsatisfactory term, used in Applied Kinesiology and some of its offshoots. It refers to systemic energetic interferences—which are indeed often involved in subtle brain dysfunction.

Palm-over-head test to check our energy system: A simple muscle testing procedure to check for correct polarity of the energy system. Placing the palm down over the head should test strong—(the palm and top of the head having opposite bioelectrical charges.) Placing the palm upwards over the head should test weak—it is somewhat like batteries, where, if you put them into a device the wrong way, the energy doesn't flow. A simple mnemonic is 'palm is power; back is slack'.

Psychoanalytic Energy Therapy (PEP): Developed by Phil Mollon from his extended experience as a psychoanalyst and his thorough exploration of other energy psychology modalities. PEP includes working with both meridians and chakras in a sequence which is discerned for each client and there is no fixed protocol.

Psychological reversals/see also 'Reversals'

Quantum methods: These methods work with the subtle energy system, intention/consciousness and the Unified field within the fifth dimension. New forms are emerging all the time. A few examples include: Sandi Radomski, and Tom Altaffer's *Ask and Receive*; Jo Dunning's *The Quick Pulse Technique*; Phil Mollon's *Blue Diamond*; *Quantum Touch*; Tara Love Perry's I Love You, Me; Meg Benedict, *Access Consciousness*; and energy psychotherapy generally.

Reversals (see also Psychological reversals): Energy psychotherapy identifies and clears 'reversals'. When there is an objection to change there is a reversal of the body's energy system. Instead of the energy moving forward—the life flow of *libido*—the energy flows backwards—like Freud's 'death instinct'. This is the energetic equivalent of psychodynamic resistances known as psychological reversal. There are three kinds of problems that completely block the process of healing until corrected:

- *Psychological reversals* (PR) which express the self-sabotaging psychodynamics of the mind. The main motives behind PR are
  - It is not safe
  - I do not deserve
  - I will not still be me/identity violated
  - I am too angry to heal/I want to keep expressing my suffering through my symptom
- *Energy reversals: sometimes caused by a physical illness or an 'energy toxin'.*
- *Systemic energy disturbances* such as 'neurological disorganisation'. Sometimes termed 'polarity reversal' these are not the same as PR, although they are sometimes confused with them. System energy disturbances occur when the flow of energy either down the vertical axis or across the body ('homolateral energy flow') becomes disorganised or out of alignment

Reversals can be cleared by tapping on the side of the hand on the karate-chop point while naming the conflict followed by a phrase affirming positive energy such as *I love and accept myself.*

Scope of practice: This is an important legal boundary for energy psychotherapists to consider, which will vary from country to country. It refers to a practitioner's legitimate and legal area of 'Code of Practice' and denotes their professional limits based on their professional training. For example, at the present time in the UK, a psychotherapist is not considered qualified to claim to treat allergies or food sensitivities under their psychological licence, although somatic aspects of psychological experience can be addressed in the course of the primary psychological task. On the other hand, a trained kinesiologist or medical doctor is fully entitled to treat allergies. In energy psychotherapy the boundaries between these different realms of work can become somewhat blurred—it is well known for example that tapping can be quite effective in pain relief.

Soul: Our soul is infinite, an aspect of the divine, the one who *experiences* at an incarnate level and helps us be grounded in our physical reality on earth. Our soul also holds the akashic record of all our incarnations and all the experiences we have been through in our physical bodies throughout all our lifetimes. As souls, we are the owners of our own experience, our inner truth, and have our own unique energetic signature.

Star seeds: 'Star seeds' have incarnated on the planet to anchor in the frequencies for New Earth. They are said to have a galactic component having originated from other star systems such as Sirius, The Pleiades, Arcturus, Andromeda and so on. Some are 'channels', some have extraordinary technological gifts with extremely high levels of intelligence, others simply carry their own high frequencies, raising the energies to help the plant ascend to the fifth dimension. There are said to be three main 'wave' of Star seeds including: Indigo, Star, Rainbow, Crystals, Divine and Hybrid Star seeds. All act as antennas of high vibrational energy.

Subjective units of distress (SUDs): A commonly used indicator of subjective levels of distress, on a scale of zero to ten.

Subtle energy: A term proposed by material scientist William Tiller. Such energy has also been known as Qi, Chi, bio energy, orgone energy, Elan Vitale, life energy, and many other names.

Subtle energy system: The main components of the subtle energy system include the meridians, the chakras/energy centres, and biofields or thought Field. Energy psychotherapy works with this subtle energy to clear trauma out of the body through these various systems.

Systemic energetic interferences: Disturbances of the energy system that prevent it functioning coherently or providing clear signals in muscle testing/energy testing. This is also sometimes called 'neurological disorganisation'.

Tapas Fleming: A Californian acupuncturist who developed Tapas Acupressure Technique.

TAT (Tapas Acupressure Technique): The approach developed by Tapas Fleming.

Tearless Trauma Techniques: A very useful technique within Emotional Freedom Techniques, making use of intentional dissociation, for resolving severe trauma that would be hazardous to approach directly.

'Tell the Story Technique': The core procedure in EFT, where the client is guided to give a detailed account of trauma, stopping at each point of distress to tap on acupoints until calm.

Third dimension: This is one of the twelve dimensions. The third dimension is the domain of dualism, Newtonian physics, and cause and effect. Ego's dualistic mind operates in this realm of 'ordinary reality'.

Thought field: A term used by Roger Callahan to denote an information-holding energetic field, comprising thoughts and their expression in the body's subtle energy system.

Thought Field Therapy (TFT): The mode of therapy developed by Roger Callahan, addressing the information-holding thought field as expressed in meridian acupoint sequences.

Yin and yang meridians: The following meridians are thought to be yin in nature: lung; spleen; heart; kidney; heart protector/circulation sex; liver. The following are considered yang in nature: large intestine; stomach; small intestine; bladder; triple heater; gall bladder.

Zero point field: This is the point of balance neutrality and stillness in the unified field. In Buddhism this is referred to as the heart—based space of compassionate awakened consciousness, sometimes referred to as 'emptiness'.

References

Ainsworth, M. D. S., Blehar, M. C., Waters, E., & Wall, S. (1978). *Patterns of Attachment: A Psychological Study of the Strange Situation*. New York: Psychology Press/Lawrence Erlbaum Associates, Inc.

Almaas, A. H. (2004). Self and self-representation. In: *The Point of Existence—Transformations of Narcissism in Self-Realization* (Chapter 5). Boston: Shambala.

Alvarez, A. (1992). *Live Company*. London: Routledge.

Anan, M. (2013). Resonance and harmony webinar, Darius Barazandeh. Available at: https://liveshow. youwealthrevolution.com (last accessed 29 April 2013).

Ashbrook, J. B. (1995). *Minding the Soul: Pastoral Counselling As Remembering*. Minneapolis: Fortress Press.

Assagioli, R. (1961). *Self-Realization and Psychological Disturbances*. Literary Licensing LLC, 2011.

Assagioli, R. (2008). *Transpersonal Development: The Dimension Beyond Psychosynthesis*. Findhorn, Scotland. Smiling Wisdom, 2007.

Aurobindo, S. (1950). *Supramental Light and the Supramental Manifestation upon Earth. Bulletin, Aug 1950*.

Bache, C. M. (2008). *The Living Classroom: Teaching and Collective Consciousness*. New York: Suny Series in Transpersonal and Humanistic Psychology.

Bair, P. (1998). *Living from the Heart*. New York: Rivers Press.

Baniel, A. (2012). *Kids Beyond Limits: The Anat Baniel Method for Awakening the Brain and Transforming the Life of Your Child with Special Needs*. USA: Perigree, Penguin.

Barnes, M., & Berke, J. (1973). *Mary Barnes: Two Accounts of a Journey Through Madness*. London: Pelican.

Bateman, A., & Fonagy, P. (2004). *Psychotherapy for Borderline Personality Disorder: Mentalization-based Treatment*. Oxford: Oxford University Press.

Bateson, G., Jackson, D. D., Haley, J., & Weakland, J. (1956). Toward a theory of schizophrenia. *Behavioral Science, 1*: 251–264.

Beesley, R. P. (1978). *Creative Ethers*. Los Angeles: DeVorss & Company.

Benedicte, M. (2019). Creator of the healing method '*Quantum Access*'. 'Living in 5D' webinar '*Beyond The Ordinary*', John Burgos. Available at: https://beyondtheordinaryshow.com (last accessed 5 October 2019).

Benedicte, M. *Quantum Access* information on Meg Benedicte's website www.megbenedicte.com (last accessed in 2017).

Bentov, I. (1977). *Stalking the Wild Pendulum*. London: Wildwood House.

Bick, E. (1968). The experience of the skin in early object-relations. *International Journal of Psychoanalysis, 49*: 484–486.

Bion, W. R. (1962). *Learning from Experience*. London: Karnac.

Bion, W. R. (1967). *Second Thoughts*. London: Karnac.

Bohm, D. (2002). *Wholeness and the Implicate Order*. London: Routledge.

Bollas, C. (1987). *The Shadow of the Object*. London: Free Association Books.

Boon, S., Steele, K., & Van Der Hart, O. (2011). *Skills Training for Patients and Therapists*. New York: W. W. Norton.

Bowlby, J. (1988). *A Secure Base*. London: Routledge.

Braden, G. (1997). *Walking Between the Worlds: The Science of Compassion*. Radio Bookstore Press.

Braden, G. (2004). *The God Code. The Secret of our Past, the Promise of our Future*. Carlsbad, CA: Hay House.

Braden, G. (2007). *The Divine Matrix: Bridging Time, Space, Miracles, and Belief*. Carlsbad, CA: Hay House.

Brockman, H. (2006). *Dynamic Energetic Healing: Integrating Core Shamanic Practices with Energy Psychology Applications and Processwork Principles*. New York: Colombia Press.

Brown, G., Batra, K., Dorin, E., Bakhru, R., Han, A., Palermini, A., Sottile, R., Khanbijian, S., & Hower, M. (2023). Comparing AIT and EFT in reduction of negative emotions associated with a past memory: A randomized control study. *Psychology, 14*(12): 1868–1887. https://doi.org/10.4236/psych.2023.1412111

Brown, G. W., Hilderbrand, J., & Harris, T. O. (1978). *Social Origins of Depression: A Study of Psychiatric Disorder in Women*. London: Tavistock.

Byrne, R. (2006). *The Secret*. New York: Astria Books.

Callahan, R. (1985). *Five Minute Phobia Cure: Dr. Callahan's Treatment for Fears, Phobias and Self-Sabotage*. Henderson, NV: Enterprise Publishing Inc.

Callahan, R. (1995). A thought field therapy (TFT) algorithm for trauma: a reproduceable experiment in psychotherapy. Paper presented at the annual meeting of the American Psychological Association, New York, August 1995.

Cannon, D. (2011). *The Three Waves of Volunteers and the New Earth*. Ozark Mountain Publishing Inc.

Castaneda, C. (1968). *The Teachings of Don Juan: A Jaqui Way of Knowledge*. Berkeley, CA: University of California Press.

Childre, D. L., Martin, H., Rozman, D., & McCraty, R. (2016). *Heart Intelligence: Connecting with the Intuitive Guidance of the Heart*. CA: Waterford Press, Heartmath.

Chopra, D. (1989). *Quantum Healing: Exploring the Frontiers of Mind/Body Medicine*. New York: Bantam Books.

Chopra, D. (2019). *Metahuman—Unleashing Your Infinite Potential*. UK: Random House.

Church, D. (2018). *Mind to Matter*. Carlsbad, CA: Hay House.

Clarke, I. (2010). *Psychosis and Spirituality: Consolidating the New Paradigm* (2nd edn). Sussex: Wiley-Blackwell.

Cori, P. (2000). *The Cosmos of the Soul, A Wake-up Call for Humanity*. Gateway, imprint of Gill and MacMillan.

Cozolino, L. (2006). *The Neuroscience of Human Relationships: Attachment and the Developing Social Brain.* New York: W. W. Norton.

Currivan, J. (2017). *The Cosmic Hologram: In-formation at the Center of Creation.* Rochester, VT: Inner Traditions.

Damasio, A. (2003). *Looking for Spinoza: Joy, Sorrow, and the Feeling Brain.* New York: Random.

Damasio, A. (2010). *Self Comes to Mind: Constructing the Conscious Brain.* New York: Vintage.

Dana, D. (2018). *Polyvagal Theory in Therapy: Engaging the Rhythm of Regulation.* New York: W. W. Norton.

Davies, J. M., & Frawley, M. G. (1994). *Adult Survivors of Childhood Sexual Abuse: A Psychoanalytic Perspective.* New York: Basic Books.

Dawkins, R. (2006). *The God Delusion.* London: Black Swan.

Dent, A. (2019). *Using Spirituality in Psychotherapy: The Heart Led Approach to Clinical Practice.* New York: Routledge.

De Shazer, S. (1994). *Words were Originally Magic.* New York: W. W. Norton.

Dispenza, J. (2012a). *You are the Placebo: Making Your Mind Matter.* London: Hay House.

Dispenza, J. (2012b). *Breaking the Habit of Being Yourself: How To Lose Your Mind And Create A New One.* London: Hay House.

Dispenza, J. (2017). *Becoming Supernatural: How Common People are Doing the Uncommon.* Carlsbad, CA: Hay House.

Dispenza, J. (2019). DMT, pineal gland and the piezoelectric effect. *YouTube,* 26 November 2019.

Divband, S. (2020). *Divinely Guided: A Guide for Teens, Parents and Young Adults to Become Spiritually Centred in an Ever-changing World.* IntuitiveWellnessCenter.com

Doidge, N. (2007). *The Brain That Changes Itself: Stories of Personal Triumph from the Frontiers of Brain.* New York: Viking.

Dossey, L. (2013). *One Mind: How our Individual Mind is Part of a Greater Consciousness, and Why it Matters.* London: Hay House.

Eden, D. & Feinstein, F. (2008). *Energy Medicine: How to Use Your Body's Energies for Optimum Health and Vitality.* London: Piatkus.

Eisenhower, L. (2022). Newsletter, https://cosmicgaia.org (last accessed February 2022).

Elkins, D. N. (1995). Psychotherapy and spirituality: Toward a theory of the soul. *Journal of Humanistic Psychology, 35*(2): 78–98. https://doi.org/10.1177/00221678950352006

Emoto, M. (2008). *The Healing Power of Water.* London: Hay House.

Erikson, E. H. (1950). *Childhood and Society.* New York: W. W. Norton.

Essonne, C. (2022). La physique des particules expliquée par l'ether/particle physics explained by the Aether(ST) Science Interdite. YouTube, 5 June 2022 (last accessed 7 June 2022).

Fairbairn, W. R. D. (1944). Endopsychic structure considered in terms of object relationships. *International Journal of Psychoanalysis, 25:* 70–93.

Farrer, F. (2002). *Sir George Trevelyan and the New Spiritual Awakening.* UK: Floris Books.

Feinstein, D. (2019). Energy psychology. Efficacy, speed, mechanisms. *Explore, 15:* 340–351. Open access: https://doi.org/10.1016/j.explore.2018.11.003

Feinstein, D. (2021a). Six empirically-supported premises about energy psychology: mounting evidence for a controversial therapy. *Advances, 35*(2): 17–32.

Feinstein, D. (2021b). Applications of energy psychology in addressing the psychological roots of Illness. *OBM Integrative and Complementary Medicine, 6*(2). Open Access. doi:10.21926/obm.icm.2102014

Felitti, V. J., Anda, R. F., Nordenberg, D., Williamson, D. F., Spitz, A. M., Edwards, V., Koss, M. P., & Marks, J. S. (1998). Relationship of childhood abuse and household dysfunction to many of the leading causes of death in adults: The Adverse Childhood Experiences (ACE) Study. *American Journal of Preventive Medicine*, *14*(4), 245–258. https://doi.org/10.1016/S0749-3797(98)00017-8

Freud, S. (1895d). *Studies on Hysteria. S. E.,* 2: London: Hogarth.

Freud, S. (1920g). *Beyond the Pleasure Principle. S. E., 18*: 1–64. London: Hogarth.

Freud, S. (1923b). *The Ego and the Id. S. E., 19*: 1–66. London: Hogarth.

Freud, S. (1926d). *Inhibitions, Symptoms And Anxiety. S. E., 20*: 75–176. London: Hogarth.

Freud, S. (1933a). *New Introductory Lectures on Psycho-Analysis. S. E., 22*: 1–182. London: Hogarth.

Frost, G. (2020). *The Girls Within: A True Story of Triumph over Trauma and Abuse.* Bicester: Phoenix.

Gerhardt, S. (2004). *Why Love Matters: How Affection Shapes a Baby's Brain.* London & New York: Routledge, 2015.

Gilfillan, C., & Scott, A. (2022). *Hail Sisters of the Revolution.* UK: Cowslip Press.

Glennie, E. (2015). Hearing essay, Evelyn Glennie, Teach the World to Listen, evelyn.co.uk

Grand, S., & Salberg, J. (2016). *Trans-generational Trauma and the Other: Dialogues Across History and Difference.* London & New York: Routledge.

Greenberg, J., & Mitchell, S. A. (1984). *Object Relations in Psychoanalytic Theory.* Cambridge, MA: Harvard University Press.

Greene, D. (2021). How do energy psychology modalities work? An energy-based theoretical perspective. *International Journal of Healing and Caring, 21*(1).

Grotstein, J. S. (2007). *A Beam of Intense Darkness: Wilfred Bion's Legacy to Psychoanalysis.* London & New York: Routledge.

Gump, J. (2016). *The Presence of the Past: Transmission of Slavery's Traumas.* London & New York: Routledge.

Hagelin, J. (1993). Effects of group practice of the transcendental meditation program on preventing violent crime in Washington DC. https://abundance.org.au/washington-meditation-project/

Hammond, M., & Crowley, C. (2008). *Living Your Soul's Purpose: Wellness and Passion with Energy Psychology.* Global Healing Press.

Harari, Y. N. (2011). *Sapiens: A Brief History of Humanity.* New York: Random House.

Harari, Y. N. (2017). *Homo Deus: A Brief History of Tomorrow.* New York: Random House

Hawking, S. (2018). *Brief Answers to the Big Questions.* Audible Audiobook.

Hawkins, D. R. (2014). *Power Vs. Force.* Carlsbad, CA: Hay House.

Hawkins, D. R. (2015). *Transcending the Levels of Consciousness: The Stairway to Enlightenment.* London: Hay House.

Hebb, D. O. (1949). *The Organization of Behavior.* New York: Wiley & Sons.

Heflin, J. (2017). *The Quantum Business Model: A New Paradigm.* Embracing Master. https://medium.com/embracing-mastery/the-quantum-business-model-a-new-paradigm-6795bc248d56

Herman, J. (1992). *Trauma and Recovery: From Domestic Abuse to Political Terror.* New York: Basic Books, 2015.

Hicks, E., & J. (2006). *The Law of Attraction: The Basics of the Teachings of Abraham.* Carlsbad, CA: Hay House.

Hillman, J. (1967). *Insearch: Psychotherapy and Religion.* Thompson, CT: Spring Publications.

Hillman, J. (1997). *The Soul's Code: In Search of Character and Calling.* London: Bantam Books.

Hillman, J. (2010). *A Blue Fire: Selected Writings.* Harper-perennial.

Horowitz, L. G. (2011). *The Book of 528 Prosperity Key of Love.* Rockport, MA: Tetrahedron.

Hover-Kramer, D. (2002). *Creative Energies: Integrative Energy Psychotherapy for Self-Expression and Healing.* New York. W. W. Norton.

Huxley, A. (1954). *The Doors of Perception.* London: Chatto & Windus.

Jacobi, M. (2022). S5 E45 *Quantum Manifestation,* 11-19-22, https://rumble.com

James, W. (1902). *Varieties of Religious Experience: A Study in Human Nature*. London: Longman's, Green & Co.

James, W. (2010). *Pragmatism: A New Name for Some Old Ways of Thinking*. Whitefish, MT: Kessinger Publishing.

Judith, A. (1987). Wheels of life. Woodbury, MN: Llewellyn, 1999, 2007.

Judith, A. (1996). *Eastern Body, Western Mind: Psychology and the Chakra System as a Path to the Self*. Berkeley: Celestial Arts, 2004.

Jung, C. G. (1973a). *Memories, Dreams, Reflections*. New York: Pantheon.

Jung, C. G. (1973b). *Letters (Vol. 1)*. Princeton, NJ: Princeton University Press.

Jung, C. G., & Shamdasani, S. (Ed.) (2009). *The Red Book: Liber Novus*, M. Kyburz & J. Peck (Trans.). New York: W. W. Norton.

Kaehr, S. A. (2019). *Edgar Cayce's Egyptian Energy Healing*. ARE Press.

Kahn, M. (2015). Demystifying ascension: Part 2: Entering the 5th dimension. *Newsletter Energy Update*, April 2015.

Kalsched, D. (1996). *The Inner World of Trauma*. London & New York: Routledge.

Kalsched, D. (2013). *Trauma and the Soul*. London: Routledge.

Kenyon, T. (2012). *Non-Duality and the Matrix of Creation: A Hathor Planetary Message Through Tom Kenyon*. www.tomkenyon.com (last accessed January 2013).

Kingsley, C. (1863). *The water babies: A fairy tale for a land-baby*. Macmillan Collector's Library, 72, 2016.

Klein, M. (1940). Mourning and its relation to manic-depressive states. *International Journal of Psychoanalysis, 21*: 125–153.

Klein, M. (1946). Notes on some schizoid mechanisms. *International Journal of Psychoanalysis, 27*: 99–110.

Kopp, S. B. (1976). *If You Meet the Buddha on the Road, Kill Him! The Pilgrimage of Psychotherapy Patients*. New York: Bantam.

Krszowski, S. (1988). *In Our Experience: Workshops at the Women's Therapy Centre*. London, Ontario. Attic Books.

Laing, R. D. (1960). *The Divided Self: An Existential Study in Sanity and Madness*. London: Tavistock.

Lanza, R., & Berman, B. (2008). *Biocentrism: How Life and Consciousness are the Keys to Understanding the True Nature of the Universe*. Dallas, TX: Benbella Books.

Lao Tzu (1973) *Tao Te Ching*. New York: Vintage Books/Random House.

Leary, T. (1999). *Turn On, Tune In, Drop Out*. Berkeley, CA: Ronin Publishing.

Levin, M. (1998). *The Pool of Memory: The Autobiography of an Unwilling Intuitive*. Dublin: Newleaf.

Levy, P. (2018). *Quantum Revelation: A Radical Synthesis of Science and Spirituality*. New York: Select Books.

Lie, S. (2015). Learning/remembering to read light language. Webinar on Lauren Galey's 'Acoustic Health' (last accessed August 2015).

Lillas, C., & Turnbull, J. (2011). *Infant/Child Mental Health, Early Intervention, and Relationship-Based Therapies: A Neuro-Relational Framework for Interdisciplinary Practice*. New York: W. W. Norton.

Linville, W. (2021). Mastering creator consciousness. Video Webinar and Teleconference series, Williamlinville.com (last accessed September 2021).

Lipton, B. (2010). *The Biology of Belief: Unleashing the Power of Consciousness, Matter and Miracles*. London: Hay House.

Lipton, B. (2016). Invisible biology: An introduction to quantum biophysics. In: *The Science of Energy Healing*. Association for Comprehensive Energy Psychology, energypsych.org

Lipton, B. (2022). Belief change. https://www.brucelipton.com/belief-change/ (last accessed 13 June 2022).

Little, M. L. (1977). *Psychotic Anxieties and Containment: A Personal Record of an Analysis with Winnicott*. New York: Jason Aronson.

Lorimer, D. (1990). *Whole in One: The Near-Death Experience and the Ethics of Interconnectedness*. New York: Penguin.

Luna, A. (2022). *What is the Ego? Should it be Destroyed?* Lonerwolf.com (last accessed online 17 April 2022).

Maclean, P. (1990). *The Triune Brain in Evolution: Role in Paleo Cerebral Functions*. Portland, OR: Book News.

Main M., & Solomon J. (1986). Discovery of a new, insecure-disorganized/disoriented attachment pattern. In Yogman M. & Brazelton T. B. (Eds.), *Affective Development in Infancy* (pp. 95–124). Norwood, NJ: Ablex.

Mars, I. (2021). *Unity Theory*. Crimson Eagle Publishing e-book. https://thecrimsoneagle.com

Maslow, A. H. (1943). A theory of human motivation. *Psychological Review*, 50(4).

Mate, G. (2003). *When the Body Says No: The Cost of Hidden Stress*. Toronto: Knopf.

Mayers, M. (2018). *Blessed with Energy: The Mystery of Energy Medicine Explained Through Science and Scripture*. Carlsbad, CA: Balboa Press, Hay House.

McCraty, R. (2004). The energetic heart: Bioelectromagnetic communication within and between people. In: P. J. Rosch & M. S. Markov (Eds.), *Clinical Applications of Bioelectromagnetic Medicine* (pp. 541–562). New York: Marcel Dekker.

McTaggart, L. (2001). *The Field*. London: Harper Collins.

McTaggart, L. (2017). *The Power of Eight: Harnessing the Miraculous Energies of a Small Group to Heal Others, Your Life and the World*. New York: Atria (Simon and Schuster).

Miller, L. (2024). *The Oxford Handbook of Psychology and Spirituality* (2nd edn). Oxford: Oxford University Press.

Mitchell, S. (1988). *Relational Concepts in Psychoanalysis*. Cambridge, MA: Harvard University Press.

Moacanin, R. (1986). *Jung's Psychology and Tibetan Buddhism: Western and Eastern Paths to the Heart*. London: Wisdom Publications.

Mollon, P. (2002). *Shame and Jealousy: The Hidden Turmoils*. London & New York: Routledge.

Mollon, P. (2005). *EMDR and the Energy Therapies: Psychoanalytic Perspectives*. London: Karnac.

Mollon, P. (2008). *Psychoanalytic Energy Psychotherapy*. London: Karnac, 2015.

Mollon, P. (2015). The porous personality. In: *The Disintegrating Self: Psychotherapy of Adult ADHD, Autistic Spectrum and Somato-psychic Disorders* (Chapter 7). London: Karnac.

Mollon, P. (2022). *Blue Diamond Healing: Exploring Transpersonal and Trans-dimensional Aspects of Energy Psychotherapy*. London: Karnac.

Mooji, S. (2022). A simple and profound introduction to self-inquiry. *YouTube* (last accessed 16 June 2022).

Moore, T. (1992). *Care of the Soul: An Inspirational Programme to Add Depth and Meaning to Your Everyday Life*. London: Piatkus, 2012.

Music, G. (2013). Stress pre-birth: How the fetus is affected by a mother's state of mind. *International Journal of Birth & Parent Education*, 1. http://repository.tavistockandportman.ac.uk/602/1/Music.pdf

Newberg, A., & Waldman, R. W. (2009). *How God Changes Your Brain: Breakthrough Findings from a Leading Neuroscientist*. New York: Ballantine Books.

Newland, T. (2019). *Fallout: Recovering from Abuse in Tibetan Buddhism*. Amazon.

Ogden, P., Minton, K., & Pain, C. (2006). *Trauma and the Body: A Sensorimotor Approach to Psychotherapy*. New York: Norton Series on Interpersonal Neurobiology.

Padmasambhava & Kongtrul, Jamgon (1998). *Light of Wisdom Vol II: A Collection of Padmasambhava's Advice to the Dakini Yeshe* (pp. 45–51). ISBN 962-7341-33-9.

Paramahansa Yogananda (2006). *Autobiography of a Yogi*. Reprint of the Philosophical Library 1946, First Edition. US: Crystal Clarity.

Pearl, E. (2004). *The Reconnection: Heal Others, Heal Yourself*. Carlsbad, CA: Hay House.

Perez, I. (2021). *Our Cosmic Origin* (new edn). London: Amazon.

Pert, C. B. (1999). *Molecules of Emotion: The Science Behind Mind-Body Medicine*. London: Simon & Schuster.

Pixie, M. (2020). *Science Mysticism and Beyond: Insights from Beyond the Veil for 2020 and 2021*. Webinar Episode 68 on Inspire Health Podcasts with Dr Jason Loken.

Pixie, M. (2022). Posting in Telegram Channel, 11 June 2022 (accessed 12 June 2022).

Planck, M. (1944). *Das Wesen der Materie* [*The Nature of Matter*], speech at Florence, Italy (from Archiv zur Geschichte der Max-Planck-Gesellschaft, Abt. Va, Rep. 11 Planck, Nr. 1797).

Pollan, M. (2018). *How to Change Your Mind: The New Science of Psychedelics*. New York: Random House.

Porges, S. W., & Dana, D. (2018). *Clinical Applications of the Polyvagal Theory. The Emergence of Polyvagal-Informed therapies*. New York. W. W. Norton.

Radin, D. (2006). *Entangled Minds*. New York: Paraview.

Redfield, J. (1994). *The Celestine Prophecy*. New York: Bantam.

Reschel, A. (2016). Science proves meridians exist. *Medical Veritas, The Journal of Truth*. Online journal.

Rinpoche, S., Gaffney, P., & Harvey, A. (2002). *The Tibetan Book of Living and Dying*. London: Rider.

Rizzolatti, G., & Sinigaglia, C. (2008). *Mirrors in the Brain: How Our Minds Share Actions and Emotions*. Oxford: Oxford University Press.

Rodwell, M. (2016). *The New Human: Awakening to our Cosmic Heritage*. Australia: New Mind Publishers.

Rössler, W. (2012). Stress, burnout, and job dissatisfaction in mental health workers. *European Archives of Psychiatry and Clinical Neuroscience, 262*: 65–69. https://doi.org/10.1007/s00406-012-0353-4

Rothschild, B. (2000). *The Body Remembers: The Psycho-physiology of Trauma and Trauma Treatment*. New York: W. W. Norton.

Sanders, K. (1984). Bion's 'protomental system' and psychosomatic illness in general practice. *British Journal of Medical Psychology, 57*(2): 167–172.

Sandler, J. (2003). On attachment to internal objects: Role responsiveness, and unconscious wish-fulfilling life 'scripts'. *Psychology – Psychoanalytic Enquiry* (article).

Schatzman, M. (1973). *Soul Murder: Persecution in the Family*. New York: Random House.

Schore, A. N. (2003). *Affect Regulation and the Repair of the Self*. New York: W. W. Norton.

Schore, A. N. (2019a). *Right Brain Psychotherapy*. New York: W. W. Norton.

Schore, A. N. (2019b). *The Development of Unconscious Mind*. New York: W. W. Norton.

Schwartz-Salant, N. (1989). *The Borderline Personality: Vision and Healing*. Wilmette, IL: Chiron.

Scott Peck, M. (1978). *The Road Less Traveled*. London: Arrow, New Age.

Shadid, T. (2021). QM and Paul MacLean's triune brain model. *Quadrune Mind: A Neurospiritual Guide to a Purposeful Life* (posted 28 June 2021).

Shah, I. (1978). *Learning How to Learn: Psychology and Spirituality in the Sufi Way*. London: Octagon Press.

Shaw, D. (2014). *Traumatic Narcissism: Relational Systems of Subjugation*. New York: Routledge.

Sheldan, M. (2019). *Mentoring the Higher Self*. Lightworker Circle No 9, online course.

Sheldrake, R. (1981). *A New Science of Life*. London: Icon, 2009.

Sheldrake, R. (2023). *On Morphic Resonance: Telepathy, Resistance from Scientific Establishment, The Religion of Science*. Merging Science and Spirituality. Youtube /BSP 4. Video Before Skool https://www.youtube.com/watch?v=68fjlUuvOGM

Siegel, D. (1999). *The Developing Mind: Toward a Neurobiology of Interpersonal Experience*. New York: Guilford.

Siegel, D. (2010). *Mindsight: Transform Your Brain with the New Science of Kindness*. London: Oneworld Publications.

Siegel, D. (2016). *Invisible Biology—An Intro to Quantum Biophysics*. Module 1 of 'The Science of Energy Healing: The Energetic Nature of the BodyMind'. *Association for Comprehensive Energy Psychology*. Available at: https://acep.mykajabi.com/store/SG5TEQqT

Stein, A. (2017) *Terror, Love and Brainwashing: Attachment in Cults and Totalitarian Systems*. New York: Routledge.

Stern, D. (1985). *The Interpersonal World of the Infant: A View from Psychoanalysis and Developmental Psychology*. New York: Basic Books.

Stern, D. et al. [The Process of Change Study Group] (1998). Non-interpretive mechanisms in psycho-analytic therapy. *International Journal of Psychoanalysis, 79*: 903.

Suzuki, S. (1973). *Zen Mind Beginner's Mind*. Toronto: Penguin Canada.

Symington, N. (1994). *Emotion and Spirit*. London: Cassell.

Taylor, S. (2018). *Spiritual Science Why Science Needs Spirituality to Make Sense of the World*. London: Watkins.

Teicholz, J. G., & Kreigman, D. (Eds.) (1998). *Trauma, Repetition, and Affect Regulation: The Work of Paul Russell*. New York: Other Press.

Tiller, W. (1993). What are subtle energies? *Journal of Scientific Exploration, 7*(3): 293–304.

Tiller, W. (2004). Personal disclosure. In: J. Diepold (Ed.), *Evolving Thought Field Therapy*. New York: W. W. Norton.

Tiller, W. (2007). *Psychoenergetic Science: A Second Copernican-Scale Revolution*. Available from the Tiller Foundation website www.tillerfoundation.org

Tolle, E. (1999). *The Power of Now*. London: Hodder & Stoughton.

Tolle, E. (2005). *A New Earth: Awakening to Your Life's Purpose*. New York: Random House, 2018.

Trungpa, C. (1973). *Cutting Through Spiritual Materialism*. Boston, MA: Shambhala Publications.

Van der Kolk, B. (2015). *The Body Keeps the Score: Mind, Brain and Body in the Transformation of Trauma*. New York: Penguin.

Walker, P. (2013). *Complex PTSD: From Surviving to Thriving (A Guide and Map for Recovering from Childhood Trauma)*. Lafayette, CA: Azure Coyote.

Walsch, N. D. (1995). *Conversations with God: Book One*. London: Hodder & Stoughton.

Wamser, N. R., & Vanderberg, B. R. (2013). Empirical support for the definition of a complex trauma event in children and adolescents. *Journal of Traumatic Stress*, 25 November 2013 (Wiley).

Ward, C. (2021), In life there are no coincidences. Newsletter, 16 March 2021 (last accessed January 2022).

Watts, A. (1989). *The Book: On the Taboo Against Knowing Who You Are*. New York: Random House.

Weiss, B. (1994). *Many Lives, Many Masters: The True Story of a Prominent Psychiatrist, His Young Patient and the Past-Life Therapy That Changed Both Their Lives*. London: Piatkus.

White, J. (2006). *Generation: Preoccupations and Conflicts in Contemporary Psychoanalysis*. London: Routledge.

White, J. (2018). Death and resurrection: enlightenment and the body of light. *Journal of Conscious Evolution, 1*(1): Article 7. Available at: https://digitalcommons.ciis.edu/cejournal/vol1/iss1/7

Wilber, K. (2000). *Integral Psychology: Consciousness, Spirit, Psychology*. Boston: Shambala.

Wilbur, K. (1977). *The Spectrum of Consciousness*. Wheaton, IL: Quest.

Willoughby, R. (2001). The petrified self: Esther Bick and her membership paper. *British Journal of Psychotherapy, 18*(1): 3–6.

Winnicott, D. W. (1960). Ego distortion in terms of true and false self. In: *Maturational Processes and the Facilitating Environment* (pp. 140–152). London: Hogarth, 1965.

Wood, E. (1989). *The Seven Rays*. Whitefish, MT: Kessinger.

Yeomans, T. (1994). Conference on 'Spirituality and psychotherapy' at the Kripalu Center in Lenox, MA (paper presented May 1994).

Zepf, S. (2008). Libido and psychic energy: Freud's concepts reconsidered. *International Forum of Psychoanalysis*, 19(1). https://doi.org/10.1080/08037060802450753

Zukav, G. (1979). *The Dancing Wu Li Masters*. London: Hutchinson.

Appendix

The *Nine Yanas* (Nyingma School of Buddhism)

Sutra/Tantra	Three yanas classification	Tantras	Nine yanas classification	Description
Sutrayana	Hinayana	n/a	1. Sravakayana	Vehicle of listening and hearing
			2. Pratyekabuddhayana	Vehicle of the solitary realiser
	Mahayana		3. Bodhisattvayana	Vehicle of the bodhisattva
Tantrayana	Vajrayana	Outer tantras	4. Kriya tantra yana	Concerned mainly with external conduct, the practices of ritual purification and cleanliness and so on.
			5. Charya tantra yana	Places an equal emphasis on the outer actions of body and speech and the inner cultivation of samadhi.
			6. Yoga tantra yana	Emphasises the inner yogic meditation upon reality, combining skilful means and wisdom.
		Inner tantras	7. Mahāyoga yana	Focuses mainly on the development stage (Tib. kyérim), and emphasises the clarity and precision of visualisation as skilful means.
			8. Anuyoga yana	Focuses mainly on the completion stage (Tib. dzogrim), and emphasises the inner yoga of channels, winds-energies and essences (Tib. tsa lung tiklé). Visualisation of the deities is generated instantly, rather than through a gradual process as in Mahayoga.
			9. Atiyoga yana (Dzogchen)	The highest of all vehicles. It involves the realisation that all phenomena are nothing other than the appearances of the naturally arising primordial wisdom which has always been beyond arising and ceasing.

https://encyclopediaofbuddhism.org/wiki/Nine_yanas

A new high heart twelve-chakra system

For bringing us to zero point[1] Raquel Spencer

Raquel Spencer wrote the account below specifically for this book, informing how the chakra system is evolving and changing the way it operates.

As our consciousness rises, our chakra system is returning to the original design; the way our bodies were intended to process energy and Light as information: a chakra system which is fuelled by Source energy through the high heart. We are returning to our original organic functionality. The high heart chakra is located at the thymus gland and referred to as the eighth chakra. This chakra is the 'Zero Point' access to Source energy, through which a self-rejuvenating and infinitely expansive field of Life Force Energy flows into your personal energy system.

This upgraded chakra system helps to protect/remove the influences of the collective programmes, that continuously impacts our personal energy system, in order to support a new level of direct connection to Source energy and wisdom. The system is similar to our current one in many ways, but very different in others. Here are some key elements:

- It is circular in nature. Each chakra is an energetic loop/circle connected directly into the heart chakra, in addition to connecting up/down with the others through an upgraded central channel or column of Light.
- The system is self-sustained, with much less influence from the environment which often drains our energy.
- This shift in the functionality of the chakras makes it much easier to sustain higher frequencies of Light. In addition, it provides more of a 'closed-circuit' system, fuelled by Source energy. This is key, as we disconnect from the distorted matrix/mass consciousness grids and amplify the energy flowing from our Zero Point access.
- This shift in the way our chakra system functions, enhances your natural ability to rejuvenate your physical body and achieve a more direct connection to Universal Life/ Light Force Energy.
- This self-sustained circular flow of Source Life Force Energy allows our chakras to be less vulnerable, less impacted by the energy of other people and the environment at large.
- Our ability to run Source energy through our main chakras and central column via the high heart is paramount to achieving higher states of awareness.

---

[1] The high heart is located just below the collar bones, where a tie knot would be.

HEALING AND TRANSFORMATIVE MEDITATIONS

The following are various healing and meditative practices which I have found helpful on the path of transformation.

Vajrasattva mantra (one-hundred-syllable mantra)

VAJRASATTVA is the Buddha for purification and healing of the body emotions and spirit, and also the Buddha for the moment of death. When the Dalai Lama gave an empowerment of the Vajrasattva practice in England he emphasised the universal application of the Vajrasattva principle, whatever our faith or particular spiritual connection. For instance, Christians can perceive Vajrasattva as representing the healing energy of Christ, whereas Buddhists will see him as a healing Buddha and those who feel connected with spirituality but are not aligned with a specific religion may see Vajrasattva as representing universal healing energy.

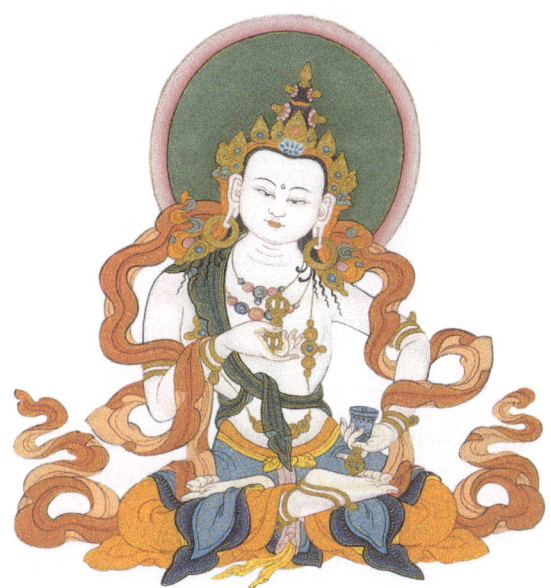

Figure 15 Vajrasattva, Buddha of healing and purification

The one-hundred-syllable mantra is the embodiment in sound of Vajrasattva, and chanting it cleanses and purifies all our peaceful and wrathful emotions which represent all the energies in the universe. As you chant—or listen to the chant—consider that brilliant white light pours down through your crown chakra, through every cell of your body like a waterfall of light, cleansing and healing. The liquid light passes into the ground, continuing to heal all who receive it.

This one-hundred-syllable mantra is chanted twenty-one times in the recording.

OM VAJRASATTVA SAMAYA
MANUPALAYA VAJRASATTVA TENOPA
TISHTHA DRIDHO ME BHAWA
SUTOKHAYO ME BHAWA SUPOKHAYO ME BHAWA
ANURAKTO ME BHAWA
SARWA SIDDHI ME PRAYACCHA)
SARWA KARMA SU TSA ME
TSITTAM SHREYANG KURU
HUNG : HA HA HA HA : HO :
BHAGAWAN SARWA TATHAGATA
VAJRA MA ME MUNCA VAJRI BHAWA
MAHA SAMAYASATTVA AH

NB pronunciation in the recorded chant uses Benza (Tibetan) instead of Vajra (Sanskrit)
The chant can be downloaded for free on the Flame website www.theflamecentre.co.uk

Invocation of the violet flame for transformation

With thanks to Troika Saint Germain who gave permission to me to share the following meditation in this book before her passing

Note from Ruthie Smith: I am on the violet ray myself and Saint Germain is one of my guides. The sacred flame—of all colours—is very important to me—hence establishing 'The Flame Centre' in London. I see the violet flame when I meditate, which is why I am including this meditation. This invocation is a powerful vehicle for transformation. You can also invoke the protective force of Arch Angel Michael

Troika Saint Germain's Introduction to the Meditation
(her emphases have been maintained in the following text)

'The Violet Flame is a Divine gift and tool for everyone, given to us by Ascended Master Saint Germain. It is a sacred fire that exists in the Higher Dimensions. People with the gift of inter-dimensional sight have seen it. Cameras have captured it when it was not visible to the person taking the photo. The violent Flame is REAL and I invite you to use it to your great advantage.'

The Violet Flame is Spiritual Alchemy in action. Just as Alchemy is said to turn lead into gold, the ultimate purpose of the Violet Flame is to turn the Human into the Divine Human. Its action is to TRANSMUTE denser feelings, actions, deeds, karma etc into a higher vibrational frequency, which helps us prepare for Ascension. Ascension means becoming a Divine Human, also known as a Christed Being—a level of consciousness obtainable by any person. You may use the Violet Flame in perfect harmony with any belief system, religion or practice. It is a neutral too with absolutely no conditions attached to it.

Saint German has always told me that the words themselves are not so important—the really important point of using the Flame is the feelings in your heart, your desire, your intention, and sincerity. Use the words from your own heart.

Ways to use the violet flame

This is the basic method Saint Germain taught me over thirty years ago and he wishes everyone to use as a foundation for Violet Flame work. It is simple with only four steps. Once you understand the principles behind this practice, you can adapt it and use it in unlimited ways.

Step 1. Bring the Violet Flame into your body. Ask your Higher Self, a Master, Guide or Angel to assist you to do so, or just ask the Flame to 'be made manifest'. It is helpful to visualise (doesn't matter if you can or cannot actually see it) or pretend that there is a ball of violet fire above your head. Then ask that ball of fire to come into your body and fill every speck of your entire body.

Step 2. Spin the flame in and around your body. Keep the Flame inside your body while asking it to also come out through your heart chakra and spin around or encircle the outside of your body so that it's encompassing your emotional, mental and spiritual bodies.

Step 3. Ask the Violet Flame to transmute everything you wish to be changed or eliminated from your life. You can do this like a shopping list—all karma, negative feelings such as anger, poverty, frustration, sadness, physical illnesses, etc.—of simply use a catch-all phrase, such as 'transmute anything and everything standing in the way of my ascension, or of becoming a Christed Being.' One important phrase to add is, 'on all dimensions, on all levels, through all time and space, past, present and future' to your request.

Step 4. Change negativity into Divine Light and fill your body. Energy is never lost, nor can it be 'deleted', however, it can be CHANGED into a higher frequency. That is why it is important to ask the Violet Flame to do so. You can specify what the energy is to become and then call that new energy into your body and aura. For example: 'Please transmute everything into love, prosperity, abundance, peace and happiness.' Or you can ask for specific Colour Rays, which are pure energy. Example, Pink is unconditional love. Blue is peace and tranquillity. Green is health and abundance. Deep dark blue is spiritual knowledge and intuition. Violet is spiritual advancement and knowledge. Either way works fine. The Violet Flame Invocation below turns everything into the Golden Platinum light of the Christ Consciousness, which encompasses all the qualities of the other colors.

The following Invocation was given to me directly by Saint Germain as an example of the four-step Alchemical Violet Flame Meditation, which will transmute your karma and negative thoughts, actions and emotions. Once you understand the process, **please individualise the Invocation using words from your heart and say them with great feeling and intention.** Saying the words out loud is best because the power and vibration of the spoken word has energy. However, if you are among people that would not understand your words, you can say it quietly in your mind.

THE INVOCATION

Centre yourself. Take a few deep breaths to prepare, and then say:

Mighty I AM Presence, Beloved God, My Heavenly Source, Please make manifest in me now the Sacred Violet Flame of Transmutation. Bring the Violet Flame into every cell, molecule and atom of my body filling me totally and completely.

Blessed Violet Flame blaze into my Heart and expand out and around all of my bodies, physical, emotional, mental and spiritual, surrounding my entire Being with your Divine Grace, Love, Mercy and Forgiveness.

Transmute all karma, negative thoughts, actions, deeds and energy that I have ever created at any time, in all dimensions, on all levels, in all bodies, through all time and space, past, present and future, for all Eternity. Transmute anything and everything that stands in my way of embodying the Ascended Christ Being That I AM.

Beloved Violet Flame turn all that has been transmuted Into the Golden Platinum Light of God, the Christ Consciousness, The Light of God that never fails.

Send this Golden Platinum Light to me now, filling and surrounding my entire body with its Divine Radiance. Raise my vibration and frequency to the highest level possible for me at this time.

So Be It and So It Is. Thank You God. Amen.

It is suggested that you do this first thing in the morning and last thing at night, or anytime you feel a little overwhelmed or upset. Just Violet Flame what is going on, right then and there.

Troika Saint Germain, 2007

Magenta Pyramid Meditation for raising your vibration

With thanks to Judy Sartori

The Magenta Pyramid is used as a vehicle of energy transformation. The colour magenta is a combination of rose pink (the love vibration) and purple (the spiritual enlightenment vibration). When they are combined in the colour magenta, they become a powerful transformative force.

VISUALISE a magenta pyramid. The top of it is about 18 inches above your head. The base of it is below your shoulder line. In the meditation:

PEACE is at the left-hand side of the base of the triangle
LOVE is on the right side of the triangle
JOY is above the crown at the apex of the triangle

Breathe in the energy of each of the vibrations of Peace, Love and Joy, as you move round the triangle. This will help you to build your connection with these vibrations.

Advice on meditation H.H. Dudjom Rinpoche

HH Dudjom Rinpoche, a Dzogchen Master, was my first meditation teacher. His 'Advice on Meditation' is a well-known classic meditation instruction within Buddhism. It is from traditional teachings such as this that the generic form of 'Mindfulness' meditation developed.

Since everything originates in the mind, this being the root cause of all experience, whether 'good' or 'bad', it is first of all necessary to work with your own mind, not to let it stray and lose yourself in its wandering. Cut the unnecessary build-up of complexity and fabrications which invite confusion in the mind. Nip the problem in the bud, so to speak.

Allow yourself to relax and feel some spaciousness, letting mind be to settle naturally. Your body should be still, speech silent, and breathing as it is, freely flowing. Here, there is a sense of letting go, unfolding, letting be.

What does this state of relaxation feel like? You should be like someone after a really hard day's work, exhausted and peacefully satisfied, mind contented to rest. Something settles at gut level, and feeling it resting in your gut you begin to experience a lightness. It is as if you're melting.

The mind is so unpredictable—there's no limit to the fantastic and subtle creation which arise, its moods, and where it will lead you. But you might also experience a muddy, semi-conscious drifting state, like having a hood over your head—a kind of dreamy dullness. This is a manner of stillness, namely stagnation, a blurred, mindless blindness. And how do you get out of this state? Alert yourself, straighten your back, breathe the stale air out of your lungs, and direct your awareness into clear space in order to bring about freshness. If you remain in this stagnant state you will not evolve, so when this setback arises clear it again and again. It is important to develop watchfulness, to stay sensitively alert.

So, the lucid awareness of meditation is the recognition of both stillness and change, and the quiet clarity of peacefully remaining in our basic intelligence. Practice this, for only by actually doing it does one experience the fruition or begin to change.

View in action

During meditation one's mind, being evenly settled in its own natural way, is like still water, unruffled by ripple or breeze, and as any thought or change arises in that stillness it forms, like a wave in the ocean, and disappears back into it again. Left naturally, it dissolves; naturally. Whatever turbulence of mind erupts- if you let it be—it will of its own course play itself out, liberate itself; and thus the view arrived at through meditation is that whatever appears is none other than the self display or projection of the mind.

In continuing the perspective of this view into the activities and events of everyday life, the grasp of dualistic perception of the world as solid, fixed and tangible reality (which is the root cause of our problems) begins to loosen and dissolves. Mind is like the wind. It comes and goes; and through increasing certainty in this view one begins to appreciate the humour of the situation. Things start to feel somewhat unreal, and the attachment and importance which one signifies to events begin to seem ridiculous, or at any rate light-hearted.

Thus one develops the ability to dissolve perception by continuing the flowing awareness of meditation into everyday life, seeing everything as the self-manifest play of the mind. And immediately after sitting meditation, the continuation of this awareness is helped by doing what you have to do calmly and quietly, with simplicity and without agitation.

So in a sense everything is like a dream, illusory, but even so humorously one goes on doing things. If you are walking, for instance, without unnecessary solemnity or self-consciousness, but light-heartedly walk towards the open space of suchness, truth. When you eat, be the stronghold of truth, what is. As you eat, feed the negativities and illusions into the belly of emptiness, dissolving them into space; and when you are pissing consider all your obscurations and blockages are being cleansed and washed away.

So far I have told you the essence of the practice in a nutshell, but you must realise that as long as we continue to see the world in a dualistic way, until we are really free of attachment and negativity, and have dissolved all our outer perceptions into the purity of the empty nature of mind, we are still stuck in the relative world of 'good' and 'bad', 'positive' and 'negative' actions, and we must respect these laws and be mindful and responsible for our actions.

Post meditation

After formal sitting meditation, in everyday activities continue this light spacious awareness throughout and gradually awareness will be strengthened and inner confidence will grow.

Rise calmly from meditation; don't immediately jump up or rush about, but whatever your activity, preserve a light sense of dignity and poise and do what you have to do with ease and relaxation of mind and body. Keep your awareness lightly centred and don't allow your attention to be distracted. Maintain this find thread of mindfulness and awareness, just flow.

Whether walking, sitting, eating or going to sleep, have a sense of ease and presence of mind. With respect to other people, be honest, gentle and straightforward; generally be pleasant in your manner, and avoid getting carried away with talk and gossip.

Whatever you do, in fact, do it according to the *dharma* which is the way of quieting the mind and subjugating negativities.

Index

Page numbers in **bold** indicate Glossary entries